GUY'S, ST THOMAS' AND LEWISHAM HOSPITALS

Paediatric Formulary

5th Edition

Revised January 1999

WARNING

We have endeavoured to ensure that the information and drug dosages in this paediatric formulary are correct at the time of publication, but errors may have occurred and the therapeutic regimes may have been altered. Where there is any doubt, information should be checked against manufacturers summary of product characteristics (data sheets), published literature or other specialist sources.

The paediatric formulary is intended for rapid reference and cannot always contain all the information necessary for prescribing and dispensing. It should be supplemented as necessary from specialist publications and also manufacturers summary of product characteristics (data sheets).

The formulary is intended for the guidance of medical practitioners, pharmacists, dentists, nurses and others who have the necessary training and experience to interpret the information it provides.

ISBN 0 9534812 0 4

CONTENTS

FOREWORD

INTRODUCTORY NOTES

The fifth edition of the paediatric formulary has been fully revised. It has been produced with the assistance of expert opinions from the paediatric departments of the 3 hospitals. Although not all views relating to drug treatment concur, the formulary committee has sought to incorporate the majority of opinions received in order to present a consensus view.

The **drug monographs** included are presented in alphabetical order and are indexed and cross referenced.

Use of recommended International Non-proprietary Names (rINNs) and British Approved Names (BANs).
The rINN should be used as the approved name. For a small number of medicines marketed in the UK, the rINN differs significantly from the BAN. In order to enable prescribers to familiarise themselves with the rINNs in these cases prior to full changeover, the BAN has been used in the formulary with the rINN stated in brackets; for example adrenaline (epinephrine), trimeprazine (alimemazine).

Treatment guidelines are included for some aspects of drug therapy. These should be tailored where necessary to individual patient needs. They do not replace the need for consultation with senior staff and/or referral for expert advice.

Prescribing a drug not included in the formulary
Occasionally it will be considered necessary to prescribe a drug not included in the formulary. These are not stocked routinely but can usually be obtained within 48 hours.

A non-formulary form is available from your clinical pharmacist or charge nurse in paediatric outpatients for this purpose.

Consultants will be advised at regular intervals of all "non-formulary" items prescribed on their behalf:

a)   **Treatment initiated by hospital staff**
       Pharmacy staff will suggest and encourage the use of a similar drug that is included in the formulary.

b)   **Patient admitted on regular therapy with a non-formulary drug**
       If it is inappropriate to change therapy (e.g. admitted for a surgical procedure), where possible, patients' own medications should be used. These will be checked by the ward pharmacist.
       When patients have an inadequate supply of their own drugs, a supply will be bought by the pharmacy specifically for that patient.
       If the patient is admitted for a review of current treatment, prescribers will be encouraged to change to a formulary preparation where appropriate.

Health Authorities do not encourage General Practitioners (GPs) to prescribe outside their own practice formulary and as a result may refuse to prescribe certain therapies based on clinical grounds but not cost grounds.
Shifting the prescribing of hospital non-formulary items to the GP is discouraged.

Shared Care

Under certain circumstances some drug therapies are part of a shared care arrangement with the General Practitioner (GP). Where this is the case it is good practice to encourage prescribing using an agreed guideline or protocol with agreement on the total number of days supply. Clinical responsibility will be shared between the hospital clinician and the GP. Shared care and the associated prescribing responsibility cannot occur if the GP is unable to take on the clinical responsibility for the management of the patient receiving a named therapy. In such instances the clinical and prescribing responsibility remains with the hospital clinician.

Some "high tech" therapies are only prescribable from hospitals e.g. TPN, ganciclovir infusions (check with pharmacy).

THE USE OF MEDICATION IN CHILDREN

Many drugs used in children are used outside the recommendations of the Summaries of Product Characteristics (Data Sheets). We have therefore endeavoured to highlight the unlicensed products and indications.

Unlicensed medicinal products are indicated in the text where appropriate. Those included within the formulary have been approved for use in the specific clinical setting by the Drug and Therapeutics Committees of the 3 hospitals. Prescribers must take full responsibility for prescribing unlicensed products.

The use of **named patient** refers to unlicensed products available from pharmaceutical companies on an individual named patient and consultant basis. **Manufactured special** preparations are made by a manufacturing unit holding a manufacturer's licence. **Extemporaneously prepared** preparations are made on an individual basis in pharmacy and are not subjected to full quality assurance.

Prescribers also take full responsibility for prescribing products outside the license which is stated in the Summary of Product Characteristics (Data Sheets) i.e. use in indications or age range outside the manufacturers' recommendations.

FOREWORD

ACKNOWLEDGEMENTS

The formulary committee would like to thank all paediatricians, nurses, dietitians and pharmacists who have given their time and expertise during the production of this edition. We would like to extend special thanks to Leonie Duke and Claire Eldridge for their enthusiasm and dedication which has enabled production of the fifth edition to be completed.

We hope you will find the paediatric formulary useful. If you have any comments please direct these to:

Stephanie Barnes/Philip Moore	or	Steve Tomlin
FORMULARY PHARMACIST		PAEDIATRIC PHARMACIST
GUY'S HOSPITAL		GUY'S HOSPITAL
ST THOMAS STREET		ST THOMAS STREET
LONDON SE1 9RT		LONDON SE1 9RT
Tel: 0171-955-5000 ext 3591		Tel:0171-955-5000 blp1348

ADMINISTRATION OF MEDICINES TO CHILDREN

PRESCRIBING IN CHILDREN

DOSES

The doses in the monographs are either stated on a specific dose per weight/surface area basis or by an age/weight range.

In some circumstances other methods may be required for calculating the appropriate dose in children.

The following method of calculating doses should only be used if a specific dose can not be found since it assumes the child is 'average'.

PERCENTAGE METHOD OF CALCULATING DOSES

Age	Mean weight for age		Mean surface area for age (m^2)	% of adult dose
	kg	lb.		
New-born (full term)	3.5	7.7	0.23	12.5
2 months	4.5	10	0.27	15
4 months	6.5	14	0.34	20
1 year	10	22	0.47	25
3 years	15	33	0.62	33.3
7 years	23	50	0.88	50
10 years	30	66	1.05	60
12 years	39	86	1.25	75
14 years	50	110	1.50	80
16 years	58	128	1.65	90
Adult	68	150	1.73	100

Wherever possible, to avoid confusion and errors, doses have been expressed in whole numbers of units. This means that less familiar units, such as nanograms have been used. This table may help with conversion between units.

1kg	=	1000g
1g	=	1000mg
1mg	=	1000micrograms
1microgram	=	1000nanograms

DEFINITIONS OF AGE

As a guideline only:

Premature baby	Born before 37 weeks gestation
Term baby	Born at 37-42 weeks gestation
Neonate	First 4 weeks of life
Infant	Up to 1 year of age
Child	From 1 - 12 to 16 years of age

CALCULATION OF BODY SURFACE AREA

Many nomograms underestimate the body surface area in infants and small children, therefore separate nomograms for infants (figure 1) and children and adults (figure 2) have been included (Haycock et al 1978).

FIGURE 1: NOMOGRAM REPRESENTING THE RELATIONSHIP BETWEEN HEIGHT, WEIGHT AND BODY SURFACE AREA IN INFANTS.

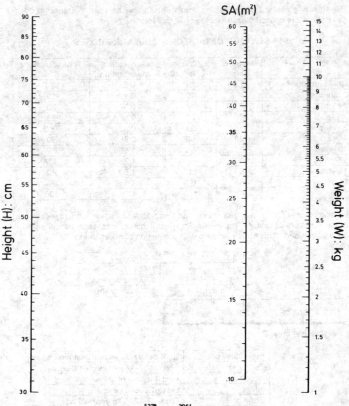

$$SA = W^{.5378} \times H^{.3964} \times .024265$$

FIGURE 2: NOMOGRAM REPRESENTING THE RELATIONSHIP BETWEEN HEIGHT, WEIGHT AND BODY SURFACE AREA IN CHILDREN AND ADULTS.

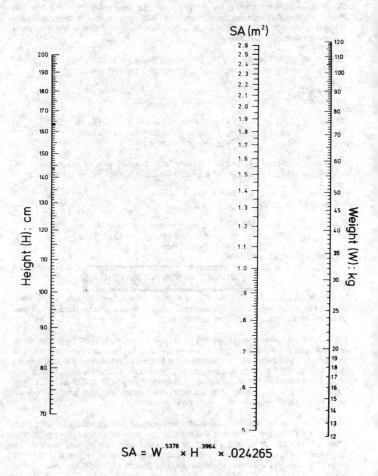

$$SA = W^{.5378} \times H^{.3964} \times .024265$$

DOSAGE ADJUSTMENT IN RENAL IMPAIRMENT

Where applicable the monographs contain dosage adjustments for renal function based on normalised clearance of creatinine. Adjustments should be made using the glomerular filtration rate (GFR), if determined, or by calculating the estimated creatinine clearance, see below.

Use the equation, calculated by Morris et al (1982), for children aged 1-18 years. This equation may be used for infants although it is not a reliable method.

"Estimated" Cl_{CR} (ml/minute/1.73m^2) $= \dfrac{40 \times ht}{S_{CR}}$

Where
Cl_{CR} = Creatinine clearance in ml/minute/1.73m^2
S_{CR} = Serum creatinine in micromol/litre
ht = Height in cm

Calculated creatinine clearances are not reliable below 1 year of age however the following equation may be helpful as a guide to dosage adjustments in neonates.

"Estimated" Cl_{CR} (ml/minute/1.73m^2) $= \dfrac{30 \times ht}{S_{CR}}$

Where
Cl_{CR} = Creatinine clearance in ml/minute/1.73m^2
S_{CR} = Serum creatinine in micromol/litre
ht = Height in cm
(Adapated from Schwartz et al)

ADMINISTRATION IN CHILDREN

The parenteral route for children is the most reliable with regard to obtaining predictable blood levels. The intramuscular route should only be used in children when the intravenous route is not appropriate.

Care should be taken when preparing parenteral doses as many of the preparations are produced for adult use. Small volumes should be measured using graduated syringes or, in some cases, by dilution of the injection. When reconstituting freeze-dried injections, the displacement value is important. Displacement values are given in the text under "Administration" and are the volume of fluid displaced by the powder. It must be taken into account where part vials are used otherwise significant errors in the dose drawn up may result.

The oral route is usually the easiest and most convenient, especially for long term treatment. Problems can occur because of the lack of suitable dosage forms. Therefore the use of named patient or specialist preparations may need to be considered. It is important when planning discharges to allow for this and to notify pharmacy as soon as possible so arrangements can be made for continuity of supply.

With liquid oral preparations oral syringes should be used.

ACCIDENTAL POISONING

Accidental poisoning in the under five age group accounts for 45,500 attendances to Accident and Emergency Departments in the United Kingdom. In an effort to reduce this number, the following measures can be taken: the use of child resistant packaging, warning messages on product labels, educational campaigns and returning unused medicines to pharmacies for safe disposal.

The effectiveness of packaging has been assessed with encouraging results and the problems of accidental poisoning with drugs in children has been shown to be reduced by the use of child resistant closures (CRCs). Unit dose packaging such as aluminium strips, opaque blister and sachets are considered to be child resistant but transparent blister packs are not. Clik-loks are used for all dispensed loose tablets and liquid containers.

It is important to remember that child-**resistant** closures are not child-**proof**, and so safe storage is still of paramount importance. Often keeping medicines out of the reach of children is not enough as toddlers and young children can be very proficient at climbing. Perhaps "**keep out of sight of children**" would be a more useful directive. This is particularly true of medicines stored in the fridge e.g. antibiotic mixtures, as a fridge cannot be locked. Such medicines are often involved in accidental poisoning, and so care should be taken to keep them well hidden within the fridge.

It is still best to keep medicines in locked cupboards or drawers. If this is not possible, research shows that bathroom cabinets or kitchen cupboards are the safest places; open shelves, fridges and handbags being the most dangerous places. Overall, the kitchen is the safest room, probably because the child is more likely to be supervised there.

The group of medicines most commonly associated with accidental poisoning is analgesics, particularly paracetamol and ibuprofen. The most toxic group are tricyclic antidepressants. Oral contraceptives have a high incidence of accidental ingestion by children, probably due to storage (e.g. bed-side cabinet, handbag) and because they are packaged in transparent blister packs. Fortunately the consequences of such ingestion are minimal.

Educational and DUMP (Disposal of Unwanted Medicines and Poisons) campaigns can raise awareness amongst adults and children about the risk of accidental poisoning and encourage the removal of potential poisons from the home however whether these reduce the incidence of poisoning is debatable. Thus the use of CRCs and safe storage are of utmost importance.

The information provided is based on a personal communication with the London Medical Toxicology Unit.

CHILDREN'S DOSES

ACETAZOLAMIDE

Preparations:	TABLETS 250mg. SUSTAINED RELEASE CAPSULES 250mg.
	INJECTION 500mg. LIQUID (**Extemporaneously prepared**).
Dosage:	*RAISED INTRACRANIAL PRESSURE*

This is an unlicensed indication.

Orally or IV injection, all ages, initially 25mg/kg/day in 2-4 divided doses, increasing by 25mg/kg/day up to a maximum dose of 100mg/kg/day. Sodium bicarbonate may be required to maintain bicarbonate levels above 18mmol/L, see metabolic acidosis page 194.

GLAUCOMA, EPILEPSY

The use in glaucoma is an unlicensed indication in children.

Orally or IV injection,

Under 12 years, 5mg/kg 2-4 times a day. Maximum 750mg/day. Over 12 years, 5mg/kg 4 times a day or, if appropriate, initially one or two sustained release capsules (250mg). Maximum 1000mg/day.

Administration:	Reconstitute each vial with 5ml water for injection, and administer as a injection.
Notes:	

a) Injection can be given orally, but must be diluted first.
b) IM injection should be avoided due to the alkaline pH of the solution.
c) SR capsules are not licensed for children under 12 years old and are only licensed for use in the treatment of glaucoma.
d) Sodium content of 500mg vial is 2.36mmol.

ACETYLCYSTEINE

Preparations: INJECTION 20% (200mg in 1ml) 10ml ampoules.
LIQUID (**Extemporaneously prepared**).

Dosage: *PARACETAMOL OVERDOSE*

> **IF IN ANY DOUBT CONTACT THE MEDICAL TOXICOLOGY UNIT**
> ☎ 0171-635-9191 ☎

If the child presents within 8 hours and can be given an oral preparation, **methionine** tablets (page 146) are effective. If they present after 8 hours or cannot be given an oral preparation, give **acetylcysteine** using the following regimen:
Initially, by *slow IV injection,*
150mg/kg over 15 minutes, as loading dose
followed by *IV infusion*
50mg/kg over 4 hours,
finally by *IV infusion,*
100mg/kg over 16 hours.

Total of 300mg/kg over 20 hours to be given.

ANTIOXIDANT, ACUTE LIVER FAILURE
This is an unlicensed indication.
IV infusion, 4-8mg/kg/hour, up to 20mg/kg/hour.

MECONIUM ILEUS
This is an unlicensed indication.
Neonates, *orally,* 1-2ml two or three times a day.

MECONIUM ILEUS EQUIVALENT
This is an unlicensed indication.
Orally, doses of 2-20ml two or three times a day have been used depending on the age of the child. (See note a).

BLADDER WASHOUT
This is an unlicensed indication.
Dilute 10ml of the 20% injection solution with 40ml sodium chloride 0.9%. *Instil* into the bladder using a bladder syringe, retain for up to 1 hour. If necessary injection may be used undiluted.

Administration: Dilute loading dose to 30-50mg in 1ml with glucose 5%. Infusion should be diluted to 5mg in 1ml with glucose 5%. In fluid restricted patients dilute to 50mg in 1ml. Glucose 50% can be used to dilute acetylcysteine.

Notes:

a)   Acetylcysteine injection solution diluted to 50mg in 1ml can be given orally but is very bitter. Orange or blackcurrant syrup, or coca cola can be used to dilute the injection solution.

b)   If anaphylactoid reactions occur with IV acetylcysteine, stop infusion and give an antihistamine e.g. chlorpheniramine (see page 60). Restart the infusion at the lowest dose rate once the reaction has subsided, or give methionine if it is less than 8 hours since the overdose.

c)   Acetylcysteine (Parvolex®) contains 12.8mmol of sodium per 2000mg in 10ml.

ACICLOVIR

Preparations: DISPERSIBLE TABLETS 200mg, 400mg and 800mg. LIQUID 200mg in 5ml. INJECTION 250mg and 500mg. OPHTHALMIC OINTMENT 3%. CREAM 5% .

Dosage:

> CHECK INDICATION, IMMUNE STATUS, RENAL FUNCTION AND AGE VERY CAREFULLY BEFORE PRESCRIBING.

TREATMENT OF HERPES SIMPLEX ENCEPHALITIS AND THE TREATMENT OF SHINGLES AND CHICKENPOX IN THE IMMUNOCOMPROMISED
IV infusion,

Under 3 months	10mg/kg	3 times a day
3 months - 12 years	500mg/m^2	3 times a day
Over 12 years	10mg/kg	3 times a day

Treatment for herpes simplex encephalitis should be for a minimum of 14 days. Treatment for shingles and chickenpox is for 10 days or longer if clinically indicated.

ORAL TREATMENT OF CHICKENPOX AND SHINGLES
Treatment of shingles and chickenpox infections are unlicensed for use in infants under 3 months.
Orally,
All ages, 20mg/kg 4 times a day for 5 to 7 days. Maximum single dose is 800mg.
OR

3 months - 2 years	200mg	4 times a day
2 - 6 years	400mg	4 times a day
6 - 12 years	800mg	4 times a day
Adult	800mg	5 times a day

> THE ABOVE DOSES CAN BE USED IN THE IMMUNOCOMPROMISED TO COMPLETE COURSE OF IV THERAPY. THIS IS AN UNLICENSED INDICATION.

HERPES SIMPLEX VIRUS TREATMENT
Orally,

3 months - 2 years	100mg	5 times a day for 5 days
Over 2 years	200mg	5 times a day for 5 days

IV infusion,

Under 3 months	10mg/kg	3 times a day for 10 days
3 months - 12 years	250mg/m^2	3 times a day for 5 days
Over 12 years	5mg/kg	3 times a day for 5 days

> IN IMMUNOCOMPROMISED CHILDREN THE ABOVE DOSES CAN BE DOUBLED AND GIVEN FOR 10 DAYS EXCEPT FOR THE IV DOSE IN NEONATES AND INFANTS UNDER 3 MONTHS.

HERPES SIMPLEX VIRUS PROPHYLAXIS IN IMMUNOCOMPROMISED CHILDREN
Orally,

3 months - 2 years	100mg	4 times a day for period at risk
Over 2 years	200mg	4 times a day for period at risk

> IN SEVERELY IMMUNOCOMPROMISED CHILDREN THE ABOVE DOSES MAY BE DOUBLED.

HERPES SIMPLEX KERATITIS
Ophthalmic ointment: Apply 5 times a day until corneal re-epithelialisation has occurred; continue for a further 3 days after healing is complete.

HERPES SIMPLEX INFECTION OF THE SKIN
Cream: Apply 5 times a day for 5 days. If skin has not healed continue for a further 5 days.

IN RENAL FAILURE
IV infusion,

Creatinine clearance (ml/minute/1.73m²)	Dose	Dosage interval (hours)
25-50	Normal	12
10-25	Normal	24
CAPD	Half	24
Haemodialysis	Half	24 (and after dialysis)

Orally, for Herpes simplex virus

Creatinine clearance (ml/minute/1.73m²)	Dosage interval (hours)
Less than 10	12

Orally, for Varicella virus

Creatinine clearance (ml/minute/1.73m²)	Dosage interval (hours)
10-25	8
Less than 10	12

Administration: Reconstitute each 250mg vial with 10ml or each 500mg vial with 20ml of water for injection or sodium chloride 0.9% to give 25mg in 1ml solution (displacement volume negligible). The injection can be given undiluted, via a central line using a syringe pump, over a minimum of **1 hour**, OR dilute to 5mg in 1ml with sodium chloride 0.9% or glucose/saline and infuse over 1 hour.

Notes:

a) Aciclovir is not given as an IV injection to avoid a rapid increase in blood urea and creatinine levels.
b) Polyuric renal failure usually occurs with high doses. If renal impairment develops during treatment, a rapid response normally occurs following hydration of the patient and/or dosage reduction or withdrawal. Avoid dehydration; specific care should be taken in all patients receiving high doses to ensure they are well hydrated.
c) Concomitant administration with mycophenolate increases plasma levels of both drugs.
d) The use of the oral route in neonates is based on anecdotal evidence and the pharmacokinetics are uncertain. Diarrhoea has also been a particular problem.
e) Each 250mg of powder for injection contains 1.1mmol of sodium.
f) Aciclovir liquid (Zovirax®) is sucrose free.

15

ACTIVATED CHARCOAL

Preparations: CARBOMIX® SUSPENSION 50g.
Dosage: **TREATMENT OF POISONING**

> **IF IN ANY DOUBT CONTACT THE MEDICAL TOXICOLOGY UNIT**
> ☎ 0171-635-9191 ☎.

Orally, 1g/kg. In some cases (e.g. following ingestion of sustained release products) this dose should be repeated every 4 hours until charcoal is seen in stools or until clinical improvement.

Administration: Give as a suspension in water as soon as possible after ingestion of the poison or stomach wash-out.

Notes:

Concurrent drugs (e.g. to treat shock) should be given parenterally since absorption may be reduced.

ADENOSINE

Preparations: INJECTION 6mg in 2ml.
Dosage: **ANTIARRHYTHMIC**

This indication is unlicensed for use in children.

Fast IV bolus, initial dose 50microgram/kg increasing by 50microgram/kg every 2 minutes to 250microgram/kg. Doses as high as 400microgram/kg have been used but **seek specialist advice before prescribing.**

Administration: Fast IV bolus injection over less than 2 seconds, given centrally if possible as adenosine is both painful and rapidly metabolised in the peripheral circulation.

Notes:

a) Initial dose should be quartered (i.e. 12.5microgram/kg) if patient is on concurrent dipyridamole.
b) Aminophylline, theophylline, caffeine and other xanthines are strong inhibitors of adenosine's antiarrhythmic action.
c) Dosage adjustment of adenosine is not required in renal or hepatic impairment.
d) Adenosine is not recommended in asthmatics because it can cause bronchoconstriction in such patients.
e) Very rarely, adenosine may accelerate some tachycardias and therefore resuscitation facilities must be available before administration.
f) See also tachycardia guidelines page 239.

ADRENALINE (EPINEPHRINE)

Preparations: INJECTIONS 1mg in 1ml (1 in 1000) (1ml, 5ml, [ITU only]) and 1mg in 10ml (1 in 10,000) (**Manufactured special**) [Paediatrics only]. MINIJET 1 in 10,000, 10ml. EPI-PEN 150microgram in 1ml and 300microgram in 1ml.

Dosage: These indications are unlicensed for children under 1 year.

CARDIAC ARREST

SEE CPR GUIDELINES PAGE 234

All ages,
IV/IO injection, 10microgram/kg (0.1ml/kg of 1 in 10,000). Subsequent doses, *IV/IO injection* 100microgram/kg (0.1ml/kg of 1 in 1,000).
OR
IV/IO injection,

AGE	NEWBORN	6 MTHS	1 YR	4 YRS	8 YRS
WEIGHT	3kg	6kg	10kg	15kg	25kg
Adrenaline (Epinephrine) 1 in 10,000 10microgram/kg	0.3ml	0.6ml	1ml	1.5ml	2.5ml
Adrenaline (Epinephrine) 1 in 1,000 100microgram/kg	0.3ml	0.6ml	1ml	1.5ml	2.5ml

If vascular access not available, administer via an endotracheal tube, *endotrachaelly,* 100microgram/kg (0.1ml/kg of 1 in 1,000).

ACUTE ANAPHYLAXIS AND STATUS ASTHMATICUS
All ages,
IM or SC injection, 10microgram/kg (0.01ml/kg of 1 in 1000). Doses may be doubled and repeated twice.
OR

Age (Average weight or greater)	Volume of adrenaline (1 in 1000/1mg in 1ml)
Under 1 year	0.05ml
1 year	0.1ml
2 years	0.2ml
3 - 4 years	0.3ml
5 years	0.4ml
6 - 12 years	0.5ml
Adult	0.5-1ml

OR

Weight	Dose
15-30kg	Epipen Jr® 150microgram in 1ml
Over 30kg	Epipen® 300microgram in 1ml

IV injection, 10microgram/kg (0.1ml/kg of 1 in 10,000).

ACUTE HYPOTENSION
IV infusion, all ages, 0.1-1.5microgram/kg/minute increasing until a response obtained. Higher doses have been used.

CROUP OR STRIDOR FOLLOWING VENTILATION

This is an unlicensed indication.

All ages, *nebulised*, 1ml of 1 in 1000 adrenaline diluted with 3ml sodium chloride 0.9% has been used to acutely relieve stridor. The effect rapidly wears off.

Administration: Infusion: dilute with sodium chloride 0.9% or glucose 5%.

Via endotrachael tube: dilute with an equal volume of sodium chloride 0.9% (up to 5ml) and bag in over at least 5 minutes.

ALCOHOL (ETHANOL)

Preparations: INJECTION 100% (8g in 10ml) (**Manufactured special**).

Dosage: *TREATMENT OF ETHYLENE GLYCOL AND METHANOL POISONING*

> IF IN ANY DOUBT CONTACT THE MEDICAL TOXICOLOGY UNIT
> ☎ 0171-635-9191 ☎.

See notes below.

Initial treatment

Oral or IV injection,

Loading dose of alcohol = 0.6g/kg over 15-30 minutes.

Continuation treatment

Oral or IV infusion, 66mg/kg/hour adjusted if necessary to maintain blood ethanol concentration of 1-1.5g/L.

Administration: Where possible give orally; dilute as necessary. IV infusion, dilute to 10mg in 1ml with sodium chloride 0.9% or glucose/saline.

Notes:

a) Gastric aspiration with a narrow gauge tube should be considered where a potentially toxic amount has been recently ingested.

b) Haemodialysis may be required in very severe cases e.g. respiratory or cardiac depression.

ALFACALCIDOL (1-ALPHAHYDROXYCHOLECALCIFEROL)

Preparations: CAPSULES 250nanogram (0.25microgram) and 1microgram.

SOLUTION 200nanogram in 1ml (0.2microgram in 1ml).

INJECTION 2microgram in 1ml (renal unit only).

Dosage: *PROPHYLAXIS AGAINST EARLY NEONATAL HYPOCALCAEMIA IN PREMATURE BABIES*

Orally, 100nanogram(0.1microgram)/kg/day.

NEONATAL HYPOCALCAEMIA AND HYPOPHOSPHATAEMIC RICKETS

Full term and premature neonates, *orally*, initially 50-100nanogram(0.05-0.1microgram)/kg once a day then modify according to response. In severe cases, doses of up to 2microgram/kg/day may be needed.

HYPOPHOSPHATAEMIC RICKETS

Children less than 20kg, *orally*, initially 25-50nanogram (0.025-0.05microgram)/kg once a day, adjust according to response.

Children over 20kg, *orally*, initially 1microgram once a day then modify according to response.

TREATMENT OF AND PROPHYLAXIS AGAINST RENAL OSTEODYSTROPHY
Under 20kg, *orally*, 15-30nanogram/kg once a day.
Over 20kg, *orally*, 250-500nanogram (0.25-0.5microgram) once
a day.
Adjust dose according to response.

Notes:

a) For comparison of vitamin D preparations see 9.6.4 of Adult
Formulary.
b) Alfacalcidol solution (One-alpha®) is colouring and sucrose free. The
capsules contain sesame oil.
c) A significant risk of hypercalcaemia exists if treatment is long term.

ALLOPURINOL

Preparations: TABLETS 100mg and 300mg.
LIQUID (**Extemporaneously prepared**).

Dosage: *PREVENTION OF URIC ACID NEPHROPATHY, NEOPLASTIC DISEASE, METABOLIC
DISORDERS e.g. LESCH-NYHAN SYNDROME*
Orally,

1 month - 15 years	10-20mg/kg once a day. See maximum doses below.
Over 15 years	Initially 100mg once a day, increasing according to condition to a maximum of 900mg/day. Divide doses over 300mg.

IN RENAL FAILURE

Creatinine clearance (ml/minute/1.73m^2)	Dosage
10-50	7-14mg/kg/day
Less than 10	3-7mg/kg/day or give at longer intervals

Haemodialysis: Allopurinol and its metabolites are removed by
haemodialysis. Dose should be given after dialysis with none in
the interim.
Peritoneal dialysis: Dose as for creatinine clearance less than
10ml/minute/1.73m^2 and monitor oxypurinol levels. Levels are
measured by the Purine Research Laboratory ☎ Guy's ext 4024.

Notes:

a) If concurrent use of mercaptopurine or azathioprine is necessary, reduce
the dose of these drugs to 25% as allopurinol competes for excretion
within the renal tubule.
b) Allopurinol toxicity may be increased by thiazide diuretics.
c) If rash occurs withdraw therapy. If rash is mild reintroduce allopurinol on
resolution of rash however discontinue if rash recurs.

ALTEPLASE (t-PA)

Preparations:	INJECTION 10mg and 20mg (**Non-formulary**) and 50mg.
	INJECTION 4mg in 4ml (**Manufactured special**).
Dosage:	*OCCLUDED ARTERIOVENOUS SHUNTS, PERITONEAL DIALYSIS CATHETERS AND INDWELLING CENTRAL LINES*
	This is an unlicensed indication.
	Using the 4mg in 4ml solution, *instill* the appropriate volume into the catheter. Refer to catheter manufacturer if lumen volume is unknown. Dose into catheter should not exceed 1.5mg/kg.
Administration:	**Instillation:** 4mg in 4ml injection is stored in the freezer. Defrost thoroughly and allow solution to come to room temperature before using. Instill into the affected catheter, clamp off and retain for at least 4 hours. The lysate is then **aspirated**, DO NOT FLUSH until alteplase has been aspirated from the catheter.

Notes:

a) Alteplase is a recombinant human tissue-type plasminogen activator. Antibody formation has not been observed with alteplase and hence repeated doses may be given.

b) **Extreme caution** should be used in patients with an increased risk of bleeding and with recent traumas e.g. biopsies, venepuncture.

ALUMINIUM HYDROXIDE

Preparations:	MIXTURE 400mg in 10ml. CAPSULES 475mg.
Dosage:	*PHOSPHATE BINDING IN RENAL PATIENTS*

The mixture is unlicensed for use in children under 6 years.
Orally, initially,

4 weeks - 12 months	2.5-5ml	3-4 times a day
1 - 4 years	5-10ml	3-4 times a day
5 - 12 years	10-20ml or 1-2 caps	3-4 times a day

Dose is adjusted according to phosphate levels.

ANTACID
Orally,

6 - 12 years	up to 5ml	3 times a day
Over 12 years	5-10ml	4 times a day

Notes:

a) Calcium carbonate (see page 45) is the preferred phosphate binding agent because of the risk of aluminium toxicity.

b) 10ml (400mg) of aluminium hydroxide mixture is equivalent to 194-244mg of elemental aluminium (variable bioavailability).

c) Aluminium hydroxide mixture does not contain sucrose and has a low sodium content (1mmol in 10ml). The capsules are sodium free.

d) Converting between aluminium hydroxide and calcium carbonate as phosphate binders the following can be used as a starting guide:
One aluminium hydroxide 475mg capsule (Alucap®) is equivalent to:-
one calcium carbonate 1250mg tablet (Calcichew®).
5ml of aluminium hydroxide mixture BP is equivalent to:-
two calcium carbonate 300mg tablet
or 5ml of calcium carbonate 120mg in 1ml mixture

e) Aluminium hydroxide is very constipating, laxatives may be required.

AMIKACIN

Preparations: INJECTION 500mg in 2ml, 100mg in 2ml (**Non-formulary**).

Dosage: *TREATMENT OF INFECTION*

CONSULT MICROBIOLOGIST BEFORE PRESCRIBING

Preterm neonates,
IV injection,

Gestational age (weeks)	Dose	Interval (hours)
<30	7.5mg/kg	24
30-Term	7.5mg/kg	18

Term neonates and children,
IV or IM injection, initial loading dose of 10mg/kg followed by 7.5mg/kg every 12 hours.

IN RENAL FAILURE
Adjust dose according to blood levels (See note a).

Administration: Give by IM injection, IV injection over 3 minutes, or as an IV infusion in sodium chloride 0.9% or glucose 5% over 30 minutes.

Notes:

  a) Blood levels:
     i) Approx. time to steady state: 24 hours
     ii) Therapeutic levels: Trough   <4mg/L
                         Peak   15-30mg/L
     iii) Take trough sample, immediately prior to next dose and peak sample, 1 hour after IV and IM injection.
  b) Nephrotoxicity may be increased by concurrent administration of amphotericin and potent diuretics.
  c) Neuromuscular blockade and respiratory paralysis have occurred when aminoglycosides have been administered to patients who have received curare-like muscle relaxants, e.g. tubocurarine.
  d) Aminoglycosides interact with many drugs in infusion solutions so they should be administered as an IV injection or as a separate infusion.

AMILORIDE

Preparations: TABLETS 5mg. LIQUID 1mg in 1ml (**Non-formulary**).

Dosage: *POTASSIUM-SPARING DIURESIS*
This indication is unlicensed for use in children.
All ages, *orally*, 200microgram/kg twice a day.
Maximum dose 20mg.
IN RENAL FAILURE
Diuresis is poor in patients with renal failure, therefore amiloride is best avoided if creatinine clearance is less than 40ml/minute/1.73m^2.

Notes:

  a) Avoid concurrent use of spironolactone, ACE-inhibitors or other potassium-sparing diuretics due to the risk of hyperkalaemia.
  b) Amiloride appears particularly to cause hyperkalaemia in diabetics.
  c) Liquid is sugar-free.

AMINOPHYLLINE

Preparations:	SLOW RELEASE TABLETS 225mg and 100mg (**Non-formulary**).
	INJECTION 250mg in 10ml.
Dosage:	***ASTHMA THERAPY***

> DO NOT GIVE A LOADING DOSE IF THE CHILD WAS PREVIOUSLY ON ORAL AMINOPHYLLINE OR THEOPHYLLINE.

IV infusion, loading dose of 5mg/kg given over 20 minutes, followed by 1mg/kg/hour.

Orally, (slow release tablets - **cannot be chewed**).

Initially

Under 3 years,	see theophylline, page 212.
3 - 8 years (15-24kg)	100mg twice a day.
8 - 13 years (24-35kg)	100-225mg twice a day.

Dose is doubled after 1 week. Adjust maintenance dose according to levels. Maximum dose 40mg/kg/day.

Administration: Dilute with sodium chloride 0.9% or glucose 5%. If patient is fluid restricted, injection solution can be given undiluted.

Notes:

a) 100mg aminophylline is equivalent to 80mg theophylline.
b) Blood levels:
   i) Approx. time to steady state: 1-2 days
   ii) Therapeutic range of theophylline: 10-20mg/L
   iii) Take trough sample, immediately prior to next dose for slow release reparations or at least 8 hours after starting IV dose.
c) The bioavailability of the Phyllocontin® and Pecram® brands of slow release aminophylline may differ and therefore brand should be stated on each prescription. Pharmacy currently stocks Phyllocontin®.
d) Refer to theophylline (see page 212) for potential drug interactions.

AMIODARONE

Preparations: TABLETS 100mg and 200mg. INJECTION 150mg in 3ml.
LIQUID (**Extemporaneously prepared**).

Dosage: ***ANTIARRHYTHMIC***

SEEK EXPERT ADVICE BEFORE PRESCRIBING

The oral route is unlicensed for use in children.

All ages, *orally*, 5mg/kg 2-3 times a day for up to 14 days, then 5mg/kg once a day. Adjust the maintenance dose after 1 week, according to plasma levels.

Larger doses may be required in some patients.

Slow IV injection, 5mg/kg/dose, repeated up to total of 15mg/kg (1.2g) over 24 hours.

IV infusion, 25microgram/kg/minute for 4 hours, then 5-15microgram/kg/minute (maximum 1.2g/24hrs).

Administration: Slow IV injection, over 30 minutes or, IV infusion; via a central line, diluted in 5% glucose (**not** sodium chloride 0.9%). Do not dilute below 600microgram in 1ml.

Notes:

a) Blood levels:
   i) Steady state is achieved when ratio of desethyl-amiodarone to amiodarone is approx. 0.8 to 1.
   ii) Therapeutic range of amiodarone and metabolite: 0.6-2.5mg/L.
   iii) Take trough sample, immediately prior to next dose.
b) Severe hypotension may occur if infusion is too rapid.
c) The maintenance dose of digoxin should be halved if amiodarone therapy is introduced because it reduces digoxin excretion.
d) Amiodarone potentiates oral anticoagulants and may potentiate the effects of highly protein bound drugs such as phenytoin.
e) Corneal microdeposits usually occur during long term administration. These rarely interfere in the vision and are reversible on withdrawal of treatment.
f) Photosensitivity (sunburn) of exposed areas occur frequently. Sunblock creams are required.
g) Bluish-grey pigmentation of exposed areas may also occur after prolonged exposure and may become permanent.
h) Thyroid function tests should be checked at 6 monthly intervals.
i) Pulmonary alveolitis and pulmonary fibrosis have been reported. A baseline chest X-ray should be performed. Consider repeating at 6 monthly intervals.
j) Irreversible liver damage has been reported therefore liver function tests should be performed at 6 monthly intervals. A sample for a base line LFT should be taken before starting maintenance therapy.
k) See also tachycardia guidelines page 239.

AMITRIPTYLINE

Preparations: TABLETS 10mg, 25mg and 50mg. SUSPENSION 10mg in 5ml.

Dosage: *SEDATIVE ANTIDEPRESSANT, CO-ANALGESIA FOR NERVE PAIN*

These indications are unlicensed for use in children. Use as an analgesic is also an unlicensed indication.

Orally, 250-500microgram/kg at night.

Notes:

a) Amitriptyline is generally avoided in children due to the dangers in overdose (seizures, hypotension, arrhythmias, prolonged QRS interval, flushing, dilated pupils and coma).

b) Tricyclic antidepressants lower the seizure threshold and should be used with caution in patients with a history of convulsions. They may also increase the risk of arrhythmias and should be avoided in patients with heart block or a history of arrhythmias. Also avoid with concomitant antihistamines (especially terfenadine or astemizole). Cimetidine increases plasma levels of tricyclic antidepressants. For further information consult your clinical pharmacist or drug information (Guy's ext 3594, Lewisham ext 3202 or St Thomas' ext 3609).

c) Treatment should not exceed 3 months without further review. Treatment should be withdrawn gradually.

d) Amitriptyline suspension (Tryptizol®) is sucrose free.

AMLODIPINE BESYLATE (AMLODIPINE BESILATE)

Preparations: TABLETS 5mg and 10mg.

Dosage: *HYPERTENSION*

This indication is unlicensed for use in children.

Orally, initially, 100-200microgram/kg once a day, increased according to response. Maximum 10mg/**day**.

OR

initially,

6-15kg	1.25mg once a day
15-25kg	2.5mg once a day
over 25kg	5mg once a day

Notes:

a) Amlodipine 5-10mg/day has been shown to be comparable to nifedipine retard 40mg/day.

b) Amlodipine tablets may be dispersed in water.

AMOXICILLIN

Preparations: CAPSULES 250mg and 500mg. LIQUIDS 125mg in 5ml and 250mg in 5ml. SACHETS 3g. INJECTIONS 250mg and 500mg.

Dosage: **TREATMENT OF INFECTION**

Premature neonates, neonates up to 7 days old,
Orally or IV injection,
30mg/kg twice a day

DOSE SHOULD BE DOUBLED IN SEVERE INFECTION/MENINGITIS

Neonates over 7 days old, infants and children,
Orally,

Up to 1 year	62.5mg	}
1 - 4 years	125mg	} 3 times
5 - 12 years	250mg	} a day
Over 12 years	250-500mg	}

DOSE SHOULD BE DOUBLED IN SEVERE INFECTION

IV injection
20-30mg/kg 3 times a day up to a maximum 4g/day.

DOSE SHOULD BE DOUBLED IN MENINGITIS

PROPHYLAXIS OF INFECTIVE ENDOCARDITIS
See guidelines page 265.

IN RENAL FAILURE

Creatinine clearance (ml/min/1.73m^2)	Dosage interval (hours)
10-50	8-12
<10	12-18

Amoxicillin is significantly cleared by haemodialysis and peritoneal dialysis, give dose as per creatinine clearance of 10-50ml/minute/1.73m^2 above, ensuring a dose is given after dialysis session.

Administration: On reconstitution 250mg displaces 0.2ml. Add 4.8ml and 9.6ml water for injection to 250mg and 500mg vials respectively to give 50mg in 1ml concentration. Inject over 3-4 minutes.
May be further diluted with sodium chloride 0.9%.
During reconstitution a transient pink colour may occur, reconstituted solutions are usually a pale straw colour. Do **NOT** administer if reconstituted solution is pink.

Notes:

a) In confirmed **penicillin allergy**, cephalosporins may be an alternative treatment although approximately 10% of these patients will also be allergic to cephalosporins. Where severe allergy symptoms have occurred previously or the extent of the allergy is unknown an alternative antibiotic should be given. Contact the microbiology department for further information.
b) Amoxicillin sachets and syrups stocked in pharmacy are sucrose free.
c) Amoxicillin (Amoxil®) injection contains 3.3mmol of sodium per 1gram.

AMPHOTERICIN

Preparations:

LOZENGES 10mg.
INJECTION 50mg. LIPOSOMAL INJECTION 50mg (AmBisome®).
BLADDER WASHOUT 100microgram in 1ml (**Manufactured special**).

Dosage:

ORAL CANDIDIASIS
This indication is unlicensed for use in children.
Lozenges,
10mg dissolved slowly in the mouth 4 times a day, increased to 8 times a day if necessary. Treat for 10-15 days.

SYSTEMIC ANTIFUNGAL
This indication is unlicensed for use in neonates.
IV infusion,
Neonates, initial daily dose of 100microgram/kg/day increasing in a stepwise fashion every 1-2 days to a maximum of 1mg/kg/day.
Infants and children, give a test dose (see note b) of 12.5microgram/kg over 30 minutes, followed 1 hour later by the first daily dose of 250microgram/kg, increase gradually by 125-250microgram/kg/day every 1-2 days to a maximum of 1mg/kg/day. In life-threatening infections the dose may be increased to 1mg/kg/day over a total of 1-3 days. Maximum dose is 1.5mg/kg/day.
If therapy has been stopped for 7 days or longer, start treatment again at the lower dose of 250microgram/kg.
Liposomal IV infusion

CONSULT MYCOLOGIST BEFORE PRESCRIBING

All ages, give a test dose (see note b) of 50microgram/kg, to a maximum of 1mg, over 10 minutes, followed 1 hour later by 1mg/kg/day, increased gradually, if necessary, to 3mg/kg/day. Dose is 3mg/kg/day in febrile neutropenia.

IN RENAL FAILURE
No dosage reduction is generally required in pre-existing renal failure. However dose reduction or liposomal amphotericin should be considered if amphotericin is suspected of worsening renal function.

BLADDER WASHOUT
Use a solution of 100microgram in 1ml twice a day. Volumes up to 100ml have been used depending on the size of the bladder. A test dose is not required for bladder instillation.

Administration: IV infusion
- Add 10ml water for injection to the amphotericin to produce a 5mg in 1ml solution (displacement volume negligible).
- Add 2ml of phosphate buffer to 500ml glucose 5% to ensure a pH greater than 4.2 (no other solutions suitable) see note i.
- Take required volume of diluted amphotericin and further dilute with the buffered glucose 5% to a concentration of 100microgram in 1ml and infuse over **4-6 hours**. Infusion time maybe reduced to 2 hours if well tolerated. In fluid restricted patients concentrations up to 400micrograms in 1ml have been used. Protect from direct sunlight by covering infusion or use of an amber giving set.

Liposomal IV infusion
- Add 12ml water for injection to liposomal amphotericin to produce a 4mg in 1ml solution. SHAKE vial vigorously to disperse liposomes.
- Add the liposomal amphotericin to glucose 5% (no other solutions suitable) using the 5 micron filter provided. Liposomal amphotericin should be diluted to an appropriate concentration between 0.2mg in 1ml and 2mg in 1ml. Infuse over 30-60 minutes.

Bladder washout
- Add 10ml water for injection to the amphotericin to produce a 5mg in 1ml solution (displacement value negligible).
- Further dilute 2ml to 100ml with water for irrigation to produce a 100microgram in 1ml solution for instillation into the bladder.

Notes:

a) Adverse effects during the infusion may include fever, chills and rigors. Hydrocortisone and chlorpheniramine may be given to patients who have previously had these effects prior to starting the infusion to prevent them.

b) Give a test dose as anaphylaxis can occur with any intravenous amphotericin. A test dose is not required when converting a patient to an alternative amphotericin preparation.

c) Amphotericin is nephrotoxic; blood counts and serum potassium levels should be closely monitored. It may also decrease serum magnesium levels.

d) Other nephrotoxic drugs should not be given concurrently unless essential.

e) Amphotericin induced hypokalaemia may precipitate digoxin toxicity and enhance the effects of skeletal muscle relaxants.

f) Corticosteroids may increase the potassium loss due to amphotericin.

g) There is some evidence suggesting synergism between amphotericin and flucytosine. Concurrent administration of intravenous imidazole drugs and amphotericin may be antagonistic.

h) Amphotericin injection can be given orally for a non-systemic effect.

i) As the pH of the glucose needs to be greater than 4.2, a phosphate buffer is provided by the pharmacy department.

j) Liposomal amphotericin is indicated only when the use of conventional amphotericin is precluded because of toxicity especially nephrotoxicity or if reduced infusion time is not tolerated e.g. preterm neonates.

ANTILYMPHOCYTE GLOBULIN (ALG - HORSE)

Preparations: INJECTION 100mg in 5ml. (Merieux) **(Named patient)**.

Dosage: *PREVENTION OF RENAL GRAFT REJECTION*

> **SEEK EXPERT ADVICE.**
> THE EXACT DOSE IS DEPENDENT ON THE CURRENT TRANSPLANT REGIMEN.

All ages, *IV injection*, **test dose** 4mg (0.2ml);
then **full dose** 4mg (0.2ml)/kg/day for 4 doses.

Administration: **Test dose,** dilute to 5-10ml in sodium chloride 0.9% or glucose/saline, administered over 30 minutes. If no severe reactions are observed after 30 minutes the full dose may be commenced immediately.

Full dose, dilute to a final concentration of not more than 2mg ALG in 1ml of sodium chloride 0.9% or glucose/saline.

ALG should be administered via a central line, if possible, over a minimum of 4 hours.

Notes:

a) Chlorpheniramine and hydrocortisone injection should preferably be given 1 hour or at least 15 minutes before commencing infusion of ALG. Do not give prior to test dose.

b) If allergy develops Antithymocyte Globulin (ATG) (see below) may be considered.

ANTITHYMOCYTE GLOBULIN (ATG - RABBIT)

Preparations: INJECTION 25mg in 5ml (Merieux) **(Named patient)**.

Dosage: *PREVENTION OF RENAL GRAFT REJECTION*

> **SEEK EXPERT ADVICE.**
> THE EXACT DOSE IS DEPENDENT ON THE CURRENT TRANSPLANT REGIMEN.

All ages, *IV injection*, **test dose** 0.1mg;
then **full dose** 2mg/kg/day for 5-10 days.

TREATMENT OF APLASTIC ANAEMIA

All ages, *IV injection*, **test dose** 0.1mg; then **full dose** 10-20mg/kg/day for 8-14 days. Usual course is 10 days.

Administration: **Test dose,** dilute to 5-10ml in sodium chloride 0.9% or glucose/saline, administered over 30 minutes. If no severe reactions are observed after 30 minutes the full dose may be commenced immediately.

Full dose, dilute to a final concentration of not more than 2mg ATG in 1ml of sodium chloride 0.9% or glucose/saline.

ATG should be administered via a central line, if possible, over a minimum of 4 hours.

Notes:

a) Chlorpheniramine and hydrocortisone injection should preferably be given 1 hour or at least 15 minutes before commencing infusion of ATG. Do not give prior to test dose.

b) ATG is used when allergy to ALG has occurred.

ARGININE

Preparations:	INJECTION 10g in 50ml (**Manufactured special**).
	POWDER (**From dietitian**).
Dosage:	*TREATMENT OF UREA CYCLE DEFECTS*

> **SEEK EXPERT ADVICE FROM METABOLIC TEAM BEFORE PRESCRIBING**

Orally, all ages, 100-150mg/kg/day, usually in 3 to 4 divided doses. In citrullinaemia and arginosuccinic aciduria (ASA) doses up to 700mg/kg/day may be required.

Intravenously, all ages, total daily dose administered as a continuous infusion over 24 hours. Administer until oral route available.

GROWTH HORMONE STIMULATION TEST

Intravenously, all ages, 500mg/kg (maximum 30g), over 30 minutes.

Administration:	Dilute to 20mg in 1ml with glucose 10% or 5%, maximum concentration is 50mg in 1ml.
Notes:	

a) Injection can be given orally.
b) Blood levels should be maintained between 50-200micromol/L.
c) Citrulline is also used in the treatment of urea cycle defects and is available from the metabolic dietitian.

ASCORBIC ACID

Preparations:	TABLETS 50mg, 200mg and 500mg. 100mg (**Non-formulary**).
	INJECTION 100mg in 1ml (**Non-formulary**).
Dosage:	*TREATMENT SCURVY*

Orally,

Under 4 years	125-250mg/day
4 - 12 years	250-500mg/day
12 - 14 years	375-750mg/day
Over 14 years	500mg-1g/day

Dosage may be given in divided doses.

ASPIRIN

Preparations: DISPERSIBLE TABLETS 75mg and 300mg.
Dosage:

> WARNING: ASPIRIN SHOULD NOT BE GIVEN TO CHILDREN UNDER 12 YEARS FOR ANALGESIA OR AS AN ANTIPYRETIC BECAUSE OF THE RISK OF REYE'S SYNDROME.

Aspirin is unlicensed for use in children.
ANTI-PLATELET
All ages, *orally*, 5-10mg/kg a day.

IN RENAL FAILURE AND RENAL TRANSPLANTATION
For anti-platelet effect
Orally,
Under 20kg,   18.75mg   } on Tuesday and Friday for
20-50kg   37.5mg   } transplant patients and on three days
Over 50kg   75mg   } of the week for haemodialysis patients.
ANTI-INFLAMMATORY E.G. JUVENILE ARTHRITIS
Over 1 year, *orally*, 80mg/kg/day in 4-6 divided doses. May be increased to 130mg/kg/day in acute conditions. If monitored, keep trough blood levels of salicylate in the region of 250-300mg/L.
KAWASAKI SYNDROME
Orally,
20-25mg/kg 4 times a day for approximately 14 days (until afebrile) then 3-5mg/kg once a day for 6 to 8 weeks (until echocardiogram normal).

Notes:

To give doses less than 75mg, dissolve one tablet in 5-10ml of water and use a proportion to obtain correct dose. Use immediately and discard remainder.

ATENOLOL

Preparations: TABLETS 25mg, 50mg and 100mg. SYRUP 25mg in 5ml.
Dosage: *HYPERTENSION*
This indication is unlicensed for use in children.
Orally, all ages, 1-2mg/kg once a day. Maximum 8mg/kg/day. Dose may be given twice a day if necessary.
IN RENAL FAILURE
No dosage adjustment is required in patients with creatinine clearance above 35ml/min/1.73m^2. If creatinine clearance is below 35ml/min/1.73m^2 use the lower of the above doses and adjust according to response. Avoid in haemodialysis patients.

Notes:

a) Caution, may induce bronchospasm; do not use in asthmatics.
b) May precipitate heart failure, use with caution.
c) Atenolol syrup (Tenormin®) is sucrose free but does contain 40% w/v of sorbitol.

ATRACURIUM BESILATE

Preparations:	INJECTION 25mg in 2.5ml and 50mg in 5ml.
Dosage:	**NEUROMUSCULAR BLOCKADE FOR VENTILATION AND SURGERY**

This indication is unlicensed for use in neonates.

> NEUROMUSCULAR CONDUCTION, USING A NERVE STIMULATOR, SHOULD BE MONITORED IF REPEATED DOSES OR INFUSIONS ARE ADMINISTERED.

Over 1 month, *IV injection,* initially 300-600microgram/kg with supplementary doses of 100-200microgram/kg.

IV infusion, 200-600microgram/kg/hour. Larger doses have been used in intensive care.

Administration: Dilute to 500microgram in 1ml or above with sodium chloride 0.9%. Glucose solutions may be used however these infusions are only stable for 8 hours.

Notes:

a) Neonates show increased sensitivity to atracurium.
b) Aminoglycosides increase or prolong paralysis caused by atracurium.
c) Elimination of atracurium is by Hofmann degradation, a non enzymatic process, which occurs at physiological pH and temperature. Decreased efficacy may be seen in pyrexic patients.
d) Drug of choice for patients with renal and/or hepatic failure as elimination is independent of function.
e) Cardiovascular effects are caused by significant histamine release.

ATROPINE SULPHATE

Preparations: INJECTION 600microgram in 1ml. TABLETS 600microgram.
EYE OINTMENT 1%. EYE DROPS 1%.
LIQUID 120microgram in 1ml (**Manufactured special**).

Dosage: **PREMEDICATION**

This indication is unlicensed for the oral route.
Administer dose 45 minutes prior to procedure.
SC or IM injection, approximately 10-20microgram/kg up to maximum of 30microgram/kg.
Orally, 20-30microgram/kg

SINUS BRADYCARDIA

This indication is unlicensed for use in children.
Over 1 year, *IV injection*, 15- 30microgram/kg.

REFLEX ANOXIC SEIZURES, HYPERSALIVATION

These are unlicensed indications.
Orally, initially, 10microgram/kg three times a day.

TO PARALYSE ACCOMMODATION IN YOUNG CHILDREN

Eye ointment applied twice a day for 3 days prior to the examination. If eye ointment unavailable drops can be used.

Notes:

a) Injection can be given orally.
b) Neonates may require higher doses on a microgram/kg basis as they are more resistant to atropine.
c) Can cause constipation if given regularly.
d) Atropine liquid is sugar free.

AZATHIOPRINE

Preparations: TABLETS 10mg (**Named patient**) and 50mg. INJECTION 50mg.
LIQUID (**Extemporaneously prepared**).

Dosage: *PREVENTION OF RENAL GRAFT REJECTION, SYSTEMIC LUPUS
ERYTHEMATOSUS*

SEEK EXPERT ADVICE BEFORE PRESCRIBING

Orally or IV injection, 60mg/m^2 (approx. 2mg/kg) once a day.
PREVENTION OF LIVER GRAFT REJECTION, CARDIOMYOPATHY

Orally or IV injection, all ages, 1.5mg/kg once a day.

Administration: Reconstitute vial with 5ml of water for injection (displacement
value negligible).
IV injection, see note c), give over at least 1 minute and flush
thoroughly with sodium chloride 0.9% or glucose/saline **or**
further dilute to at least 0.5mg in 1ml with glucose/saline and
infuse over 30-60 minutes.

Notes:

   a)   If allopurinol is administered concurrently, reduce dose of azathioprine
to 25% as it is potentiated by allopurinol.
   b)   Monitor total and differential white blood cell count and platelets.
   c)   Use the intravenous route **only** when the oral route is not feasible as
the injection solution is alkaline (pH 10-12) and very irritant.

AZLOCILLIN

Preparations: INJECTION 500mg, 1g and 2g.

Dosage: *TREATMENT OF INFECTION*
IV injection,

Premature neonates	50mg/kg twice a day
Full term neonates less than 7 days	100mg/kg twice a day
Neonates over 7 days - 1 year	100mg/kg 3 times a day
Children 1 - 14 years	75mg/kg 3 times a day, up to 5g 3 times a day

IN RENAL FAILURE

Creatinine clearance (ml/min/1.73m^2)	Dosage interval (hours)
less than 30	12

Haemodialysis, give the full dose twice a day on non-dialysis
days, with an additional dose prior to dialysis.
Peritoneal dialysis, dose as for creatinine clearance of less than
30ml/minute/1.73m^2.

Administration: On reconstitution each 500mg displaces 0.4ml.
Add 4.6ml water for injection to 500mg vial giving 500mg in 5ml.
Give doses of 2g or less by IV injection without further dilution.
Doses over 2g should be given by IV infusion, diluted with
glucose 5% or sodium chloride 0.9%, over 20-30 minutes.

Notes:

   a)   Azlocillin should only be used on the advice of microbiology. Use is
generally restricted treatment of cystic fibrosis and febrile neutropenia.
   b)   Azlocillin should **NOT** be mixed with aminoglycosides in infusion fluids.
   c)   Each 1g of powder contains 2.17mmol sodium.

AZTREONAM

Preparations:	INJECTION 500mg, 1g, 2g (**Non-formulary**).
Dosage:	**TREATMENT OF INFECTION**

This indication is unlicensed for premature neonates and neonates less than 7 days old.

IV injection,

Premature neonates	30mg/kg	twice a day
Full term neonates less than 7 days	30mg/kg	2-3 times a day
Neonates over 7 days to 2 years	30mg/kg	3 to 4 times a day
Over 2 years	30-50mg/kg	3 to 4 times a day

The total daily dose should not exceed 8g.

IN RENAL FAILURE

The initial dose should be the normal dose and the following doses adjusted according to creatinine clearance. Dosage intervals should remain the same.

Creatinine clearance (ml/min/1.73m^2)	Dosage interval (hours)
10-30	50% of dose
< 10	25% of dose

Haemodialysis:

The initial dose should be the normal dose and the following doses 25% of the initial dose. A supplementary 12.5% of the initial dose should also be given after each dialysis session.

Administration: On reconstitution each 500mg displaces 0.6ml. Addition of 1.9ml of water for injection to each 500mg of Aztreonam gives 500mg in 2.5ml.

IV injection, further dilute with sodium chloride 0.9% or glucose 5% to maximum of 100mg in 1ml and give as a injection, over 3-5 minutes or an infusion, over 20-60 minutes.

Notes:

a) There is evidence suggesting synergism between aztreonam and aminoglycosides for treatment of serious pseudomonal infections.
b) Reconstituted aztreonam injection solution may vary from colourless to light straw yellow which may develop a slight pink tint on standing; however this does not affect potency.
c) Aztreonam injection vials are sodium free.

BACLOFEN

Preparations: TABLETS 10mg. LIQUID 5mg in 5ml.

Dosage: **SPASTICITY AND FLEXOR/EXTENSION SPASM**

Under 1 year, probably of little use in this age group as neuronal transmissions are underdeveloped.

Over 1 year, *orally*, 0.25mg/kg three times a day increasing at 3 day intervals to 2mg/kg/**day**. Over 10 years, maximum dose is 2.5mg/kg/**day** or 100mg/**day**.

Recommended daily maintenance doses:

12 months - 2 years	10-20mg/day
2 - 6 years	20-30mg/day
6 - 10 years	30-60mg/day

POST-OPERATIVE SKELETAL MUSCLE SPASM CONTROL

Over 1 year, *orally*, initially 0.25mg/kg twice a day increasing according to spasm score; see pain management guidelines on page 251.

IN RENAL FAILURE

If creatinine clearance is <50ml/minute/1.73m^2 or in haemodialysis or peritoneal dialysis initial dose should be 0.25mg/kg/**day**.

Notes:

a) **CSM warning:** Drug withdrawal should be gradual to avoid serious side effects.
b) Baclofen should be used with caution in epilepsy.
c) Anecdotally, baclofen liquid has been administered rectally to post-operative patients.
d) Baclofen liquid (Lioresal®) is sucrose free.

B.C.G. VACCINE

Preparations: INTRADERMAL INJECTION containing ten 0.1ml doses.

PERCUTANEOUS INJECTION containing ten 0.03ml doses.

Dosage: **ACTIVE IMMUNISATION**

Percutaneously, see note a)

Neonates and infants, 0.03ml.

Intradermal, see note a)

Neonates and infants up to 3 months, 0.05ml.

Infants over 3 months and children, 0.1ml.

Administration: <u>Intradermal</u>

Reconstitute with 1ml of water for injection.

Allow to stand for 1 minute. Do **not** shake. Draw reconstituted solution into syringe once or twice to ensure homogeneity.

Should be given at insertion of deltoid muscle, i.e. not too high. Administration into the leg in neonates is associated with a higher incidence of side effects.

The vaccine should be administered by an operator competent in intradermal injection techniques.

<u>Percutaneous</u>

Reconstitute with 0.3ml of water for injection.

Administer using multiple puncture method.

Notes:

a) Currently all newborn babies will be offered selective BCG vaccination. Percutaneous administration is the preferred route for use in neonates in the Trust. Newborn babies who are contacts of a smear positive case should receive prophylactic isoniazid chemotherapy (see page 134) for 3-6 months then skin tested and vaccinated if negative.

b) Normally BCG vaccine is offered routinely to tuberculin - negative children aged 10-14 years. BCG vaccine should also be strongly recommended to those with a recent family history of tuberculosis, those living in crowded conditions in urban communities and to all immigrants and their children from countries with a high incidence of tuberculosis. They should be tuberculin-tested before vaccination with the exception of newborn babies and infants up to three months of age who should be vaccinated without delay.

c) BCG vaccine is a live vaccine and is contra-indicated in immunosuppressed patients (see immunisation guidelines page 296).

d) The injection site is best left uncovered to facilitate healing. If ulcer discharges apply a dry dressing but do not exclude air.

e) Any portion of vial not used within 4 hours should be discarded.

BECLOMETHASONE DIPROPIONATE

Preparations: AEROSOL INHALER 50microgram/metered inhalation (Becotide 50®), 100microgram/metered inhalation (Becotide 100®), 250microgram/metered inhalation (Becloforte® - not licensed for use in children); 200 dose units.
BREATH ACTIVATED INHALER 50, 100 and 250microgram/metered inhalation; 200 dose units. (Becloforte Easi-breathe® - not licensed for use in children).
AQUEOUS NASAL SPRAY 50microgram/metered spray (Beconase®).

Dosage: **ASTHMA THERAPY** (see note a).
Inhaled doses,

Under 1 year	50microgram	twice a day
1 - 4 years	50 - 100microgram	twice a day
4 - 12 years	100 - 400microgram	twice a day
Over 12 years	200 - 400microgram	twice a day

Doses should be doubled, for at least 4 weeks, after an acute asthma attack.
In severe cases inhaled doses may be given in 2-4 divided doses up to 1600microgram/day; Cushingoid effects may occur at these doses. Adrenal suppression is possible above 600microgram per day. It is unknown at what regular dose growth is inhibited.
ALLERGIC OR VASOMOTOR RHINITIS
Nasally, 6 years and over, 2 sprays (100microgram) into affected nostril(s) twice a day to a maximum of 4 times a day.

Notes:

a) Budesonide is the preferred first line inhaled corticosteroid. Beclomethasone should only be prescribed as continuation of pre-existing therapy at low doses.

b) Children under 10 years are usually incapable of using inhalers.

c) A Volumatic® spacer can be used with beclomethasone inhalers.

d) Rinse mouth and wash face (if using mask) after use.

e) See also guidelines for management of chronic asthma page 241.

BENDROFLUAZIDE (BENDROFLUMETHIAZIDE)

Preparations: TABLETS 2.5mg and 5mg. LIQUID (**Extemporaneously prepared**).
Dosage: ***DIURESIS***
Orally,

Up to 12 months	1.25mg	once a day
1 - 4 years	1.25 - 2.5mg	once a day
5 - 12 years	2.5mg	once a day
Over 12 years	2.5 - 5mg	once a day

Doses as high as 400microgram/kg once a day have been used initially and then the dose reduced to the above maintenance doses.

Notes:

a) Monitor serum potassium levels as required.
b) Caution, may exacerbate systemic lupus erythamatosus.

BENZHEXOL (TRIHEXYPHENIDYL)

Preparations: TABLETS 2mg and 5mg. SYRUP 5mg in 5ml (**Non-Formulary**).
Dosage: ***ANTISPASMODIC***
This indication is unlicensed for use in children.
Children under 7 years, *orally*, initially 0.5mg a day, increased by 0.5-2mg a day every 10 days until there is a clinical effect.
Children over 7 years, *orally*, initially 2mg a day, increased by 0.5-2mg a day every 10 days until there is a clinical effect.

Notes:

a) Use with caution in patients with hypertension, cardiac, liver or renal failure.
b) Benzhexol syrup (Rosemont®) is sugar free.

BENZYLPENICILLIN

Preparations: INJECTION 600mg (unbuffered).

Dosage: **TREATMENT OF INFECTION**

Premature and term neonates
IV injection,

Gestational age (weeks)	Postnatal age (days)	Dose	Interval (hours)
≤29	0-28	25mg/kg	12
	>28		8
30 - 36	0-14	25mg/kg	12
	>14		8
37 - Term	0-28	25mg/kg	8
	>28		6

In severe infection (meningitis) the above doses should be doubled.

1 month-12 years,
IV or IM injection, 12.5-25mg/kg 4 times a day.
In severe infection (meningitis), 50mg/kg every 4-6 hours.

IN RENAL FAILURE

Creatinine clearance (ml/min/1.73m^2)	Dosage Interval (hours)
10-50	8-12
Less than 10	12

Benzylpenicillin is moderately dialysed. For intermittent haemodialysis, CVVHD and CAVH/CVVH, dose as for creatinine clearance of 10-50ml/minute/1.73m^2.

Administration: On reconstitution 600mg displaces 0.4ml.
For IM injection add 1.6ml water for injection to 600mg vial to give 600mg in 2ml.
For IV injection add 4.6ml water for injection to 600mg vial to give 600mg in 5ml.
Further dilute with sodium chloride 0.9% and give as an IV injection over 5-30 minutes. Longer administration time is particularly important when using doses of 50mg/kg as too rapid administration has been associated with CNS toxicity and convulsions.

Notes:

a) In confirmed penicillin allergy, cephalosporins may be an alternative treatment although approximately 10% of these patients will also be allergic to cephalosporins. Where severe allergy symptoms have occurred previously or the extent of the allergy is unknown an alternative antibiotic should be given. Contact the microbiology department for further information.

b) 1 mega unit is equivalent to 1,000,000 units or 600mg.

c) **Caution:** benzylpenicillin **is not to** be given via the intrathecal route.

d) Each 600mg vial contains 1.68mmol of sodium.

e) See also antibiotic treatment guidelines page 259.

BERACTANT (BOVINE LUNG EXTRACT)

Preparations: VIAL 200mg in 8ml

Dosage: TREATMENT OF RESPIRATORY DISTRESS SYNDROME

This indication is unlicensed for use in term neonates and preterm neonates less than 700g.

Neonates, see notes a) and b), *intratracheally* 100mg/kg (4ml/kg). Dose may be repeated within 48 hours at intervals of at least 6 hours, maximum 4 doses.

Neonates, less than 30 weeks gestation, should be assessed to receive beractant as soon as possible after birth (i.e. within 30 minutes).

Administration: Allow vial to come to room temperature; 20 minutes on standing or 8 minutes hand held. Redisperse contents if necessary by inverting vial, DO NOT SHAKE.

Administer quickly via endotracheal tube, using a nasogastric tube which has been measured to reach the end of the E.T. tube. Dose in divided aliquots, see notes c) and d). Ventilate for 30 seconds between administration of each aliquot.

Notes:

a) Parameters for surfactant therapy are: a clinical picture and chest X-ray compatible with RDS, <72 hours old and intubated.

b) Distribution of surfactant may be improved by administering in 2 or more doses in the following positions:
1. supine with body rotated approximately 45° to the left and head to right.
2. supine with body rotated approximately 45° to the right and head to left.

c) For very unstable infants an increased number of smaller aliquots with periods of adequate ventilation in between may be of benefit.

d) Some infants may benefit from administration of surfactant via the side port. However this results in frothing and an increased incidence of blocked tubes.

e) Caution, continuous monitoring is required to avoid hyperoxaemia due to rapid improvement.

BETAINE

Preparations: TABLET 500mg (**Named patient**).

Dosage: TREATMENT OF HOMOCYSTINURIA

SEEK EXPERT ADVICE BEFORE PRESCRIBING

Orally, all ages 150-250mg/kg/day in 2-3 divided doses, adjusted according to plasma and urinary amino acid concentrations.

Notes:

Monitor methionine concentrations to avoid potentially toxic levels in classical homocystinuria.

BIOTIN

Preparations:	TABLETS 5mg (**Named patient**).
Dosage:	*METABOLIC DISORDERS*

> **SEEK EXPERT ADVICE BEFORE PRESCRIBING**

All ages, *orally*, 5-10mg 1-3 times a day. Doses up to 40mg/day may be required.

Notes:

Biotin (Vitamin H) is an essential coenzyme in fat metabolism and in other carboxylation reactions.

BISACODYL

Preparations:	TABLETS 5mg. SUPPOSITORIES 5mg (**Non Formulary**) and 10mg. ENEMA SOLUTION 2.74mg in 1ml (**Manufactured special**).
Dosage:	*CONSTIPATION*

Under 10 years	5mg *orally* at night or 5mg *rectally* in the morning.
Over 10 years	5-10mg *orally* at night increasing to 20mg in severe cases, or 10mg *rectally* in the morning.

PREPARATION FOR RADIOLOGICAL INVESTIGATION

Under 10 years	5mg *orally* on each of the 2 nights before the investigation and 5mg *rectally* (if necessary) 1 hour before the investigation.
Over 10 years	10mg *orally* on each of the 2 nights before the investigation and 10mg *rectally* (if necessary) 1 hour before the investigation.

Notes:

a) Bisacodyl is a stimulant laxative which increases intestinal motility and may be associated with abdominal cramp/colic or, in the presence of faecal impaction in the rectum, an increase of faecal overflow.

b) Many small children who experience pain or fear during defecation find rectally administered treatments very distressing and alternatives should be considered.

c) Response from rectal administration usually occurs within 30 minutes.

BOTULINUM A TOXIN

Preparations: INJECTION 500units (Dysport®).
Dosage: *DYNAMIC EQUINUS FOOT DEFORMITY IN CEREBRAL PALSY*

> **SEEK EXPERT ADVICE BEFORE PRESCRIBING**

    IM injection, over 2 years, total of 20units/kg divided equally between the muscle groups to be injected.
    A total of up to 30units/kg is required when more than four muscle bellies are injected.

Administration: Gloves must be worn when handling botulinum A toxin including during reconstitution and injecting. Reconstitute with 1.1ml of sodium chloride 0.9% to give 500 units in 1ml.
    Insert into muscle to be treated a 23G needle (blue) detached from syringe. Correct location is checked by manipulating the limb. Attach syringe to needle and draw back plunger to ensure it is not sitting in a vein followed by injection of the desired dose.

Notes:

   a)   Midazolam (page 151) is the first-line sedative for this procedure. See sedation guidelines page 247.
   b)   Discard unused botulinum A toxin vials by inactivating the residue with a 1% (10,000 parts per million (ppm)) chlorine solution. This is prepared by adding 1 Haz-tab® to 250ml of water. Botulinum A toxin spills must be wiped up with the above solution and disposable towels.
   c)   Counsel patient/carer to report any unusual/new muscle weakness not in the treated area e.g. droopy eyelids, difficulty swallowing or altered voice **or** pain or swelling at site of injection.

BOWEL CLEANSING SOLUTION

Preparations: ORAL POWDER SACHET containing polyethylene glycol 3350 59g, anhydrous sodium sulphate 5.685g, sodium bicarbonate 1.685g, sodium chloride 1.465g, potassium chloride 743mg. (Klean-Prep®). Each sachet is reconstituted in water to 1 litre.

Dosage: *PREOPERATIVE BOWEL CLEANSING, CONSTIPATION.*
    These indications are unlicensed for use in children. Use in constipation is an unlicensed indication.
    Orally,
    Children, (see note a), 20ml/kg/hr, increase to a maximum of 40ml/kg/hr to produce diarrhoea.
    Adults, 4 litres over 4-6 hours.

Administration: Give initial dose at least 2 hours after meal **(see note b)**. Solution should be drunk or given via a naso-gastric tube. Continue solution until anal discharge is clear. Solution can be flavoured with clear fruit cordial if required.

Notes:

   a)   Urticaria and allergic reactions have been reported.
   b)   Metoclopramide administered 30 minutes before initial dose may prevent abdominal distention and bloating, common side effects.
   c)   Reconstitute 1L at a time and store in the fridge, this improves taste.
   d)   Contra-indications are bowel obstruction, gastric retention, perforated bowel, toxic colitis, obstructive megacolon or ileus.
   e)   Klean-prep® is vanilla flavoured and contains aspartame.

BUDESONIDE

Preparations:	AEROSOL INHALER	50microgram/metered inhalation; 200 dose units
		200microgram/metered inhalation; 200 dose units
	TURBOHALER	100microgram/dose; 200 dose unit
		200microgram/dose; 100 dose unit
		400microgram/dose; 50 dose unit
	RESPIRATOR SOLUTION	500microgram in 2ml, 1000microgram in 2ml

Dosage:

ASTHMA THERAPY
Inhaled doses,

Under 1 year	50microgram twice a day
1 - 4 years	50-100microgram twice a day
4 - 12 years	100-400microgram twice a day
Over 12 years	200-400microgram twice a day

Doses should be doubled for at least 4 weeks after an acute asthma attack.
In **severe cases** inhaled doses up to 2mg/day may be required.
Nebulised,
This route is unlicensed for use in children under 3 months.

<3 months	0.25-0.5mg twice a day, reducing to 0.125-0.25mg twice a day
3 months - 12 years	0.5-1mg twice a day, reducing to 0.25-0.5mg twice a day.
Over 12 years	1-2mg twice a day, reducing to 0.5-1mg twice a day.

Initial doses may be doubled in severe cases.

CROUP
Nebulised,
All ages, 2mg administered as a single dose **OR** two 1mg doses administered 30 minutes apart.

CHRONIC LUNG DISEASE
This indication is unlicensed for use in children.
Nebulised,
Over 2 weeks old, 0.5mg four times a day, continue until after resolution of chronic lung disease.

Notes:

a) Children under 4 years are usually incapable of using turbohalers and children under 10 years are usually incapable of using inhalers. A Nebuhaler® spacer with a mask is available for use with budesonide inhalers.
b) Turbohalers are breath activated and are effective at low inspiratory flow rates i.e. 30L/minute. Lung deposition is also good and therefore changing to the turbohaler may allow a dose step down/better control.
c) Rinse mouth and wash face (if using mask) after use.
d) Cover eyes of neonates when using nebulised budesonide in an enclosed enviroment i.e. head box, incubator.
e) Use nebule within 12 hours of opening.
f) See also guidelines for management of chronic asthma page 241.

BUMETANIDE

Preparations: TABLETS 1mg and 5mg. LIQUID 1mg in 5ml (**Non-Formulary**).
Dosage: *DIURESIS*
This indication is unlicensed for use in children.
Orally, initially, 15microgram/kg once to four times a day to a maximum of 300microgram/kg/day.

Notes:

a) Monitor serum potassium levels regularly.
b) Bumetanide is well absorbed from the gut.
c) At low doses, Frusemide 40mg ≡ bumetanide 1mg however at higher doses this ratio falls.
d) Encephalopathy may be precipitated in patients with pre-existing hepatic impairment.
e) Bumetanide may enhance the nephrotoxicity or ototoxicity of other drugs, particularly if patients are in renal failure.
f) Bumetanide liquid (Burinex®) is sugar-free.

BUPIVACAINE

Preparations: INJECTION 0.25%, 0.5% and 0.75%; 10ml.
INJECTION 0.25% with adrenaline (epinephrine) 1 in 200,000; 10ml.
INJECTION 0.5% with adrenaline (epinephrine) 1 in 200,000; 10ml.
INJECTION 0.5% with glucose 8% in 4ml (bupivacaine heavy)
Dosage: *CAUDAL ANALGESIA*
Maximum dose: 2.5mg/kg/4 hours of 0.25% bupivacaine plain.

Up to lower thoracic (T10) (e.g. orchidopexy), 1ml/kg (maximum) of 0.25% bupivacaine plain. Dilute to 0.2% with sodium chloride 0.9% if over 20ml.

SACRAL ROOTS (e.g. circumcision, hypospadias), 0.5ml/kg of 0.25% bupivacaine plain.

LUMBAR ROOTS (e.g. inguinal hernia), up to 0.75ml/kg of 0.25% bupivacaine plain.

ILIO-INGUINAL BLOCK
0.5ml/kg of 0.5% bupivacaine plain. Maximum dose in any 4 hours not to exceed 1ml/kg.

Notes:

In children, particularly neonates and infants, the 0.25% strength provides very good pain relief and avoids dilution or difficult-to-administer infusion volumes.

BUPRENORPHINE - (CD)

Preparations: SUBLINGUAL TABLETS 200micrograms.
Dosage: **ANALGESIA FOR MODERATE TO SEVERE PAIN**
Sublingually,

16-25kg	100microgram	every 6-8 hours.
25-37.5kg	100-200microgram	every 6-8 hours
37.5-50kg	200-300microgram	every 6-8 hours
over 50kg	200-400microgram	every 6-8 hours

Notes:

a) Buprenorphine is a strong opioid mu receptor partial agonist that is not completely reversed by naloxone.
b) It is a long acting drug and may take up to 1 hour to work. The side effects are also long lasting.
c) See also pain management guidelines page 251.

CAFFEINE (BASE)

Preparations:	LIQUID 5mg in 1ml (**Manufactured special**). INJECTION 5mg in 1ml (**Manufactured special**).
Dosage:	**NEONATAL APNEOA** Premature neonates, *orally, IV injection*; Loading dose 10mg/kg followed 24 hours later by maintenance dose 5mg/kg/day; may increase to a maximum of 5mg/kg twice a day (see note b).
Administration:	Loading dose: IV infusion, dilute with sodium chloride 0.9% or glucose 5%. Give over 20 minutes. Slow IV injection, give over 3-5 minutes diluted further if needed
Notes:	

a) Caffeine base 1mg = caffeine citrate 2mg. All products from Guy's and St Thomas' pharmacy manufacturing department are labelled as the base and so doses should be prescribed, as above, as the base.
b) Neonates over 28 days of age who are still apnoeic may benefit from maintenance caffeine doses administered twice a day. Neonates on phenobarbitone should receive maintenance caffeine doses administered twice a day.
c) Therapeutic drug monitoring:
    i) Blood levels are not routinely monitored as caffeine has a wide therapeutic margin, however if required, a trough sample (just before the next dose) should be taken once the patient has been stabilised on a maintenance dose.
    ii) Therapeutic range: 5-40mg/L. Toxicity: ≥80mg/L.
d) Caffeine has a weaker diuretic action than theophylline.
e) Caffeine is a weak bronchodilator. Where this effect is desired, theophylline may be the drug of choice.

CALCITRIOL (1,25 DIHYDROXYCHOLECALCIFEROL)

Preparations:	CAPSULES 250nanogram (0.25microgram) and 500nanogram (0.5microgram) (**Non-formulary**). INJECTION 1microgram in 1ml and 2microgram in 1ml (**Both non-formulary**).
Dosage:	**PROPHYLAXIS AGAINST RENAL OSTEODYSTROPHY** This indication is unlicensed for use in children. Initially, *orally*, 15nanogram/kg (approximately 250-500 nanogram) once a day, (see note d) then titrate to response.
Notes:	

a) For a comparison of vitamin D preparations see section 9.6.4 of Adult Formulary.
b) There is a significant risk of hypercalcaemia if treatment is continued long term.
c) Calcitriol injection is available and may be indicated for hypocalcaemia in chronic dialysis, although this indication is unlicensed for use in children.
d) For doses other than 250 or 500nanogram the contents of the capsules can be syringed out.
    250nanogram capsules contain 250nanogram in 0.168ml.
    500nanogram capsules contain 500nanogram in 0.168ml.
e) Injection solution can be given orally.

CALCIUM (ORAL SUPPLEMENTS)

Preparations: LIQUID (Calcium Sandoz®) containing calcium glubionate 3.27g and calcium lactobionate 2.18g in 15ml (1ml contains 0.54mmol calcium).

EFFERVESCENT TABLETS (Sandocal-400®) each containing calcium lactate gluconate 930mg, calcium carbonate 700mg, anhydrous citric acid 1.19g, providing calcium 400mg (10mmol calcium).

Dosage: **HYPOCALCAEMIA**

Orally, up to 4 years	0.25mmol/kg	4 times a day.
Orally, 5 - 12 years	0.2mmol/kg	4 times a day.

Notes:

a)   Sandocal tablets are citrus flavoured and sucrose free but contain aspartame. Calcium-Sandoz® syrup is fruit flavoured and contains 1.5g sucrose in 5ml. They are both lactose free, and contain no added sodium or potassium or azo dyes.

b)   Tablets must be dissolved in 1/3 to 1/2 tumblerful of water.

c)   1.85ml of Calcium-Sandoz® syrup contains 1mmol of calcium.

d)   High oral doses of calcium may cause constipation.

CALCIUM CARBONATE

Preparations: TABLETS 300mg (**Manufactured special**), 1250mg (Calcichew®) and 2500mg (Calcichew Forte®)

LIQUID 600mg in 5ml (**Manufactured special**).

Dosage: **PHOSPHATE BINDING IN RENAL PATIENTS**

See notes below.

Orally, initially

Under 1 year	120mg	with feeds
1 - 6 years	300mg	3-4 times a day
6 - 12 years	600mg	3-4 times a day
Over 12 years	1250mg	3-4 times a day

Dose is adjusted according to phosphate levels.

Notes:

a)   Calcium carbonate is the preferred phosphate binding agent and should be taken immediately prior to or with food to bind dietary phosphate.

b)   Calcium carbonate is not suitable as a calcium supplement as only very small amounts of calcium are absorbed.

c)   Converting between aluminium hydroxide and calcium carbonate as phosphate binders the following can be used as a starting guide:
One aluminium hydroxide 475mg capsule (Alucap®) is equivalent to:-
one calcium carbonate 1250mg tablet (Calcichew®)
5ml of aluminium hydroxide mixture BP is equivalent to:-
two calcium carbonate 300mg tablet
or 5ml of calcium carbonate 120mg in 1ml mixture

d)   300mg tablets can be dispersed in water. 1250mg and 2500mg tablets can be chewed. The liquid can be added to feeds but must be mixed thoroughly to avoid precipitation.

e)   Calcichew® preparations are orange flavoured are sugar-free and contain 1mg of aspartame per 1250mg tablet.

CALCIUM CHLORIDE

Preparations: PREFILLED SYRINGES 10% of the dihydrate, 10ml (0.68mmol of calcium in 1ml). INJECTION 10% of the **hexahydrate**, 10ml (0.5mmol of calcium in 1ml).

Dosage: *ACUTE HYPOTENSION*

All ages, *slow IV injection* 0.2ml/kg.

> CALCIUM CHLORIDE SHOULD NOT BE USED FOR ANY OTHER INDICATION AS IT PRODUCES SEVERE TISSUE NECROSIS ON EXTRAVASATION.

Notes:

a)   Do NOT add to sodium bicarbonate.

b)   Given too rapidly IV calcium may cause cardiac arrhythmias or arrest, hypotension and vasomotor collapse, sweating, hot flushes, nausea and vomiting.

CALCIUM FOLINATE (FOLINIC ACID)

Preparations: TABLETS 15mg.

INJECTION 15mg, 30mg (St Thomas') and 350mg in 35ml.

Dosage: *TREATMENT OF MEGALOBLASTIC ANAEMIA*

Orally, 0.25mg/kg, up to 15mg, once a day.

DHPR DEFICIENCY (BIOPTERIN RECYCLING DEFECT)

Orally, initially 15mg once a day. Dose is determined by clinical response and C.S.F folate concentrations.

FOLATE RESCUE AFTER METHOTREXATE THERAPY

> DOSAGE REGIMENS VARY DEPENDING ON THE PROTOCOL USED, DOSE ADMINISTERED AND THE RESULTING BLOOD LEVELS OF METHOTREXATE.

In general doses are:

10kg and under

Orally, IV/IM injection, IV infusion; 0.5mg/kg every 4-6 hours for 36-48 hours.

Over 10kg

Orally, IV/IM injection, IV infusion, **10-15mg/m^2** every 4-6 hours for 36-48 hours.

Administration: Reconstitute each vial with 3ml of water for injection.

IV injection over 2 minutes.

Slow IV infusion, dilute with sodium chloride 0.9% or glucose 5% and give over 30 minutes.

Notes:

a)   Calcium folinate is not indicated for pernicious anaemia or other megaloblastic anaemias where vitamin B_{12} is deficient as it may improve haematological parameters but neurological symptoms may still occur or deteriorate.

b)   Injection solution can be given orally.

CALCIUM GLUCONATE

Preparations:	INJECTION 10%, 10ml (0.225mmol of calcium in 1ml).
Dosage:	*CALCIUM MAINTENANCE*
	IV infusion, 1mmol/kg/day added to the maintenance infusion.
	ACUTE HYPOTENSION, ACUTE CALCIUM SUPPLEMENTATION
	Slow IV injection, 0.5ml (0.113mmol)/kg with ECG monitoring.
	HYPERKALAEMIA

> **FOR EMERGENCY USE ONLY.**

	This is an unlicensed indication.
	For potassium levels of 6-7.5mmol/L, 0.5ml(0.1125mmol)/kg by slow *IV injection* with ECG monitoring. If potassium is greater than 7.5mmol/L give 5ml(1.125mmol)/kg.
Administration:	IV infusion: Dilute to at least 0.045mmol in 1ml (i.e. 1 in 5) with glucose 5% or sodium chloride 0.9% and administer at a rate not exceeding 0.0225mmol/minute.

> **DO NOT ADD TO SODIUM BICARBONATE**

Notes:
  a) Subcutaneous and intramuscular injections are not recommended.
  b) **Caution:** Avoid extravasation as calcuim salts cause tissue necrosis.

CALCIUM POLYSTYRENE SULPHONATE

Preparations:	POWDER for oral and rectal use. ENEMA 30g in 100ml (**Manufactured special**)
Dosage:	USE ONLY WHEN ALTERNATIVES NOT SUITABLE AND IN MILD TO MODERATE HYPERKALAEMIA WITHOUT ECG CHANGES.
	HYPERKALAEMIA
	Neonates: *rectally*, 0.125-0.25g/kg 4 times a day. *Oral* route should NOT be used.
	Children: *orally or rectally*, 0.25g/kg 4 times a day.
Administration:	Rectally: use pre-prepared enema or prepare enema solution by mixing each 1g of powder with 5-10ml of methylcellulose gel (see page 147) as inadequate dilution may result in faecal impaction. Administer immediately, once mixed. The enema should be retained and the colon should be irrigated prior to administration of next dose to ensure removal.

Notes:
  a) Administration of calcium polystyrene sulphonate should be stopped before serum potassium falls below 5mmol/L.
  b) Serum calcium levels should be monitored at weekly intervals.
  c) Give orally with a drink - **NOT SQUASH OR FRUIT JUICE** (as they are high in potassium).
  d) Bowel obstruction may occur and prophylactic laxatives (e.g. lactulose) should be prescribed.
  e) Calcium content is about 1.6 to 2.4mmol in 1g.
  f) Treatment of overdose: Give a laxative or enema to remove resin. Restore potassium levels with supplements, and lower calcium levels if raised.
  g) Exchanges 1-2mmol of potassium per g of resin.

CAPTOPRIL

Preparations:	TABLETS 2mg (**Named patient**),12.5mg and 25mg.
	LIQUID (**Extemporaneously prepared**).
Dosage:	*HYPERTENSION, CONGESTIVE CARDIAC FAILURE, PROTEINURIA*

Use in proteinuria is unlicensed for use in children.

Orally, children, initially, 100-500microgram/kg 3 times a day. Increasing to a maximum of 2mg/kg 3 times a day.

Orally,

Premature and full term neonates (see note a) initially 10-50 microgram/kg 3 times a day. Increasing to a maximum of **2mg/kg/day**.

> KEEP THE DOSE AS LOW AS POSSIBLE IN RENAL FAILURE AND IF A DIURETIC IS INDICATED, USE A LOOP DIURETIC RATHER THAN A THIAZIDE.

Notes:

a) Captopril should be avoided whenever possible in neonates, particularly preterm neonates due to the risk of renal failure, anuria and hypotension.

b) ACE inhibitors reduce glomerular filtration rate leading to severe and progressive renal failure in patients with severe bilateral renal artery stenosis (or severe stenosis in a single kidney).

c) Patient should be observed every 15 minutes for the first hour after the initial dose for effects of severe hypotension.

d) Concomitant diuretic dosages may need to be reduced or not administered concurrently to avoid severe hypotension.

e) Neutropenia is rarely reported but incidence is increased in renal failure, therefore monitor WBC every 2 weeks for first 3 months. Parent/patients should be encouraged to report any persistent sore throats or raised temperatures. Urine should be tested for protein every month for first 9 months.

f) Hyperkalaemia may occur particularly in renal failure.

g) Rashes may occur but usually disappear if dose is reduced.

h) Persistent dry cough, although rare, is sometimes alleviated by reducing dose however it is rapidly reversible upon withdrawal of drug.

i) Initiation of captopril has been associated with unexplained hypoglycaemia in severe diabetics.

j) The 2mg tablets can be dissolved in water immediately prior to use.

CARBAMAZEPINE

Preparations: TABLETS 100mg, 200mg and 400mg. CONTROLLED RELEASE TABLETS 200mg and 400mg. LIQUID 100mg in 5ml.
SUPPOSITORIES 125mg and 250mg.

Dosage: ***EPILEPSY, CO-ANALGESIA FOR NERVE PAIN***

Co-analgesia for nerve pain indication is unlicensed for use in children.

Initially, *orally*, 2.5mg/kg twice a day. Increase by 2.5-5mg/kg/day every 3-4 days until maintenance dose achieved. See note b).

TYPICAL MAINTENANCE DOSE: 5-10mg/kg twice a day,

OR

Up to 1 year	50-100mg twice a day.
1 - 5 years	100-200mg twice a day.
5 - 10 years	200-300mg twice a day.
10 - 15 years	300-500mg twice a day.
Controlled release tablets;	use doses above

Rectally, use only when the oral route is not available. Increase the required/established oral dose by 25% and give as rectal dose. Adjust according to response.

Notes:

a) Blood levels: Therapeutic range 4-14mg/L. Ideally levels to assess efficacy should be taken immediately prior to the next dose.

b) As carbamazepine induces its own metabolism, the half life falls with repeated dosing therefore the dose may have to be increased after initial treatment. Maximal induction of metabolism occurs after 4 weeks.

c) A full blood count and liver function test may be performed before and 4-6 weeks after starting treatment. Counsel patients or their carers to report any fever, sore throat, mouth ulcers, bruising or any other symptoms of blood, hepatic or skin disorders.

d) Carbamazepine can affect the metabolism of many hepatically metabolised drugs due to enzyme induction. Also carbamazepine blood levels may be increased or decreased by drugs which alter its metabolism. For further information contact your clinical pharmacist, drug information (Guy's ext. 3594, Lewisham ext. 3202, St Thomas' ext. 3069) or consult the Adult Formulary Chapter 4.8 or British National Formulary Appendix 1.

e) Anti-convulsants should be prescribed by generic AND trade name to ensure continuity of the same preparation for the patient as NOT ALL PRODUCTS ARE BIOEQUIVALENT. Tegretol® is the brand stocked by the Pharmacy Departments.

f) Controlled release tablets may be halved **BUT** must not be chewed.

g) Carbamazepine liquid and 100mg chewable tablets (Tegretol®) are sucrose free.

CARBIMAZOLE

Preparations: TABLETS 5mg and 20mg. LIQUID (**Extemporaneously prepared**).
Dosage: *HYPERTHYROIDISM*

Initially, *orally*,

Up to 1 year	250microgram/kg 3 times a day
1 - 4 years	2.5mg 3 times a day
4 - 12 years	5mg 3 times a day

Notes:

a)   Give as above until the patient is euthyroid, then progressively reduce.
b)   Monitor total and differential white blood cell count every 3 to 6 months.
c)   Counsel carer/patient to report the onset of sore throats, mouth ulcers, bruising and other indicators of bone marrow suppression and agranulocytosis.

L-CARNITINE

Preparations: LIQUID 3g in 10ml. INJECTION 1g in 5ml. (**Guy's only**).
Dosage: *TREATMENT OF PRIMARY OR SECONDARY CARNITINE DEFICIENCY.*

> **SEEK EXPERT ADVICE BEFORE PRESCRIBING**

All ages, *orally or IV injection*, 25-50mg/kg 2-4 times a day. May be increased up to 400mg/kg/day or 3g/day (see note b).

Administration: Slow IV injection over 2-3minutes.
Notes:

a)   L-Carnitine is an amino acid derivative which is an essential co-factor of fatty acid metabolism.
b)   Dose over 100mg/kg/day may cause diarrhoea.
c)   Can be diluted in fruit juice or water if required.
d)   L-Carnitine liquid (Carnitor®) contains 140mg of sucrose in 5ml.

CEFADROXIL

Preparations: CAPSULES 500mg.
                LIQUIDS 125mg in 5ml, 250mg in 5ml and 500mg in 5ml.
Dosage: *TREATMENT OF INFECTION*

Orally,

Under 1 year	12.5mg/kg twice a day
1 - 6 years	250mg twice a day
7 - 12 years	500mg twice a day
Over 12 years	500mg-1g twice a day

PROPHLAXIS OF URINARY TRACT INFECTION

Orally,

Under 1 year	6.25mg/kg at night
1 - 6 years	125mg at night
7 - 12 years	250mg at night
Over 12 years	250-500mg at night

IN RENAL FAILURE	
Creatinine clearance (ml/minute/1.73m^2)	Dosage Interval (hours)
10-25	24
Less than 10	36

Haemodialysis and peritoneal dialysis, normal doses should be given after dialysis.

Notes:

a) In confirmed cephalosporin allergy an alternative antibiotic should be prescribed. Contact Microbiology department for further advice.
b) Cefadroxil is more expensive and usually has no advantage over amoxicillin or erythromycin, unless these agents are contraindicated.
c) Cefadroxil liquid contain 2.7g of sucrose in each 5ml.

CEFOTAXIME

Preparations: INJECTIONS 500mg and 1g.
Dosage: *TREATMENT OF INFECTION*
Neonates: *IV injection,*
Less than 7 days old   30mg/kg every 12 hours
Over 7 days old   50mg/kg every 12 hours
Increase dose to 150-200mg/kg/day in 2-4 divided doses in severe infections, including neonatal meningitis.
Infants and children: *IM or IV injection,* 50mg/kg twice a day. Up to 50mg/kg 4 times a day in meningitis and other severe infections. Maximum 12g/**day**.
IN RENAL FAILURE
No dose reduction is required until the creatinine clearance is less than 5ml/minute/1.73m^2 when, following a single normal dose, the dose should be halved, keeping same frequency.
It is significantly removed by peritoneal dialysis and haemodialysis, dose as for normal renal function.

Administration: IM injection:
Reconstitute with water for injection by adding

1.8ml to	500mg vial to give	500mg in 2ml
3.5ml to	1g vial to give	1g in 4ml
8.8ml to	2g vial to give	2g in 10ml

Shake well until dissolved.
IV injection: Reconstitute as above and give over 3-5 minutes.
IV infusion: Dilute appropriate dose with glucose 5% or sodium chloride 0.9% to 20mg in 1ml and administer over 20-60 minutes.

Notes:

a) In confirmed cephalosporin allergy an alternative antibiotic should be prescribed. Contact Microbiology department for further advice.
b) Although highly effective against enterobacteria and *H. influenzae*, it is unreliable against *B. fragilis* and *Pseudomonas aeruginosa*.
c) Cefotaxime may be associated with reversible, late-onset neutropenia and eosinophilia.
d) Each 1g of powder contains 2.09mmol of sodium.
e) See antibiotic treatment guidelines page 259.

CEFTAZIDIME

Preparations: INJECTION 250mg, 500mg, 1g and 2g.

Dosage: **TREATMENT OF INFECTION**

IV or IM injection,

Under 2 months	12.5-30mg/kg twice a day.
Over 2 months	15-50mg/kg twice a day.

Doses up to 50mg/kg 3 times a day, maximum of 6g/**day**, may be given in severe infection, the immunocompromised, or children with cystic fibrosis.

IN RENAL FAILURE

Creatinine clearance (ml/minute/1.73m^2)	Dose	Dosage Interval (hours)
30-50	50-100% of dose	12
15-30	50-100% of dose	24
5-15	25-50% of dose	24
Less than 5	25-50% of dose	48

Haemodialysis: the normal dose should be given after dialysis. Peritoneal dialysis: 50% of the normal dose should be given initially, then 25-50% of the normal dose once a day. 125-250mg may be added to 2L of dialysis fluid.

CVVHD or high flux haemofiltration, dose is 25-50% of normal dose twice a day.

Administration: On reconstitution a 250mg (Fortum®) vial displaces 0.2ml; Kefadim® vials displace 0.6ml per 1g.

For Kefadim®:

IM injection: Add 1.7ml water for injection to 500mg vial or 3.4ml to 1g vial, to give 250mg in 1ml.

IV injection: Add 4.7ml water for injection to each 500mg to give 100mg in 1ml.

IV infusion: Dilute reconstituted vial with sodium chloride 0.9% or glucose 5% and give over a maximum of 30 minutes.

Notes:

a) In confirmed cephalosporin allergy, an alternative antibiotic should be prescribed. Contact the Microbiology department for further advice.

b) Ceftazidime may cause *C. difficile* associated diarrhoea and its only clear advantage over other cephalosporins is increased activity against *Pseudomonas aeruginosa*. It should be reserved for infections confirmed to be sensitive which have failed to respond to alternative antibiotics. It may be used as first line treatment in neonatal meningitis in combination with amoxicillin.

c) Neurological sequelae have been seen in renal failure where the dose has not been adjusted.

d) Each 1g of powder contains 2.3mmol of sodium.

e) See antibiotic treatment guidelines page 259.

CEFTRIAXONE

Preparations: INJECTIONS 250mg and 2g. 1g (**Non-formulary**).

Dosage: *TREATMENT OF MENINGITIS*

IM injection,
All ages, 20-50mg/kg once a day.
IV injection,
All ages, 20-50mg/kg once a day.
In severe infection up to 80-100mg/kg once a day may be given in infants and children (see note d). Maximum dose 4g/day.

PROPHYLAXIS OF MENINGOCOCCAL MENINGITIS

This is an unlicensed indication.
IM injection,
less than 12 years   125mg single dose
over 12 years   250mg single dose

IN RENAL FAILURE

No dosage reduction is required until creatinine clearance is less than 10ml/minute/1.73m^2 and then dose should not exceed 40mg/kg (2g). Ceftriaxone is generally not removed during haemodialysis or peritoneal dialysis, dose as for creatinine clearance less than 10ml/minute/1.73m^2.

Administration: On reconstitution 250mg displaces 0.2ml.

Deep IM injection: Dissolve 250mg in 0.8ml 1% lignocaine to give 250mg in 1ml. Dosages greater than 1g should be divided and injected in more than one site.
IV injection: Add 4.8ml water for injection to 250mg to give 50mg in 1ml and give over 2-4 minutes. Doses in neonates or over 50mg/kg should be given by IV infusion.
IV infusion: Dilute reconstituted dose with sodium chloride 0.9% or glucose 5% and give over 60 minutes in neonates (see note b) and 30 minutes for doses over 50mg/kg in infants and children.

Notes:

a) In confirmed cephalosporin allergy an alternative antibiotic should be prescribed. Contact Microbiology department for further advice.
b) The administration time of ceftriaxone is neonates is over 60 minutes to reduce the displacement of bilirubin from albumin thus reducing the risk of bilirubin encephalopathy.
c) Ceftriaxone should not be administered to jaundiced neonates or those with impaired or reduced bilirubin binding (e.g. prematurity, acute or chronic liver failure).
d) **Caution:** Doses over 80mg/kg may increase the risk of biliary precipitates.
e) Incompatible with calcium containing solutions i.e. Hartmann's solution.
f) Each 1g of powder contains 3.6mmol sodium.

CEFUROXIME

Preparations: INJECTION 250mg and 750mg.

Dosage: **TREATMENT OF INFECTION**

Neonates: *IV injection*, 30mg/kg twice a day.

Infants and children: *IM or IV injection*, 10-30mg/kg 3 times a day. 20mg/kg 3 times a day is the usual dose for most infections.

MENINGITIS, SEVERE INFECTION

Neonates: *IV injection*, initially, 50mg/kg twice a day. Reduce dose to 25mg/kg twice a day, on clinical improvement.

Infants and children: *IV injection*, 50-60mg/kg 3-4 times a day. Reduce dose to 100mg/kg/**day** after 3 days or on clinical improvement.

IN RENAL FAILURE

Creatinine clearance (ml/minute/1.73m^2)	Dose interval (hours)
Over 20	Not less than 8
10-20	12
Less than 10	24

Haemodialysis, normal dose once a day on non dialysis days and twice a day on dialysis days ensuring a dose is given after dialysis session.

CAVHD, high flux haemofiltration, normal dose every 12 hours.

Peritoneal dialysis, normal dose every 12 hours ensuring one dose given prior to and one dose post dialysis session.

Administration: On reconstitution 250mg displaces 0.2ml and 750mg displaces 0.5ml.

IM injection: Add 0.8ml water for injection to 250mg vial to give 250mg in 1ml and 2.5ml to 750mg vial to give 750mg in 3ml. Shake gently to produce a suspension.

IV injection: Add 2.3ml of water for injection to 250mg vial or 7ml of water for injection to 750mg vial to give 100mg in 1ml, then dilute reconstituted dose to 10ml with sodium chloride 0.9% or glucose 5% and give over 3-5 minutes.

IV infusion: Dilute reconstituted dose with sodium chloride 0.9% or glucose 5% and give over 30 minutes.

Notes:

a) In confirmed cephalosporin allergy an alternative antibiotic should be prescribed. Contact Microbiology department for further advice.

b) In the first weeks of life the serum half-life can be 3-5 times that of an adult.

c) Cefuroxime can be added to metronidazole infusion immediately prior to use.

d) Cefuroxime is a 2nd generation cephalosporin and has good activity against Gram positive organisms **except** Enterococcus (Streptococcus). It may cause *C. difficile* associated diarrhoea.

e) See also antibiotic treatment guidelines page 259.

f) Each 1g of powder contains 2.4mmol of sodium.

CETIRIZINE

Preparations:	LIQUID 5mg in 5ml. TABLETS 10mg.
Dosage:	***ANTIHISTAMINE***

This indication is unlicensed for use in children between 2 and 6 years except for seasonal rhinitis, and unlicensed in children under 2 years.

Orally,	under 2 years		0.25mg/kg	twice a day
	2 - 6 years		2.5mg	twice a day
		or	5mg	once a day
	over 6 years		5mg	twice a day
		or	10mg	once a day

IN RENAL FAILURE

If creatinine clearance below 20ml/minute/1.73m^2 or in haemodialysis or peritoneal dialysis reduce dose by 50%.

Notes:

Cetirizine liquid (Zirtek®) is banana flavoured and sugar free but does contain sorbitol.

CHLORAL HYDRATE

Preparations:	LIQUID 500mg in 5ml.
	LIQUID 200mg in 5ml (**Lewisham only**). SUPPOSITORIES 100mg and 500mg (**Manufactured specials**).
Dosage:	***SEDATIVE***

See notes below.

All ages, *orally, rectally,* 30-50mg/kg/dose (maximum single dose 1g), up to 3 times a day. It may be given more frequently in intensive care areas.

SEDATION FOR SCANS E.G. MRI

See notes below.

All ages, *orally,* single doses up to 100mg/kg have been used. If used in conjunction with trimeprazine (2mg/kg) doses of 75mg/kg or 50mg/kg (4mg/kg trimeprazine) have been used.

Notes:

a) Triclofos is the preferred sedative for procedures, see page 217. For sedation guidelines see page 247.
b) Use chloral hydrate with extreme caution in patients with severe hepatic or renal impairment.
c) All chloral hydrate liquids above are manufactured specials.
d) Take with plenty of water.
e) Chloral hydrate liquids contain sucrose.
f) Chloral liquid (St Thomas' Manufacturing) contains approximately 3g sugar in 5ml.

CHLORAMPHENICOL

Preparations:	INJECTION containing 1g of chloramphenicol (as succinate). CAPSULES 250mg. EYE DROPS 0.5%. EYE OINTMENT 1%.
Dosage:	*EYE PREPARATIONS*

Use drops or ointment hourly initially in acute infections and then 4 times a day. Continue for 2 days after infection clears (see note b).

TREATMENT OF INFECTION

> **CHLORAMPHENICOL IS NOT A FIRST LINE ANTIBIOTIC**
> **ONLY USE AFTER POSITIVE SENSITIVITIES AND ON MICROBIOLOGY ADVICE**

Neonates: In severe infection e.g. meningitis,
IV injection,

Up to 14 days	12.5mg/kg	every 12 hours
14 - 28 days	25mg/kg	every 12 hours

Orally or IV injection,

1 month - 1 year	12.5mg/kg	every 6-8 hours

In severe infection e.g. meningitis 25mg/kg every 6 hours
Over 1 year, *orally or IV injection* 25mg/kg every 6 hours
In severe infections, give a loading dose of 50mg/kg by *IV injection* followed by maintenance dose *IV injection* or orally, 25mg/kg every 6 hours.

IN LIVER OR RENAL FAILURE

Dosage reduction is not required in liver impairment and only required in severe renal impairment. Avoid unless no alternative available. Monitor levels.
Chloramphenicol is not removed by peritoneal dialysis but is removed by haemodialysis. Monitor levels.

Administration: On reconstitution 1g displaces 0.8ml. Add 9.2ml water for injection to 1g vial to give 100mg in 1ml.
IV injection: Give over 3-5 minutes.
IV infusion: Dilute with sodium chloride 0.9% or glucose 5%.

Notes:

a) Chloramphenicol use in paediatrics is generally restricted to treatment of severe infection and where a less toxic antibiotic is not available.

b) Fusidic acid 1% viscous eye drops (see page 197) are recommended for initial treatment except in neonates where chloramphenicol seems more effective. Chloramphenicol eye preparations are only indicated when sensitivities show that fusidic acid is not appropriate.

c) Blood levels:
   i) Sample should be taken immediately prior to 5th dose.
   ii) Trough less than 10mg/L.

d) Neonates are unable to metabolise the drug rapidly and accumulation can occur causing **grey syndrome** i.e. pallor, abdominal distension, vomiting and collapse. **Lower doses** are therefore required at this age, and should be controlled by blood levels. Also, chloramphenicol should only be given parenterally to neonates as they cannot adequately metabolise the palmitate.

e) High blood levels are associated with reversible bone marrow suppression. Irreversible bone marrow suppression is very rare and idiosyncratic.

f)   Chloramphenicol inhibits the metabolism of many drugs including oral anticoagulants and phenytoin. Phenobarbitone and rifampicin reduce the blood concentration of chloramphenicol. For further information contact your clinical pharmacist or drug information (Guy's ext 3594, St Thomas' ext 3069, Lewisham ext 3202).

g)   1g of chloramphenicol sodium succinate contains 3.14mmol of sodium.

CHLORHEXIDINE

Preparations: MOUTHWASH 0.2%. BLADDER WASHOUT 0.02%.

Dosage: ***ORAL HYGIENE***
Mouthwash:
Rinse mouth with 5-10ml for about 1 minute twice a day.

ANTISEPTIC BLADDER WASHOUT
The volume is dependent on the bladder size and should be retained for 10-15 minutes. Washout is not complete until returning fluid is clear.
Under 7 years,
Instill via catheter, 15-30ml at a time.
Over 7 years,
Instill via catheter, 30-50ml at a time.

Notes:
a)   Chlorhexidine mouthwash should not be swallowed. It may also cause reversible brown staining of the teeth; however this may be prevented by brushing the teeth **before** use.

b)   Ensure solution is at body temperature before instilling to avoid discomfort and bladder spasms.

CHLOROQUINE

Preparations:	TABLETS chloroquine sulphate 200mg (equivalent to 150mg chloroquine base). LIQUID chloroquine sulphate 68mg in 5ml (5ml is equivalent to 50mg chloroquine base). INJECTION chloroquine sulphate 54.5mg in 1ml (5ml) (equivalent to 40mg chloroquine base in 1ml) (**Non-formulary**).
Dosage:	**_RHEUMATOID ARTHRITIS, SYSTEMIC LUPUS ERYTHEMATOSUS_**

All ages, _orally_, 2.5mg/kg up to 3mg/kg (as chloroquine base) once a day (see note f). To avoid excessive dosages in obese or grossly oedematous patients use ideal body weight. Treatment should be discontinued if no improvement is seen in 6 months.

PROPHYLAXIS OF MALARIA

All ages, _orally_, 5mg/kg (as chloroquine base) at weekly intervals.
Start treatment 1 week before entering an endemic area and continue for 4 weeks after returning (see note e).

OR

Age	Dose (base)	
0 - 5 weeks	37.5mg	once a week
6 weeks - 1 year	75mg	once a week
1 - 5 years	150mg	once a week
6 - 11 years	225mg	once a week
12 years and over	300mg	once a week

TREATMENT OF BENIGN MALARIA
Orally,

Age		Dose (as chloroquine base)
Up to 12 years	Day 1	10mg/kg up to 600mg, then 5mg/kg up to 300mg, 6-8 hours later.
	Day 2-3	5mg/kg up to 300mg once a day (see note c).
Over 12 years	Day 1	600mg once then 300mg 6-8 hours later.
	Day 2-3	300mg once a day (see note c).

Course may need to be extended to 4-7 days (see note c).
Continuous IV infusion (see note a),
Over 4 weeks, 10mg/kg (of base) initially followed by 3 further doses of 5mg/kg (of base) i.e. Total dose of 25mg/kg (of base) in 32 hours (see note c).
SC/IM injection (see note b),
Over 4 weeks, 3.5mg/kg (of base) every 6 hours or 2.5mg/kg (of base) every 4 hours (see note c).

IN RENAL FAILURE

Dosage reduction of treatment doses may be required in renal failure due to increased unbound chloroquine in the circulation. Measure unbound chloroquine levels.

Creatinine clearance (ml/minute/1.73m^2)	Dosage
10-50	Half of the dose
< 10	One quarter of the dose

Chloroquine is not dialysed.

Administration: Slow IV infusion, diluted in sodium chloride 0.9%, over 8 hours.

Notes:

a)   IV infusion should **only** be used if oral route is impossible. **Slow** infusion is necessary to avoid arrhythmias, peripheral circulatory failure or acute encephalopathy.

b)   SC/IM route should only be used in exceptional circumstances where IV or oral route is not possible.

c)   Chloroquine alone is suitable for *P.malariae*; however a **radical cure** is required for *P.vivax* and *P.ovale*. Primaquine should be given for a radical cure.

d)

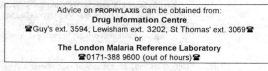

> Advice on PROPHYLAXIS can be obtained from:
> **Drug Information Centre**
> ☎Guy's ext. 3594, Lewisham ext. 3202, St Thomas' ext. 3069☎
> or
> **The London Malaria Reference Laboratory**
> ☎0171-388 9600 (out of hours)☎

> Advice on TREATMENT can be obtained from the duty doctor at:
> **The Hospital for Tropical Disease:**
> ☎0171-387 4411 (all hours)☎

e)   Retinopathy becomes more common with prolonged malaria prophylaxis for more than 1 year or after a total dose of 1.6g/kg. Specialist advice should be sought for long term prophylaxis.

f)   Before starting long term therapy a base line eye examination should be performed. Ocular toxicity is not normally seen with doses not exceeding 2.5mg/kg/day although monthly monitoring maybe considered necessary.

g)   Chloroquine liquid contains 1.8g of sucrose in 5ml, but is dye free.

CHLOROTHIAZIDE

Preparations: LIQUID 250mg in 5ml (**Named patient**).
TABLETS 500mg (**Non-formulary**).

Dosage: *DIURESIS*
Orally,

Under 6 months	12.5-17.5mg/kg	twice a day.
Over 6 months	12.5mg/kg	twice a day, increasing to a maximum of 40mg/kg/day.

Notes:

a)   Hypokalaemia and hyperuricaemia may occur.

b)   Chlorothiazide liquid (Diuril) contains 2g of sugar in 5ml.

CHLORPHENIRAMINE MALEATE
(CHLORPHENAMINE MALEATE)

Preparations:	TABLETS 4mg. LIQUID 2mg in 5ml. INJECTION 10mg in 1ml.
Dosage:	***SEDATIVE ANTIHISTAMINE***

Chlorpheniramine is unlicensed for use in children under 1 year.
Orally,

Up to 1 year	1mg	twice a day
1 - 5 years	1-2mg	3 times a day
6 - 12 years	2-4mg	3-4 times a day
Over 12 years	4mg	3-6 times a day

IV, SC or IM injection,
These routes are unlicensed for use in children.

4 weeks - 1 year	250microgram/kg
1 - 5 years	2.5-5mg
6 - 12 years	5-10mg
Over 12 years	10mg

Repeat up to 4 times in 24 hours if necessary.

> For *anaphylaxis* the injection should be given IV, as SC or IM injections rarely act more quickly than oral doses.

Administration:	IV injection, dilute in the syringe with 5-10ml of sodium chloride 0.9%, water for injection or blood and inject slowly over 1 minute.
Notes:	

a) IV injection may be associated with transient drowsiness, giddiness and hypotension particularly if administration is too rapid.
b) Paradoxical excitation can be seen in children.
c) Injection can be given orally.
d) Chlorpheniramine liquid (Piriton®) contains 1.8g of sucrose in 5ml and 6.5% v/v of alcohol but is tartrazine free.

CHLORPROMAZINE

Preparations: TABLETS 10mg (**Non-formulary**), 25mg, 50mg and 100mg.
SYRUP 25mg in 5ml. SUSPENSION 100mg in 5ml.
INJECTION 25mg in 1ml.

Dosage:

> THE IV ROUTE IS UNLICENSED AND CAN RESULT IN SEVERE HYPOTENSION,
> USE THIS ROUTE WITH EXTREME CAUTION.

PREMEDICATION
This is an unlicensed indication.
All ages, *IM injection* 1mg/kg.

CHILDHOOD SCHIZOPHRENIA, AUTISM

> SEEK EXPERT ADVICE BEFORE PRESCRIBING

Orally, IV injection, 500microgram/kg every 4-6 hours.
IM injection, 500microgram/kg every 6-8 hours.
1 - 5 years   Maximum total daily dose 40mg/**day**.
6 - 12 years   Maximum total daily dose 75mg/**day**.

NARCOTIC WITHDRAWAL IN THE NEONATE
This is an unlicensed indication.
Orally or IV injection, 550-750microgram/kg 4 times a day.
Dose can be doubled if withdrawal is severe. Once stable
reduce dose by not more than 2mg/kg/**day** on every third day.

Administration: Dilute to at least 2.5mg in 1ml in sodium chloride 0.9% and give
over 20-60 minutes. Keep patient supine and monitor BP
regularly, as **severe hypotension** may occur.

Notes:

a)   Chlorpromazine should only be used where alternatives are not
available due to the risk of side effects. Side effects include
antimuscurinic effects, photosensitivity, occasionally abnormal liver
function, agranulocytosis and rarely neuroleptic malignant syndrome
and lupus erythematosus like syndrome.

b)   Extrapyramidal side effects may also occur, especially in young
children. Chlorpromazine should not generally be used in infants
under 1 year except for narcotic withdrawal in neonates.

c)   **Caution:** Do not crush tablets and minimise handling of preparations
due to risk of contact sensitisation.

d)   The injection must be protected from light. Any solution which
develops a pink or yellow colouration should be discarded.

e)   Chlorpromazine (Largactil®) suspension is sucrose free. The syrup
(Rosemont) contains 2.25g of sucrose in 5ml.

CHOLESTYRAMINE (COLESTYRAMINE)

Preparations: SACHETS 5g containing 4g of cholestyramine (Questran Light®).
POWDERS (**Extemporaneously prepared**).

Dosage: *DIARRHOEAL DISORDERS, HYPERLIPIDAEMIA, PRURITUS ASSOCIATED WITH CHOLESTASIS.*

These indications are unlicensed for use in children under 6 years.
Orally, initially,

Under 6 years	2g (½ sachet)/day
Over 6 years	4g (1 sachet)/day

Increase dose according to response. Maximum dose is 36g/**day**. Give as a single dose or in up to 4 divided doses.

Notes:

a)   All other drugs should be administered at least 1 hour before or 6 hours after cholestyramine to reduce possible interference with absorption, especially digoxin and warfarin.
b)   Fat soluble vitamin malabsorption may occur.
c)   Cholestyramine should **only** be used to lower cholesterol in conjunction with an appropriate diet.
d)   Each sachet of Questran Light® is orange flavoured, contains 30mg aspartame and 0.72g sugar.

CHORIONIC GONADOTROPHIN

Preparations: INJECTION 5,000 units. (St Thomas' only).
Dosage: *HUMAN CHORIONIC GONADOTROPHIN STIMULATION TEST*

SEEK EXPERT ADVICE BEFORE PRESCRIBING

Intramuscularly, 1500units on days 1 to 4.

Notes:

Gonadotrophins should be employed only by those particularly experienced in their use, and then only when a thorough preliminary investigation of the problem and its underlying cause has been undertaken. Treatment of cryptorchidism and delayed puberty with such agents **may** be quite inappropriate.

CICLOSPORIN

Preparations:	ORAL LIQUID 100mg in 1ml. CAPSULES 10mg, 25mg, 50mg, 100mg. INJECTION 50mg in 1ml.
Dosage:	***PREVENTION OF RENAL GRAFT REJECTION AND STEROID RESISTANT NEPHROTIC SYNDROME***

> **CAUTION: STATE BRAND WHEN PRESCRIBING**
> **AS NEORAL® AND SANDIMMUN® ARE NOT BIOEQUIVALENT**

Initial dose, 150mg/m^2 *orally* twice a day (see current paediatric renal transplant protocol). Dosage should then be adjusted according to trough blood levels. If converting from the oral to the intravenous route, give one-third of the previous oral dose.

STEROID DEPENDENT NEPHROTIC SYNDROME

Initial dose, 75mg/m^2 *orally* twice a day. Dosage should then be adjusted according to trough blood levels.

Administration: IV injection, dilute to between 0.5mg in 1ml and 2.5mg in 1ml with sodium chloride 0.9% or glucose 5% and give over 2-6 hours.

Notes:

a) Limited to use in specialised units.
b) Ideal trough whole blood levels are 70-180 microgram/L. The therapeutic range is dependant on the assay used.
c) Blood levels of ciclosporin may be **increased** by the concurrent administration of grapefruit juice, erythromycin, cimetidine, methylprednisolone, metoclopramide, sex hormones (oral contraceptives), diltiazem, nicardipine, verapamil, tacrolimus, ketoconazole, itraconazole and fluconazole.
d) Blood levels of ciclosporin may be **reduced** by concurrent administration of rifampicin, phenobarbitone, phenytoin, carbamazepine, or heparin.
e) Concurrent administration of nephrotoxic drugs such as aminoglycosides, co-trimoxazole, amphotericin, ciprofloxacin, diclofenac, frusemide or metolazone may enhance nephrotoxicity.
f) Concurrent administration with digoxin can cause elevated plasma digoxin levels.
g) The immunological response to vaccines may be reduced in patients taking ciclosporin.
h) The oral liquid has an unpleasant taste which can be masked by milk or orange juice. Do NOT administer via a nasogastric tube.
i) Do not refrigerate oral liquid and discard two months after opening bottle.
j) After opening, the contents of the ampoule should be used immediately.
k) Ciclosporin injection contains polyethoxylated castor oil which has been reported to cause anaphylactic reactions.

CIPROFLOXACIN

Preparations:	TABLETS 100mg and 250mg. LIQUID 250mg in 5ml. INJECTION 2mg in 1ml (50ml, 100ml and 200ml).
Dosage:	**TREATMENT OF SEVERE INFECTIONS**

This indication is unlicensed for use in children under 1 year. In children and growing adolescents ciprofloxacin is only recommended where the benefits outweigh the risk of arthropathy.

All ages,

Orally,	4-7.5mg/kg twice a day.
IV infusion,	3-5mg/kg twice a day.

PROPHYLAXIS OF MENINGOCOCCAL MENINGITIS

This is an unlicensed indication but is the preferred treatment at Guy's & St Thomas'.

6 - 12 years	250mg as a single dose.
Over 12 year	500mg as a single dose.

IN RENAL FAILURE

In renal failure reduce the total daily dose by 50% if creatinine clearance is less than 20ml/minute/1.73m^2.

Administration: Infuse directly over 30-60 minutes. Dilute if required with sodium chloride 0.9%.

Notes:

a) **CSM Warning:** At the first sign of pain or inflammation, patients should discontinue treatment and rest the affected limb until tendon symptoms have resolved.

b) **Seizure threshold** may be reduced by ciprofloxacin therefore it should be used with caution where there is a history of convulsions. This risk may be increased with concomitant NSAIDs.

c) Ciprofloxacin may enhance effect of oral anticoagulants, increase theophylline levels and increase risk of nephrotoxicity with ciclosporin.

d) Ciprofloxacin absorption is very good, use the oral route whenever practicable. Antacids, iron and sucralfate however may reduce absorption.

e) The tablets can be dispersed in water immediately before taking, although the taste is very bitter. The liquid has an initial pleasant taste but still has a bitter after taste. It is not suitable for administration down a nasogastric tube as it may block the tube.

f) The liquid contains 0.57g of sucrose in 5ml.

CISAPRIDE

Preparations:	LIQUID 1mg in 1ml. TABLETS 10mg.
	SUPPOSITORIES 30mg (**Named patient**).
Dosage:	*GASTRO-OESOPHAGEAL REFLUX, GASTRIC STASIS*
	These indications are unlicensed for use in children.

> **CSM Warning:** Cisapride is contraindicated in premature neonates (less than 36 weeks gestation) for up to 3 months after birth due to increased reports of QT interval prolongation. See notes below for additional cautions and warnings.

Orally,

Premature neonates of post conceptual age ≤32 weeks, 0.1mg/kg twice a day.

Premature neonates of post conceptual age >32 weeks and neonates, 0.1mg/kg three times a day.

1 month - 12 years,	0.2mg/kg	3 or 4 times a day
Over 12 years,	10mg	3 or 4 times a day

Rectally,

1 month - 12 years,	0.6mg/kg	3 or 4 times a day
Over 12 years,	30mg	3 or 4 times a day

RENAL OR HEPATIC IMPAIRMENT (INCLUDING DIALYSIS)

Initially dose should be halved and then adjusted according to response. See notes below.

Notes:

a) Cisapride should not be prescribed first line for use in any children, (see gastro-oesophageal reflux guidelines, page 232) except where alternatives would not be appropriate. Seek expert advice. In premature neonates (<36 weeks gestation) for up to 3 months after birth where it is clinically indicated, written consent should be obtained prior to prescribing cisapride, and documented in the patients notes.

b) **WARNING:** Cisapride is not recommended in conditions leading to QT prolongation (e.g. hypokalaemia, hypomagnesaemia, renal and respiratory failure), congenital QT prolongation and with concomitant drugs which prolong QT interval (e.g. amiodarone, amitriptyline, sotalol).

c) Where cisapride is clinically indicated, a baseline ECG should be performed. A repeat ECG should be performed after 3 days of therapy in all neonates and children and then again after 7 days of therapy in premature infants (gestational age <36 weeks) up to 3 months after birth and term neonates up to 1 month of age.
Cisapride should not be started if QT interval is above 440 msec and therapy discontinued if QTc interval is 450 msec or greater.

d) **CAUTION:** Risk of ventricular arrhythmias, due to inhibition of metabolism of cisapride, may be increased with concomitant itraconazole, ketoconazole, clarithromycin, erythromycin, fluconazole, miconazole (not topical), terfenadine, ritonavir and indinavir. Patient/carer should be advised to inform health care workers that they/their child is on cisapride before the initiation of new drug therapy.

e) As cisapride accelerates gastric emptying, absorption of drugs from the stomach may be reduced whilst absorption from the small intestine may be accelerated. Plasma levels of anticonvulsants should be monitored. In patients receiving anticoagulants, prothrombin time may be prolonged with concurrent administration of cisapride. Clotting times should be checked within a week of initiating or discontinuing cisapride.

f) Cisapride suspension is cherry flavoured and contains colourings and 1g of sucrose in 5ml.

CITRATE SOLUTIONS

Preparations: LIQUID 3g in 10ml (**Manufactured special**) containing 2.8mmol potassium and 1.16mmol citrate in 1ml.

LIQUID Polycitra® and Polycitra LC® (**Named patient**) containing 1mmol sodium, 1mmol potassium and 1mmol citrate in 1ml.

Dosage: *RENAL ACIDOSIS, PRIMARY HYPEROXALURIA, URINARY ALKALISATION*

Orally, all ages, 0.5-1mmol citrate/kg/day or see note a).

Notes:

a) 1mmol of citrate is approximately equivalent to 2mmol of bicarbonate.
b) Potassium levels should be monitored.
c) Potassium citrate mixture contains sucrose.
d) Polycitra® is orange flavoured and contains 2.25g of sucrose in 5ml. Polycitra LC® is lime flavoured and is sugar free.

CLARITHROMYCIN

Preparations: LIQUID 125mg in 5ml. TABLETS 250mg; 500mg (**Non-formulary**). INJECTION 500mg (**Non-formulary**).

Dosage: **TREATMENT OF INFECTION**

The intravenous route is unlicensed for use in children.

USE IV ROUTE ON CONSULTANT ADVICE ONLY

Orally, IV injection, 7.5mg/kg twice a day. Maximum dose 500mg twice a day for severe infection.

OR, *orally*,

1 - 2 years	62.5mg	twice a day
3 - 6 years	125mg	twice a day
7 - 9 years	187.5mg	twice a day
over 10 years	250mg	twice a day

IN RENAL FAILURE

Reduce dose by 50% if creatinine clearance is less than 30ml/minute/1.73m^2. No dosage adjustments are necessary in haemodialysis or peritoneal dialysis.

Administration: Reconstitute vial with 10ml of water for injection to give 50mg in 1ml concentration. Dilute reconstituted dose to 2mg in 1ml with sodium chloride 0.9% or dextrose 5% and give over 1 hour via a **large** vein.

C

Notes:

a) **CSM Warning:** Avoid concomitant administration with astemizole, terfenadine and cisapride due to increased risk of arrhythmias.
b) Clarithromycin as with other macrolide antibiotics, increases theophylline and carbamazepine blood levels and may increase ciclosporin and digoxin levels.
c) Each 1g of powder contains less than 1mmol of sodium.
d) Clarithromycin liquid is fruit punch flavoured and contains 2.75g of sucrose in 5ml.

CLINDAMYCIN

Preparations: CAPSULES 150mg. LIQUID 75mg in 5ml.
INJECTION 300mg in 2ml.

Dosage:

CONSULT MICROBIOLOGIST BEFORE PRESCRIBING

TREATMENT OF INFECTION
Over 1 month of age,
Orally, 3-6mg/kg every 6 hours depending on severity of infection. Children less than 10kg, minimum recommended dose is 37.5mg every 8 hours.
IM or IV injection **15-25mg/kg/day** in 3-4 divided doses.

SEVERE INFECTIONS
Over 1 month of age, *IM or IV injection* **25-40mg/kg/day** in 3-4 divided doses.

ENDOCARDITIS PROPHYLAXIS
See guidelines page 265.

IN HEPATIC FAILURE
Dose should be reduced in hepatic failure and liver function tests should be monitored.

Administration: IM injection: Maximum 600mg (4ml) per dose.
IV injection: Clindamycin must be diluted before IV administration to at least 6mg in 1ml with sodium chloride 0.9% or glucose 5% and infused over at least 10-60 minutes. Maximum rate 20mg/kg over 1 hour.

Notes:

a) Monitor liver function tests and blood counts in neonates and infants. Clindamycin is not recommended in neonates under 4 weeks old.
b) Clindamycin should only be used in consultation with the microbiology department because of serious side effects.
c) Growth of *Clostridium difficile* may cause pseudomembranous colitis. This should be treated with metronidazole or **oral** vancomycin.
d) Clindamycin suspension (Dalacin C®) contains 1.8g of sucrose in 5ml.

CLOBAZAM

Preparations: TABLETS 10mg.
LIQUID 1mg in 1ml (**Manufactured special**).

Dosage: *EPILEPSY*
This indication is unlicensed for use in children less than 3 years.
Orally,
Under 3 years   initially 150microgram/kg twice a day
3 years and over   initially 500microgram/kg at night
Increase doses at 5 day intervals until satisfactory response or maximum of 1mg/kg twice a day.

Notes:

a)   Not all liquid preparations are bioequivalent. Continuation supplies should be obtained from the same manufacturer.

b)   Clobazam is on the government "black list" for all indications except epilepsy. Prescriptions should be endorsed "SLS".

c)   Clobazam liquid (St Thomas' Manufacturing) contains 1.5g of sugar in 5ml.

CLOMETHIAZOLE EDISYLATE

Preparations: CAPSULES clomethiazole base 192mg. LIQUID clomethiazole edisylate 250mg in 5ml. INTRAVENOUS INFUSION clomethiazole edisylate 0.8%, 8mg in 1ml.

Dosage: *STATUS EPILEPTICUS*
All ages, *IV infusion,* 5-10mg(0.6-1.25ml)/kg/hour. Titrate rate of infusion to response, increasing rate every 2-4 hours. Up to 18mg(2.25ml)/kg/hour has been used. After seizures are controlled, rate of infusion should be gradually decreased every 4-6 hours.

EPILEPSY
This is an unlicensed indication.
Orally, all ages, 20mg(0.4ml)/kg/day (of edisylate) in divided doses given every 2-4 hours. Tachyphylaxis occurs quickly.

Notes:

a)   Paradoxical worsening of epilepsy in Lennox Gastaut Syndrome may occur.

b)   During IV administration full observations should be completed every 4 hours, because of the risk of cardiovascular and respiratory depression which can be severe if infusion is continued for longer than 12 hours.

c)   Chlormethiazole infusion interacts with plastic (PVC) giving sets. This increases the risk of thrombophlebitis and may alter the drop rate. The giving set must be changed every 24 hours. PVC giving sets should be checked regularly during administration to ensure no softening of tubing occurs, particularly during low drip rates.

d)   Daily fluid requirements should be monitored as IV infusion of chlormethiazole can result in large volumes and sodium concentrations in excess of daily requirements being infused. Intravenous infusion sodium content is 32mmol/L.

e)   One capsule is approximately equivalent to 5ml of liquid.

f)   Chlormethiazole liquid (Heminevrin®) is sucrose free.

CLONAZEPAM

Preparations:	TABLETS 500microgram and 2mg. INJECTION 1mg in 1ml. LIQUID 2.5mg in 1ml (**Named patient**).
Dosage:	**STATUS EPILEPTICUS**

Slow IV injection, over 30 seconds, 50microgram/kg up to 500microgram. Repeat if necessary.

IV infusion, 10 microgram/kg/hour following IV injection. Adjust dose according to response, up to 60microgram/kg/hr has been used.

EPILEPSY

Orally, all ages, 50-200microgram/kg/**day** in 3-4 divided doses. Increase dose every 4-5 days.

OR

Age	Initial dose per **day**	Maintenance dose per **day**
Up to 1 year	250microgram	500microgram-1mg
1 - 5 years	250microgram	1-3mg
5 - 12 years	500microgram	3-6mg
Over 12 years	1mg	4-8mg

Administration: IV injection, dilute with 1ml water for injection immediately before use and give slowly over 2-3 minutes. IV infusion, dilute with sodium chloride 0.9% or glucose 5%. Watch infusion for signs of precipitation and change every 12 hours. Clonazepam can be infused undiluted (i.e. 1mg in 1ml).

Notes:

a) Blood levels: Therapeutic range 25-85microgram/L. Although this does not appear to correlate with either efficacy or side effects.

b) Impaired swallowing and respiratory depression are possible with IV administration. Salivary and bronchial hypersecretion may also occur, particularly if there is mental impairment. This may lead to feeding difficulties in the mentally handicapped and supervision of the airway may be necessary.

c) Prolonged infusion may lead to accumulation and delay recovery.

d) Tolerance to clonazepam may develop in some patients. If this occurs control may be re-established by increasing the dose or interrupting therapy for 2 to 3 weeks. If interrupting therapy, withdraw drug slowly and consider addition of other drugs.

e) Injection can be given orally.

f) To prevent withdrawal symptoms after prolonged maintenance therapy, withdraw clonazepam by reducing dose by approximately 40microgram/kg/**week**.

g) Clonazepam injection contains 20% v/v ethanol and 30mg of benzylalcohol per 1ml ampoule.

CLONIDINE

Preparations: TABLETS 25microgram and 100microgram.

Dosage: *ATTENTION DEFICIT HYPERACTIVITY DISORDER WITH OR WITHOUT OPPOSITIONALITY, OR WITH TIC DISORDER*

SEEK EXPERT ADVICE BEFORE PRESCRIBING

This is an unlicensed indication.

Orally, initially, 25microgram at night for 1-2 weeks then increase to 50microgram at night.

If required dose can be further increased by 25microgram every 2 weeks, side effects permitting.

Maximum dose **5microgram/kg/day** (or up to a maximum of 200microgram/day).

Notes:

a) Blood pressure and pulse must be monitored on initiating treatment and after each dosage increase. Patients on concomitant methylphenidate should have a base line and then three monthly ECGs.

b) Patients should be monitored at least weekly for side effects whilst dose is being established.

c) Abrupt withdrawal of clonidine can result in rebound hypertension.

d) Clonidine can be used as an adjunct to methylphenidate if insomnia is a significant problem e.g. methylphenidate in the morning and mid-day and clonidine in the evening.

CO-AMOXICLAV

Preparations:

	Amoxicillin		Clavulanic acid
TABLETS	250mg	plus	125mg
LIQUIDS	125mg	plus	31mg
	250mg	plus	62mg
INJECTIONS	1g	plus	200mg
	500mg	plus	100mg

Dosage:

ONLY USE AFTER POSITIVE SENSITIVITIES

TREATMENT OF INFECTION

Orally, 20mg/kg/day (based on **amoxicillin** content) in 3 divided doses, **OR**

1 - 6 years	5ml of 125/31 liquid	3 times a day
6 - 12 years	5ml of 250/62 liquid	3 times a day
Over 12 years	1 tablet (250/125)	3 times a day

In severe infections dosage may be doubled if suspension is prescribed. Extra amoxicillin only should be given if the tablets are prescribed to avoid excessive doses of clavulanic acid.

Slow IV injection,
Dosage is based on **amoxicillin** content:

Premature and neonates <7 days	25mg/kg every 12 hours
Neonates >7 days - 3 months,	25mg/kg every 8 hours
3 months - 12 years,	25mg/kg every 8 hours increase to every 6 hours in severe infections.
Over 12 years	1g every 8 hours, increase to every 6 hours in severe infections.

PROPHYLAXIS
Give one third of the total daily treatment dose at night.

IN RENAL FAILURE

Creatinine clearance (ml/minute/1.73m^2)	Dosage Interval (hours)
10-30	Orally: normal dose 12 hourly
	IV: normal dose initially, then half dose 12 hourly.
<10	Orally: half-normal dose 12 hourly.
	IV: normal dose initially, then half dose 24 hourly.

Haemodialysis:
Co-amoxiclav is cleared by dialysis therefore give as per creatinine clearance <10ml/minute/1.73m^2. May need to give an additional half dose during and after dialysis.
Peritoneal dialysis:
Dose as for creatinine clearance 10-30ml/minute/1.73m^2 ensuring a dose is given after dialysis session.

Administration: On reconstitution 1.2g displaces 0.9ml. Add 19.1ml water for injection to a 1.2g vial, resulting concentration is 1.2g of co-amoxiclav in 20ml i.e. 50mg of amoxicillin in 1ml. Give as a slow IV injection over 3-4 minutes or as an IV infusion over 30 minutes, further diluted to 12mg in 1ml with sodium chloride 0.9%.

Notes:

a) In confirmed penicillin allergy, cephalosporins may be an alternative treatment although approximately 10% of these patients will also be allergic to cephalosporins. Where severe allergy symptoms have occurred previously or the extent of the allergy is unknown an alternative antibiotic should be given. Contact the microbiology department for further information.

b) **CSM warning:** Cholestatic jaundice has been reported as an adverse reaction occurring either during or shortly after use of co-amoxiclav. Duration of treatment should not exceed 14 days except on specialist advice.

c) Co-amoxiclav liquids (Augmentin®) are tartrazine and sugar-free but contain aspartame.

d) 1.2g vial contains 3.1mmol sodium and 1mmol potassium.

CODEINE PHOSPHATE

Preparations:	TABLETS 15mg and 30mg. INJECTION 60mg in 1ml (**CD**).
Dosage:	***ANALGESIA FOR MILD TO MODERATE PAIN***

This indication is unlicensed for use in children under 1 year.
All ages, *orally, SC/IM injection,*
0.5-1mg/kg/dose repeated every 4-6 hours.

Notes:

a) Codeine phosphate should be avoided in children with renal impairment and used with caution in patients with hepatic impairment.

b) **Codeine phosphate injection must not be given by IV injection as it causes histamine release, resulting in reduced cardiac output.**

c) Caution in neonates and infants as they show increased susceptibility to respiratory depression.

COLISTIN

Preparations:	INJECTION 1,000,000 units. VIALS for nebulisation 1,000,000 units in 4ml (**Manufactured special**).
Dosage:	***NEBULISED DOSE IN CYSTIC FIBROSIS***

SEEK EXPERT ADVICE BEFORE PRESCRIBING

Nebulised,
Under 40kg   500,000 units every 12 hours
Over 40kg   1,000,000 units every 12 hours

Administration: Nebulised: reconstitute the dose in 2-4ml of water for injection or sodium chloride 0.9%.

Notes:

a) Nebulise after physiotherapy to allow improved lung penetration.

b) To reduce environmental contamination, colistin should be nebulised using a scavenging system or 'elephant' tubing vented via an external window or with a filter attached. Contact PICU ventilator technician on bleep 1360 for filter and advice on setting up tubing.

CORTICOTROPHIN (ACTH)

Preparations:	CORTICOTROPHIN GELATIN INJECTION 80 units in 1ml, 5ml (**Named patient**).
Dosage:	***INFANTILE SPASM AND INTRACTABLE MYOCLONIC EPILEPSY***

SEEK EXPERT ADVICE BEFORE PRESCRIBING

SC or IM injection, over 1 month, initially 20-40 units once a day for periods ranging from 2 weeks-9 months.

Notes:

a) Administer in the morning (10am) to minimise "growth interference". Rotate sites of administration.

b) Corticotrophin gel must not be given by IV injection.

c) Corticotrophin is the preferred drug however if it is not available tetracosactrin may be substituted, see page 210.   0.5mg of tetracosactrin depot is approximately equivalent to 40 units of corticotrophin gel.

CO-TRIMOXAZOLE

Preparations:

	Sulphamethoxazole		Trimethoprim
Co-trimoxazole			
ADULT TABLETS 480mg	400mg	plus	80mg
FORTE TABLETS 960mg	800mg	plus	160mg
PAEDIATRIC LIQUID 240mg/5ml	200mg	plus	40mg
IV INJECTION 480mg/5ml	400mg	plus	80mg

Dosage:

> **CSM Recommendation:** Use should be limited to drug of choice for Pneumocystis carinii pneumonia, toxoplasmosis and nocardiasis. Use for acute exacerbations of chronic bronchitis and UTIs where there is evidence of bacterial sensitivity and good reason to prefer to a single antibiotic. There must also be good reason to prefer it to a single antibiotic for use in acute otitis media.

SYSTEMIC INFECTION
Orally,
18-24mg **co-trimoxazole**/kg twice a day OR

6 weeks - 6 months	2.5ml	twice a day
6 months - 6 years	5ml	twice a day
6 - 12 years	10ml **or** 1 adult tablet	twice a day

IV infusion, over 6 weeks, 18mg **co-trimoxazole**/kg twice a day.

In severe infection IV dosage may be increased to 27mg **co-trimoxazole**/kg twice a day.

PROPHYLAXIS OF URINARY TRACT OR RESPIRATORY TRACT INFECTION
Orally, 12mg **co-trimoxazole**/kg, once a day, at night.

In impaired renal function, *orally,* 6mg **co-trimoxazole**/kg at night.

PNEUMOCYSTIS
Orally or IV injection, 60mg **co-trimoxazole**/kg twice a day for 10-14 days. The oral route is preferred unless nausea is severe.

PROPHYLAXIS OF PNEUMOCYSTIS INFECTIONS IN THE IMMUNOCOMPROMISED
Give *oral* systemic infection dose, i.e. 18-24mg **co-trimoxazole**/kg twice a day, on three days of the week.

PROPHYLAXIS OF PNEUMOCYSTIS INFECTIONS IN RENAL TRANSPLANT PATIENTS
Orally, 12mg **co-trimoxazole**/kg, up to 480mg, at night for 6 months.

CONTINUED PLEASE TURN OVER

C

IN RENAL FAILURE

Creatinine clearance (ml/minute/1.73m^2)	Dosage
15-25	Normal dose for 3 days then half the dose.
Less than 15	Avoid unless haemodialysis available, and then give half the normal dose.

Co-trimoxazole is NOT removed by peritoneal dialysis.

Administration: IV injection: Wherever possible, give centrally. In severe fluid restriction this can be given undiluted via the central route. For peripheral injection, the manufacturers recommend a 25-fold dilution, in glucose 5% or sodium chloride 0.9%. However in severe fluid restriction dilute 10-fold with glucose 5%. Dilution to less than 1 in 10 is not possible as the propylene glycol precipitates out. Infuse over 60-90 minutes. Use IV route for a maximum of 3 consecutive days unless using a central line.

Notes:

a) Sulphonamides displace bilirubin from protein binding sites, and so, because of the risk of kernicterus, **co-trimoxazole is contraindicated in neonates and also the last month of pregnancy.**

b) **CAUTION:** Treatment should be stopped if blood disorders or rashes develop. Counsel patient/parent to report all rashes, sore throats, fevers and other manifestations of agranulocytosis.

c) Severe adverse reactions to co-trimoxazole, similar to Stevens-Johnson syndrome, may occur, particularly in HIV patients. Seek expert advice.

d) Therapeutic drug monitoring:
Monitor blood levels of sulphamethoxazole when large doses of co-trimoxazole are given e.g. pneumocystis or if renal function is poor
   i) Approx. time to steady state: 2-3 days.
   ii) Therapeutic level: 100-200mg/L.
   If level is above 150mg/L stop treatment until level falls below 120mg/L than restart treatment at a lower dose.
   iii) Take a trough sample, immediately prior to next dose.

e) Co-trimoxazole may raise plasma phenytoin levels and potentiate warfarin effect. Concomitant use of trimethoprim, with or without sulphamethoxazole, and ciclosporin has shown increased risk of nephrotoxicity.

f) Co-trimoxazole injection contains 45% w/v propylene glycol together with ethyl alcohol. It also contains sulphite which in susceptible patients can cause bronchospasm or anaphylaxis.

g) Co-trimoxazole paediatric liquid (Septrin®) and dispersible tablets (Septrin®) are sucrose free.

CYCLOPHOSPHAMIDE

Preparations: TABLETS 50mg. INJECTION 100mg, 500mg and 1g.
LIQUID (**Extemporaneously prepared**).

Dosage: **NEPHROTIC SYNDROME**

> **SEEK EXPERT ADVICE BEFORE PRESCRIBING**

This is an unlicensed indication.
Orally, 3mg/kg once a day for 8 weeks **OR** 2mg/kg once a day for 12 weeks (see note a).
SYSTEMIC LUPUS ERYTHEMATOSUS

> **REFER TO RENAL UNIT PROTOCOL OR SEEK EXPERT ADVICE BEFORE PRESCRIBING.**

This is an unlicensed indication.
IV injection, (see notes below).
If GFR > 1/3 normal, initially, 750mg/m^2 once a month.
If GFR ≤ 1/3 normal, initially, 500mg/m^2 once a month.
Renal function and white blood cell count must be monitored before prescribing.
The above doses are given once a month for 6 months and then once every 3 months until patient has been in remission for 1 year.

Administration: Cyclophosphamide is a cytotoxic drug therefore it will be reconstituted by the oncology pharmacy department.

> ☎ Guy's ext. 5418, Lewisham ext. 3201, St Thomas' ext. 3851 ☎

Administer over 30 minutes.

Notes:
a) Cyclophosphamide should preferably be administered in the morning.
b) Maintain good urine output following administration. Mesna may be used to prevent haemorrhagic cystitis.
c) Check white blood cell count regularly.
d) Cyclophosphamide may also cause nausea and vomiting (see Antiemetic guidelines page 277), alopecia, amenorrhoea and azoospermia.

CYSTEAMINE

Preparations:	CAPSULES 50mg and 150mg.
	EYE DROPS 0.11% (**Manufactured special**).
Dosage:	**TREATMENT OF NEPHROPATHIC CYSTINOSIS**

Orally,

Initial dose, all ages, 200-300mg/m^2/**day** increasing over 4-6 weeks to maintenance dose (see note a).

Maintenance dose,

Under 12 year, 1.3g/m^2/**day** in 2 to 4 divided doses.

Over 12 year, 2g/**day** in 2 to 4 divided doses.

OR

Weight (kg)	Dose (given four times a day)
0-4.5	100mg
5-9	150mg
10-13	200mg
14-18	250mg
19-22	300mg
23-31	350mg
32-41	400mg
42-50	450mg
>50	500mg

Total daily dose can be given in 2 or 3 divided doses, if tolerated to aid compliance, especially in older children.

Instill, eye drops into affected eyes four to six times a day.

Notes:

a) Doses should be increased slowly to ensure they are tolerated. Larger doses may cause nausea and vomiting.

b) White cell cystine levels should be monitored regularly to assess effectiveness. A trough blood sample should be taken i.e. immediately prior to next dose.

c) Cysteamine has an unpleasant taste and smell. Patients should be advised if opening capsules, to sprinkle on or mix in strongly flavoured drink or food. Cysteamine may cause an unpleasant smell on the breath of patients taking it. This may be masked using breath fresheners including Breathasure®.

d) Cysteamine capsules contain the bitartrate salt and the eye drops are the hydrochloride salt.

DANTROLENE

Preparations: CAPSULES 25mg, 100mg. INJECTION 20mg.
              LIQUID (**Extemporaneously prepared**).

Dosage: *CHRONIC SEVERE SPASTICITY*

This indication is unlicensed for use in children.

Orally, initially, 0.5mg/kg twice a day for 4 days increasing to 0.5mg/kg three times a day for 4 days then 0.5mg/kg four times a day.

If the desired response is still not achieved then increase dose by 0.5mg/kg every 4 days.

The maximum dosage should not exceed 3mg/kg or 100mg 4 times a day.

MALIGNANT HYPERTHERMIA

IV injection, 1mg/kg repeated if necessary to maximum cumulative dose of 10mg/kg. Reversal usually requires an average dose of 2.5mg/kg.

Administration: Dissolve contents of vial with 60ml of water for injection and give as a injection. Reconstituted solution should be protected from light and used within 6 hours.

Notes:

a)   Dantrolene has been associated with symptomatic hepatitis (fatal and non-fatal). Liver function tests should be performed before starting treatment and at regular intervals during treatment.

b)   Dantrolene should be used with caution in patients with cardiac and pulmonary disorders.

c)   Therapeutic effect may take a few weeks to develop, however if effect is not seen within 4-6 weeks discontinue drug.

d)   Dantrolene 20mg injection contains 3g of mannitol and has a pH of 9.5.

DAPSONE

Preparations: TABLETS 50mg and 100mg.
Dosage:

SEEK SPECIALIST ADVICE BEFORE PRESCRIBING

TREATMENT OF PNEUMOCYSTIS CARINII PNEUMONIA
This is an unlicensed indication.
Orally, over 1 month, 1-2mg/kg/day up to 200mg.

PROPHYLAXIS
This indication is unlicensed for use in children.
Orally, over 1 month, 1mg/kg/day up to 100mg.

Notes:

a)   Dapsone Syndrome may occur after 3 to 6 weeks therapy; symptoms include rash, fever and eosinophilia - discontinue therapy immediately.

b)   Caution with use in pulmonary or cardiac disease, severe glucose-6-dehydrogenase deficiency or porphyria. Dapsone may cause haemolysis and rarely agranulocytosis. Monitor blood counts and counsel patient/carer to report any sore throats, fever, mouth ulcers, bruising or rashes.

c)   Liquid is **not** available, tablets may be crushed.

DAPSONE with PYRIMETHAMINE (MALOPRIM®)

Preparations:	TABLETS containing pyrimethamine 12.5mg, dapsone 100mg (**Non-formulary**).
Dosage:	*MALARIA PROPHYLAXIS*

This indication is unlicensed for use in children under 5 years.
Orally,

1 - 5 years	One quarter of a tablet once a week.
6 - 11 years	Half a tablet once a week.
12 years	One tablet once a week.

Treatment should be started one week prior to entering an endemic area and continued for 4 weeks after returning.

Notes:

a)

> Advice on **PROPHYLAXIS** can be obtained from:
> **Drug Information Centre**
> ☎Guy's ext. 3594, Lewisham ext. 3202, St Thomas' ext. 3069☎
> **The London Malaria Reference Laboratory**
> ☎0171-636 8636 (out of hours)☎

b) Maloprim can be used with caution in renal and hepatic impairment, however if treatment is prolonged patients should be monitored for signs of bone marrow depression.

c) Doses higher than those stated are more commonly associated with agranulocytosis. Risk is also greater in patients with glucose-6-phosphate dehydrogenase deficiency.

DESFERRIOXAMINE MESYLATE

Preparations: INJECTION 500mg.

Dosage: *PATHOLOGICAL IRON OVERLOAD*

IV or SC infusion 30-40mg/kg over about 8-12 hours 3 to 7 times a week. Dose can be increased to 180mg/kg/24 hours in severe iron overload.

IM injection initial dose 500mg-1g a day as 1-2 injections. Maintenance dose depends on iron excretion rate.

ACUTE IRON POISONING

For indications discuss with the medical toxicology unit.

In **confirmed** cases and where there is doubt about potential toxicity, *IV infusion* of 15mg/kg/hour initially. Reduce rate after a few hours to ensure maximum dose 80mg/kg in 24 hours is not exceeded.

In **serious** cases larger amounts have been used. Discuss with the medical toxicology unit. If oliguric or anuric consider peritoneal dialysis or haemodialysis to remove ferrioxamine.

> **IF IN ANY DOUBT CONTACT THE MEDICAL TOXICOLOGY UNIT**
> ☎ 0171-635-9191 ☎

ALUMINIUM OVERLOAD IN DIALYSIS PATIENTS

Haemodialysis, haemofiltration 5mg/kg via fistula once a week over the last hour of dialysis for 3 months. Remeasure aluminium levels 4 and 8 weeks after completing course.

CAPD or CCPD 5mg/kg once a week prior to the last exchange of the day. Desferrioxamine is equally effective IV, IM, SC or intraperitoneally. Aluminium levels generally fall to acceptable levels within 12-18 months.

Administration: Dissolve contents of vial in 5ml water for injection to give 500mg in 5ml (10% solution). Only a clear solution should be used for parenteral administration. For IV infusion the 10% solution can then be further diluted with sodium chloride 0.9% or glucose 5%. Up to 2g of desferrioxamine per unit of blood can be administered through the same infusion line as the blood transfusion.

Notes:

a)   Theoretically 100mg of desferrioxamine binds 8.5mg of ferric iron or 4.1mg of aluminium.

b)   Patients should be monitored for acute side effects including allergic or anaphylactic reactions, hypotension, hypokalaemia and cardiac arrhythmias.

c)   Chronic usage may be associated with auditory and visual problems and acceleration of bone disease. Hearing and vision should be monitored regularly; effects can be reversed on cessation of therapy.

DESMOPRESSIN (ADH ANALOGUE) - DDAVP

Preparations:	NASAL SPRAY 10microgram in each spray. INTRANASAL SOLUTION 100microgram in 1ml. INJECTION 4microgram in 1ml. TABLETS 100microgram (**Non-formulary**) and 200microgram.
Dosage:	***DIABETES INSIPIDUS***

IV, SC or IM injection children and infants, initially 400nanogram (0.4microgram, 0.1ml) once a day.
Adults, 1 to 4microgram once day.
Intranasally, 5-10microgram (0.05-0.1ml) once or twice a day, infants may require a smaller dose.
Orally, initially 100microgram 3 times a day.

PRIMARY NOCTURNAL ENURESIS
Over 5 years of age (see note a),
Intranasally, 10-20microgram (1-2 sprays or 0.1-0.2ml) at night. Increased to maximum of 40microgram. Taper off dose slowly.
Orally, 200microgram at night. Increased to maximum of 400microgram. Taper off dose slowly.
Therapy should be discontinued after 3 months for at least 1 week for reassessment.

WATER DEPRIVATION TEST

Under 5 years	2.5-5microgram (0.025-0.05ml) intranasally or 400nanogram (0.4microgram, 0.1ml) by IM injection.
5 - 10 years	10microgram (0.1ml or 1 spray) intranasally or 1microgram (0.25ml) by IM injection.
Over 10 years	20microgram (0.2ml or 2 sprays) intranasally or 2microgram (0.5ml) by IM injection.

Stop test if body weight is reduced by 3%. Measure urine osmolality after 0 hours, 0.5 hours, 1 hour and 2 hours.
A dramatic increase in urine osmolality indicates sensitivity to vasopressin. In diabetes insipidus urine flow is reduced.

TO TREAT/PREVENT BLEEDING
This is unlicensed for the intranasal route.
IV infusion, 0.2-0.5microgram/kg diluted in 30ml of sodium chloride 0.9% and given over 20 minutes (see note c). Doses may be repeated every 12 hours until cover no longer required or bleeding stopped.
Intranasally, 4microgram/kg.

Notes:

a) **CSM warning:** To minimise the risk of hyponatremic convulsions patients with primary nocturnal enuresis should be advised to avoid excessive fluid intake (including during swimming) and to stop desmopressin treatment during episodes of vomiting or diarrhoea.

b) Desmopressin injection must **not** be diluted in patients with diabetes insipidus requiring doses of 4microgram or less, as there is a tendancy for the peptide to adhere to surfaces when in diluted solutions, resulting in inaccuracy. A diabetic syringe should be used to measure the dose. For treatment of uraemic bleeding the dose used is much higher, and the amount of adherence less critical, therefore dilution is possible.

c) Vasodilation during intravenous infusion may occur, monitor patient's blood pressure and heart rate. Decrease infusion rate if hypotension or tachycardia occur.

d) Desmopressin intranasal solution should be used for doses less than 10microgram as it employs a calibrated plastic catheter capable of measuring doses as low as 5microgram.

DEXAMETHASONE

Preparations: TABLETS 500microgram and 2mg. INJECTION dexamethasone sodium phosphate equivalent to dexamethasone phosphate 4mg in 1ml (equivalent to 3.33mg in 1ml dexamethasone). LIQUID 2mg in 5ml (**Manufactured special**).

Dosage: Parenteral doses are given in terms of **dexamethasone phosphate** except where noted otherwise.

ANTI-INFLAMMATORY

Adjust on the basis of individual response.

Orally, 10-100microgram/kg once a day.

IV, SC or IM injection, 200-400microgram/kg once a day.

CEREBRAL OEDEMA

High IV dose schedule:

	Children below 35kg	Children over 35kg
Initial dose	20mg	24mg
1st-3rd day	4mg 3 hourly	4mg 2 hourly
4th day	4mg 6 hourly	4mg 4 hourly
5-8th day	2mg 6 hourly	4mg 6 hourly
Thereafter	decrease by daily reduction of 1mg	decrease by daily reduction of 2mg

SUSPECTED LARYNGEAL OEDEMA FOLLOWING TRAUMATIC INTUBATION OR INSTRUMENTATION OF THE AIRWAY OR SUSPECTED SUBGLOTTIC OEDEMA AFTER LONG TERM VENTILATION

IV injection, neonates, up to 1mg/kg/dose for up to 6 doses around extubation. Infants and children up to 0.5mg/kg/dose for up to 6 doses around extubation.

WEANING OFF A VENTILATOR IN BRONCHOPULMONARY DYSPLASIA

IV injection, orally, (doses expressed as dexamethasone).

1st-3rd day	0.5mg/kg/day in 2 divided doses
4th-6th day	0.3mg/kg/day in 2 divided doses
7th-9th day	0.1mg/kg/day in 2 divided doses
10-17th day	0.1mg/kg on alternate days

In some cases treatment may be necessary for up to 42 days.

Administration: IV injection, dilute if required with sodium chloride 0.9% or glucose 5%.

Notes:

a) Budesonide, nebulised, is the preferred first line corticosteroid in the management of croup.
b) Dexamethasone administration results in increased serum levels of phenytoin.
c) For relative potencies see Hydrocortisone, (page 123, note b).
d) Injection can be given orally.
e) Tablets will disperse in water.

DEXAMFETAMINE SULPHATE - (CD)

Preparations: TABLETS 5mg (**Non-formulary**).
Dosage: *ATTENTION DEFICIT HYPERACTIVITY DISORDER*

Orally, initially,

3 - 5 years	2.5mg once a day, increase by 2.5mg a day at weekly intervals. Maximum 20mg/**day**.
6 years and over	5mg once to twice a day, increase by 5mg a day at weekly intervals. Maximum 20-40mg/**day**.

Dose may need to be given in up to 3-4 divided doses.

Notes:

a) Patients should be monitored at least weekly for side effects whilst dose is being established.
b) Dexamfetamine sulphate can decrease appetite and lead to reversible growth retardation. Baseline assessment of weight and height should be performed and subsequently monitored 3 monthly.
c) If anorexia is a problem, give dose after breakfast and lunch.
d) A baseline blood pressure should be performed. Blood pressure should be monitored whilst dose being established and after any dosage increases.
e) Doses may be given in 3-4 divided doses if rebound hyperactivity occurs in the latter part of the day but because dexamfetamine sulphate may cause insomnia, the last dose should not usually be given later than 4pm.
f) Caution, use is not recommended in patients with a diagnosis or family history of tics or Tourette's syndrome. Use with caution in epilepsy.
g) Avoid abrupt withdrawal. Dexamfetamine sulphate should be withdrawn over a few weeks to avoid extreme fatigue and mental depression.

DEXTROMETHORPHAN HYDROBROMIDE

Preparations: LIQUID (Delsym®) Long acting polystirex equivalent to 30mg of hydrobromide in 5ml. (**Named patient**).

Dosage: **NON KETOTIC HYPERGLYCINAEMIA**

SEEK SPECIALIST ADVICE BEFORE PRESCRIBING

This is an unlicensed indication

Orally, initially, 2.5mg/kg twice a day of Delsym® increasing to 10mg/kg/**day**. Doses as high as 22mg/kg/**day** have been used. If using the hydrobromide salt administer total daily dose in 3 divided doses. See note c).

Notes:
a) Caution, may cause respiratory depression.
b) Delsym® is alcohol free but does contain 1.7g of sugar in 5ml.
c) Dextromethorphan hydrobromide 7.5mg in 5ml liquid (Robitussin®) is available; however it is on the government "black list". This product is not a long acting formulation. Ensure preparation is alcohol free.

DIAMORPHINE - (CD)

Preparations: INJECTION 5mg, 10mg, 30mg, 100mg and 500mg.

Dosage: **ANALGESIA FOR CHRONIC PAIN MANAGEMENT**

Over 1 month

Extradural injection	25-50microgram/kg/dose.
Extradural infusion	5-25microgram/kg/hour.
SC infusion	20-100microgram/kg/hour.

Administration: Reconstitute 5-100mg vials with 1ml of water for injection, and the 500mg vial with 2ml water for injection, to give concentrations of 5-100mg in 1ml and 250mg in 1ml, respectively.

SC infusion: Dilute with water for injection or sodium chloride 0.9% and use within 24 hours. Only use glucose 5% for infusions to be administered over 48 hours.

Notes:
a) Use with caution in infants under 1 year, because of their increased susceptibility to respiratory depression.
b) There is no advantage to using diamorphine over morphine except where high doses are required as larger concentrations can be used.
c) Hyoscine, metoclopramide and methotrimeprazine are compatible with diamorphine concentrations up to 50mg/ml, for 24 hours. Haloperidol and cyclizine are compatible but can precipitate when using high concentrations.
d) Extradural use should be performed in high dependency areas under the supervision of an appropriately trained anaesthetist.
e) See section 4.7.2 of Adult Formulary for equivalent opiate doses.
f) Premedication guidelines are on page 250, and pain management guidelines on page 251.

DIAZEPAM

Preparations: TABLETS 2mg, 5mg and 10mg. LIQUID 2mg in 5ml and 5mg in 5ml. RECTAL TUBES 2.5mg in 1.25ml, 5mg in 2.5ml and 10mg in 2.5ml. INJECTION 10mg in 2ml, for IM use. DIAZEMULS™ BRAND OF DIAZEPAM 10mg in 2ml for IV use.

Dosage: **ANXIOLYTIC**

This indication is unlicensed for use in children.

Orally, initially,

4 weeks - 1 year	50microgram/kg	twice a day
1 - 4 years	500microgram	twice a day
5 - 12 years	1-1.5mg	twice a day
Over 13 years	2mg	twice a day

PREMEDICATION AND SPASMOLYTIC DOSE

Orally, 200-300microgram/kg/dose,

OR

4 weeks - 1 year	250microgram/kg	twice a day
1 - 4 years	2.5mg	twice a day
5 - 12 years	5mg	twice a day
Over 13 years	10mg	twice a day

IV injection: 100-200microgram/kg to a maximum total daily dose of 10-20mg.

The above doses are used on an as required basis in post-operative skeletal muscle spasm; see pain management guidelines on page 251.

The above doses also may initially be used for the control of tension and irritability of cerebral spasticity, however larger doses may be required. Dose is determined by therapeutic response.

STATUS EPILEPTICUS

This indication is unlicensed for the rectal route in children under 1 year.

Slow IV injection,

200-300microgram/kg, repeated after 10 minutes if necessary.

OR

IV infusion,

initially, 1microgram/kg/minute (60microgram/kg/hour), to maximum of 3mg/kg over 24 hours.

OR

Rectally, (see note d).

Under 1 year	2.5mg via rectal tube
1 - 3 years	5mg via rectal tube
Over 3 years	10mg via rectal tube

If necessary this dose may be repeated after 5 minutes.

Administration: IV infusion, dilute to between 100microgram in 1ml and 400microgram in 1ml of glucose 5% or 10%. Discard remaining infusion after 6 hours.

Notes:

a) For slow IV injection and IV infusion Diazemuls brand should be used. Other brands of diazepam injection should not be given by the IV route because they are more irritant.

b) Beware of respiratory depression during acute use.

c) Paradoxical reactions (restlessness, agitation) are more likely in children.

d) Anecdotally, diazepam rectal tubes have been administered sublingually where the rectal route has not been practicable.

e) Injection can be given orally and rectally.

f) Diazepam liquid 2mg in 5ml (Valium®) is sugar free and diazepam liquid 5mg in 5ml contains 1.1g sucrose in 5ml.

DIAZOXIDE

Preparations: LIQUID (see note e). TABLETS 50mg (**Non-formulary**).

INJECTION 300mg in 20ml (**Non-formulary**).

Dosage: *REFRACTORY HYPOGLYCAEMIA*

SEEK EXPERT ADVICE BEFORE PRESCRIBING

Orally, initially, 1.7mg/kg three times a day up to **15mg/kg/day** according to response. Doses up to **20mg/kg/day** have been used in Leucine-sensitive hypoglycaemia.

SEVERE HYPERTENSION

SEEK EXPERT ADVICE BEFORE PRESCRIBING

Rapid IV injection **5mg/kg/dose**. Repeat after 1 hour if necessary. Maximum of 4 doses in 24 hours. Monitor blood glucose to avoid hyperglycaemia.

Administration: Give as a rapid IV injection over 30 seconds or less. Do not dilute.

Notes:

a) Diazoxide should never be given by IM or SC injection as it is very irritant, pH 11-12.

b) In hypertensive encephalopathy a rapid reduction in blood pressure to normotensive levels can result in water shed cerebral infarction, blindness or death. Diazoxide is **NOT** the first line drug in this condition.

c) A reduced dose may be required with concomitant diuretics.

d) During prolonged therapy children should be monitored for leucopenia and thrombocytopenia and have regular assessments of growth and bone and psychological maturation.

e) Liquid can be extemporaneously prepared from powder which is available on a named patient basis.

DICLOFENAC SODIUM

Preparations: TABLETS 25mg, 50mg. SUSTAINED RELEASE TABLETS 75mg, 100mg.
SUPPOSITORIES 12.5mg, 25mg, 50mg and 100mg.
DISPERSIBLE TABLETS 50mg (**Non-formulary**).

Dosage: *NON-STEROIDAL ANTI-INFLAMMATORY ANALGESIC*

This indication is unlicensed for use in children.
Orally or rectally, 0.5-1mg/kg two or three times a day.
Maximum of **3mg/kg/day**. See pain management guidelines.
The above doses are used in the treatment of Juvenile Arthritis.

Notes:

a) Diclofenac is contraindicated in patients with a history of hypersensitivity (including asthma, angioedema, urticaria or rhinitis) to aspirin or any other non-steroidal anti-inflammatory drug or with a coagulation defect.

b) Caution, use in renal, cardiac or hepatic failure may cause a deterioration in renal function; the dose should be kept as low as possible and renal function monitored.

c) Increased risk of convulsions with concomitant quinolones. Increased risk of nephrotoxicity with concomitant ciclosporin.

d) Diclofenac tablets should not be crushed as they are enteric coated. Patients unable to swallow tablets should be prescribed the rectal preparation where appropriate or naproxen liquid.

DIGOXIN

Preparations: TABLETS 62.5microgram, 125microgram, 250microgram.
PAEDIATRIC LIQUID 50microgram in 1ml. INJECTION 250microgram in 1ml. PAEDIATRIC INJECTION 100microgram in 1ml
(**Manufactured special**).

Dosage: *DIGITALISATION*

ONLY NECESSARY IN URGENT SITUATIONS

See note a)

Age	Total loading dose (microgram/kg/24hours)	
	Orally	*IV* (Only if oral not possible)
Premature neonate (<1.5kg)	25	20
Premature neonate (1.5-2.5kg)	30	30
Neonate - 2 years	45	35
2 - 5 years	35	35
5 - 10 years	25	25

Over 10 years, 750micrograms to 1.5mg.
Give 50% of loading dose immediately, then 25% at 8 hours and 16 hours assessing clinical response before giving dose.
Start maintenance (24 hours after loading).

MAINTENANCE

Orally, IV injection:

Premature neonates	2-3micrograms/kg twice a day
Neonates - 5 years	5micrograms/kg twice a day
5 - 10 years	3micrograms/kg twice a day

Total daily dose may be given once a day. Monitor levels.
Over 10 years, 125microgram to 750microgram once a day determined by clinical response and monitoring of levels.

IN RENAL FAILURE

Monitor levels carefully.

Creatinine clearance (ml/minute/1.73m^2)	Dosage
10-50	50% of dose
<10	25% of dose

Digoxin is not significantly cleared by dialysis. Give 25% of maintenance dose after haemodialysis or automated peritoneal dialysis session. Monitor levels.

Administration: Give IV injection diluted with sodium chloride 0.9%, glucose 5% or glucose/saline over 10-20 minutes for maintenance doses. Loading doses should be administered over 30-60 minutes.

Notes:

a) Reduced loading dose required if cardiac glycosides have been administered in the preceding two weeks.

b) IV route should only be used for life threatening arrhythmias or where oral route is impossible. The IM route should **never** be used.

c) Therapeutic drug monitoring:
   i) Approx. time to steady state: 5-10 days.
   ii) Therapeutic range: 0.8-2.2microgram/L.
   iii) Take sample at least 6 hours after oral or IV dose.

d) The oral bioavailability of the liquid (80%) and tablets (70%) differs. Although this may not be clinically significant, blood levels should be checked if preparation is changed. When changing from the IV to the oral preparation dose may be increased by 20% (liquid) or 30% (tablets) to maintain the same blood levels.

e) The clinical effect of digoxin is potentiated by amiodarone, diltiazem, hypokalaemia, quinidine, quinine and verapamil and the maintenance dose should be halved if any of these drugs are introduced.

f) Erythromycin, omeprazole and tetracycline may also cause blood levels of digoxin to double in approximately 10% of patients and this effect may last for several months after discontinuation of the aforementioned drugs.

g) Digoxin toxicity may occur if treatment with amphotericin or diuretics induces hypokalaemia.

h) Injection can be given orally, however bioavailability is unpredictable.

i) Digoxin liquid contains 1.5g sucrose in 5ml and is lime flavoured. Injection also contains alcohol and propylene glycol.

DIHYDROCODEINE TARTRATE

Preparations: TABLETS 30mg. LIQUID 10mg in 5ml.
                 INJECTION 50mg in 1ml (**CD**).

Dosage: ***ANALGESIA FOR MODERATE TO SEVERE PAIN***

                 This indication is unlicensed in children under 4 years of age.
                 Orally, IM or deep SC injection:

1 - 4 years	500microgram/kg	every 4-6 hours
4 - 12 years	500microgram-1mg/kg	every 4-6 hours

                 ANTITUSSIVE
                 Orally, 4 - 12 years, 200microgram/kg every 4-6 hours.

Notes:

a)   Intravenous administration is not recommended due to increased risk of respiratory depression.
b)   Dihydrocodeine causes constipation and laxatives may be required.
c)   Use cautiously in chronic liver disease and renal impairment.
d)   Dihydrocodeine liquid (Napp) contains 2.5g of sucrose in each 5ml and 7.5%v/v of alcohol.
e)   See recommended analgesics page 255.

DINOPROSTONE (PROSTAGLANDIN E2)

Preparations: INJECTION 1mg in 1ml. LIQUID (**Extemporaneously prepared**).
Dosage: ***TO MAINTAIN PATENCY OF THE DUCTUS ARTERIOSUS***

                 This is an unlicensed indication.
                 IV infusion, initially 50nanogram/kg/minute for 15-30 minutes, reducing gradually to 10-20nanogram/kg/minute, then to 5nanogram/kg/minute if possible.
                 Orally, initially 20-40microgram/kg hourly. Reduce the frequency of the dose to 4 hourly over several days.

Administration: IV infusion, dilute in sodium chloride 0.9% or glucose 5%.
Notes:

a)   IV dinoprostone can cause **respiratory depression** and **apnoea**. Facilities for intubation and ventilation must be available and should be considered for babies being transferred with a prostaglandin infusion.
b)   Injection can be given orally. Dilute first with water.

DIPYRIDAMOLE

Preparations: TABLETS 25mg and 100mg. INJECTION 10mg in 2ml.
                 LIQUID 10mg in 1ml (**Manufactured special**).
Dosage: ***MODIFICATION OF PLATELET FUNCTION***

                 Orally, all ages, 2.5mg/kg twice a day.

Notes:

a)   The effects of aspirin and dipyridamole on platelet behaviour may be synergistic.
b)   Injection can be given orally.
c)   Give before meals.

DISOPYRAMIDE

Preparations:	CAPSULES 25mg and 50mg (**Named patient**), 100mg and 150mg. INJECTION 50mg in 5ml.
Dosage:	*ANTIARRHYTHMIC*

This indication is unlicensed for use in children.

IV injection, 2mg/kg, give over 5-10minutes. Maximum dose 150mg.

IV infusion, 400microgram/kg/hour. Maximum 300mg in first hour and 800mg/**day**.

The IV route should only be used with ECG monitoring and facilities must be available for cardiopulmonary resuscitation.

Orally, initially 1-2mg/kg 3 times a day then increase to 3-5mg/kg 3-4 times a day. Dose is determined by clinical response and levels. In children under 4 years higher doses, up to 35mg/kg/**day** may be required to achieve therapeutic blood levels.

IN RENAL FAILURE

Reduce dose in severe renal failure. If creatinine clearance is <20ml/minute/1.73m² then start at lowest dose and increase according to clinical response and blood levels.

Notes:
a) **CAUTION:** Increased risk of arrhythmias with astemizole, terfenadine, amiodarone, erythromycin and phenothiazines.
b) Blood levels:
   i) Approx. time to steady state: 48 hours.
   ii) Therapeutic range: 2-5mg/L.
   iii) Take trough sample i.e. immediately prior to next dose.
c) Injection can be given orally.

DOBUTAMINE

Preparations:	INJECTION 250mg in 20ml.
Dosage:	*INOTROPIC SUPPORT*

This indication is unlicensed for use in children.

IV infusion, 2-20microgram/kg/minute.

Administration: Dilute further with sodium chloride 0.9% or glucose 5%. Concentrations as high as 5mg in 1ml have been used in patients on restricted fluids although these concentrations must be infused via a central line.

Notes:
a) Dobutamine may cause vasodilation and reduce blood pressure.
b) Dobutamine and dopamine can be mixed together in glucose 5% or sodium chloride 0.9%.
c) Solutions of dobutamine may turn pink due to a slight oxidation of the drug. Such solutions are safe to use and there is no significant loss of potency.
d) Dobutamine can **NOT** be mixed with sodium bicarbonate or other strongly alkaline solutions.

DOCUSATE SODIUM

Preparations: LIQUIDS 12.5mg in 5ml and 50mg in 5ml. CAPSULES 100mg.
        MICRO-ENEMA 120mg in 10g (approximately 8ml).

Dosage: **CONSTIPATION**

Only the 12.5mg in 5ml elixir is licensed for use in children, over 6 months of age. The micro-enemas are unlicensed for children under 3 years.

Orally,

All ages	2.5mg/kg	2-3 times a day

OR

4 weeks - 1 year	12.5mg	2-3 times a day
1 - 4 years	12.5-25mg	2-3 times a day
5 - 12 years	25-50mg	2-3 times a day

Initial doses should be large and then reduced as condition improves.

Rectally,

(See notes below).

Under 3 years: Approx. half an enema as necessary.

Over 3 years: One enema as necessary.

Notes:

a) Regular oral treatment for 1-3 days is required before stools soften.
b) Many small children who experience pain or fear during defecation find rectally administered treatment very distressing and alternatives should be considered.
c) Response from rectal administration usually occurs within 20 minutes.
d) The enema is not recommended for use in children under 3 years as a smaller volume cannot be measured accurately, and dehydration may occur.
e) Liquid may be diluted with milk or squash.
f) The liquid is sucrose and colourant free.

DOMPERIDONE

Preparations: TABLETS 10mg. SUPPOSITORIES 30mg. LIQUID 1mg in 1ml.

Dosage: **CYTOTOXIC AND RADIOTHERAPY INDUCED NAUSEA AND VOMITING**

Orally, 2 - 12 years, 200-400microgram/kg every 4-8 hours.

Rectally, 2 - 12 years, approximately 3mg/kg/**day**.

OR

10-15kg	15mg 2 times a day
16-25kg	30mg 2 times a day
26-35kg	30mg 3 times a day
36-45kg	30mg 4 times a day

GASTRO-OESOPHAGEAL REFLUX, GASTRIC STASIS

This indication is unlicensed for use in children.

Orally, all ages, 200microgram/kg 3-4 times a day.

Notes:

a) Domperidone liquid has been used in children as young as 1 month, however extrapyramidal side effects may occur in these young children.
b) Domperidone liquid (Motilium®) is sucrose free and contains sorbitol.

DOPAMINE

Preparations: INJECTION 200mg in 5ml.

Dosage: **LOW DOSE FOR RENAL EFFECT**

This is an unlicensed indication.

See note a).

IV infusion, 2-5microgram/kg/minute.

INOTROPIC SUPPORT

This indication is unlicensed for use in children.

IV infusion, 2-20microgram/kg/minute (start at 2microgram/kg/minute and titrate upwards in 5microgram/kg/minute increments).

Administration: It is preferable to dilute dopamine with sodium chloride 0.9% or glucose 5% for accuracy, although, if fluid is restricted, it can be administered undiluted via a syringe pump. Infuse via a central line. Low doses may be infused peripherally (see note d).

Notes:

a) The use of dopamine at a low dose for a renal effect remains controversial. Its use should be governed by a possible effect outweighing potential side effects.

b) Dopamine and dobutamine can be mixed together in glucose 5% or sodium chloride 0.9%.

c) Dopamine can **NOT** be mixed with sodium bicarbonate and other strongly alkaline solutions.

d) Peripheral infusions of inotropic doses should not be used as vasoconstriction and gangrene of the fingers or toes may occur.

e) Dopamine should be discarded if a brown colouration develops.

DOXAPRAM

Preparations: INJECTION 100mg in 5ml. INFUSION doxapram 2mg in 1ml of glucose 5% (500ml).

Dosage: **APNOEA IN PREMATURE INFANTS**

This is an unlicensed indication.

Continuous IV infusion, 500microgram/kg/hour, dose may be increased to 2.5mg/kg/hour (see notes below). Treatment is usually continued for 48 hours, however a repeat course may be necessary.

Notes:

a) High doses **may** result in CNS toxicity including convulsions, hypertension and an increased risk of necrotising enterocolitis, particularly if serum concentration is greater than 0.5mg/L.

b) Frequent arterial blood gas and pH measurements are necessary to ensure an appropriate dose is being administered.

c) Caution, concomitant administration of doxapram and aminophylline may cause increased agitation and skeletal muscle activity.

d) Doxapram can **NOT** be mixed with alkaline fluids such as aminophylline, frusemide, sodium bicarbonate or thiopentone sodium.

DOXAZOSIN

Preparations:	TABLETS 1mg, 2mg and 4mg.
Dosage:	**HYPERTENSION**

This indication is unlicensed for use in children.

Orally, initially,

6 - 12 years	0.5mg once a day
Over 12 years	1mg once a day

Increase dose according to response at weekly intervals. Usual daily dose between 2-4mg. Maximum dose 16mg/**day**.

IN RENAL FAILURE

No dosage reduction is required in renal failure. Doxazosin is not dialysable.

Notes:

Blood pressure should be monitored closely after the first dose as doxazosin may cause postural hypotension.

DROPERIDOL

Preparations:	INJECTION 10mg in 2ml. LIQUID 1mg in 1ml. TABLETS 10mg.
Dosage:	**PREMEDICATION IN ANAESTHESIA**

IM injection, 60 minutes before operation.

1 month - 12 years	200-500microgram/kg
Over 12 years	up to 10mg

Orally,

1 month - 12 years	300-600microgram/kg
Over 12 years	up to 10mg

NEUROLEPTANALGESIA

IV injection, 200-300microgram/kg/dose at induction.

Administration:	*IV injection*, over 2-5 minutes; dilute if required with sodium chloride 0.9% or glucose 5%.
Notes:	
a)	Droperidol liquid is sucrose free.
b)	Injection can **NOT** be given orally.

EDROPHONIUM

Preparations: INJECTION 10mg in 1ml.
Dosage:

SEEK EXPERT ADVICE BEFORE PRESCRIBING

DIAGNOSTIC TEST FOR MYASTHENIA GRAVIS
IV injection, 100microgram/kg. Initially give one fifth of the dose (ie. 20microgram/kg) followed after 30 seconds (if no reaction has occurred) by the remainder of the dose (i.e. 80microgram/kg).

TEST TO DIFFERENTIATE BETWEEN MYASTHENIC OR CHOLINERGIC CRISIS
This indication is unlicensed for use in children.
IV injection, 20microgram/kg.
Test should be performed just before next dose of anticholinesterase and only in conjunction with someone skilled in intubation.
If anticholinesterase treatment is excessive, edrophonium will either have no effect or symptoms will intensify. A transient improvement will be seen if anticholinesterase treatment is inadequate.

ANTAGONIST TO NON-DEPOLARISING NEUROMUSCULAR BLOCKADE
Slow IV injection, (over several minutes), 500-700microgram/kg of edrophonium with 7microgram/kg of atropine.

Administration: IV injection, can be diluted, immediately before use, with water for injection.

Notes:

a) Have atropine sulphate drawn up in a syringe before test, as edrophonium may cause profound bradycardia.
b) Use with extreme caution in patients with asthma.

EFORMOTEROL FUMARATE

Preparations: TURBOHALER 6microgram/metered inhalation, 60 dose unit, 12microgram/metered inhalation, 60 dose unit.
Dosage: *ASTHMA THERAPY*

ON CONSULTANT ADVICE ONLY

This indication is unlicensed for use in children under 12 years.
Inhaled, over 4 years, 6 microgram once a day.
Increase dose according to response.
Maximum 24microgram/**day** in 1 or 2 divided doses.

Notes:

a) **Note:** Eformoterol is not for immediate relief of acute attacks and existing corticosteroid therapy should not be withdrawn or reduced.
b) Turbohalers are breath activated and are effective at low inspiratory flow rates i.e. 30L/minute. Children under 4 years are usually incapable of using a turbohaler.
c) If an inhaler device is required salmeterol (page 192) should be prescribed.
d) See chronic asthma management guidelines page 241.

ENALAPRIL MALEATE

Preparations: TABLETS 2.5mg, 5mg and 10mg. WAFER 2.5mg and 5mg.

Dosage: **HYPERTENSION, CONGESTIVE CARDIAC FAILURE, PROTEINURIA**

This indication is unlicensed for use in children.

Orally, initially, 0.1mg/kg/day, adjusting according to response to a maximum of 1.0mg/kg/day. Dose is usually given once a day although twice a day doses have been used.

KEEP THE DOSE AS LOW AS POSSIBLE IN RENAL FAILURE AND IF A DIURETIC IS INDICATED, USE A LOOP RATHER THAN A THIAZIDE.

Notes:

a) Enalapril should be avoided whenever possible in neonates, particularly pre-term neonates due to the risk of renal failure, anuria, and hypotension.

b) ACE inhibitors reduce glomerular filtration rate leading to severe and progressive renal failure in patients with severe bilateral renal artery stenosis (or severe stenosis in a single kidney).

c) Enalapril has been substituted for captopril on a basis of 1mg enalapril for every 7.5mg of captopril.

d) Hyperkalaemia may occur particularly in renal failure.

e) Severe hypotension may occur particularly following the first dose. Patient should be observed every 15 minutes for the first hour.

f) Concomitant diuretic dosages may need to be reduced or not administered concurrently to avoid severe hypotension.

g) It is **NOT** possible to prepare a suspension.

h) Enalapril wafers can either be placed on the tongue and dissolved in the mouth or dissolved in water and the resultant solution used immediately.

i) Enalapril wafers (Innovace Melt®) are mint flavoured and contain aspartame (1.4mg of phenylalanine/2.5mg of enalapril).

ENOXIMONE

Preparations: INJECTION 100mg in 20ml.

Dosage: **CONGESTIVE CARDIAC FAILURE**

SEEK EXPERT ADVICE BEFORE PRESCRIBING

This indication is unlicensed for use in children.

IV Injection, all ages, loading dose of 0.5mg/kg, followed by 5-20microgram/kg/minute, according to response. Dose should not normally exceed 24mg/kg/**24 hours**.

Orally, all ages, 1mg/kg 3 times a day.

IN RENAL FAILURE

Dose should be reduced when creatinine clearance falls below 20ml/minute/1.73m^2.

Administration: Immediately before use, dilute with an equal volume of water for injection or sodium chloride 0.9%. Do **NOT** dilute further or use glucose solutions as this may result in precipitation of enoximone.

Notes:

a) Do **NOT** mix enoximone injection with dopamine, dobutamine or adrenaline due to pH incompatibility.
b) Hyperosmolality may occur with large doses of enoximone infusion as injection contains 43.4% w/v of propylene glycol.
c) Injection can be given orally, however the solution has a very alkaline pH and should therefore be mixed with milk feeds or orange juice. Once opened ampoules should be discarded after 12 hours.

EPHEDRINE

Preparations: TABLETS 30mg. NOSE DROPS 0.5%.
Dosage: **NASAL CONGESTION**

Under 3 months: if sodium chloride nose drops are ineffective, ephedrine 0.25% nose drops (extemporaneously prepared) can be used (see note b and c). Place 1-2 drops into each nostril when required, 15 minutes before feeds. Maximum 5 days treatment.

Over 3 months: 1-2 drops of 0.5% into each nostril when required, 15 minutes before feeds if appropriate. Maximum 5 days treatment.

BLADDER NECK WEAKNESS
This is an unlicensed indication.
Orally, 800microgram/kg 3 times a day. Maximum dose is 30mg 3 times a day.
OR

1 - 5 years	15mg three times a day
Over 6 years	15-30mg three times a day

Notes:

a) Avoid excessive use of nose drops as tolerance develops with rebound congestion on stopping therapy.
b) Use nose drops with caution in infants under 3 months (no good evidence of value and irritation may narrow nasal passages) - see sodium chloride nose drops (page 195).
c) Ephedrine 0.5% nose drops can be diluted with sodium chloride 0.9% to produce 0.25% nose drops.
d) Ephedrine may act as a stimulant in some children and disturb sleep. It may have a sedative effect in some children.

EPOETIN (ERYTHROPOETIN)

Preparations:	EPOETIN BETA MULTIDOSE INJECTION (Neo-Recormon®) 50,000units.
	EPOETIN ALFA PREFILLED SYRINGES (Eprex®) 1000units/0.5ml.
	EPOETIN BETA PEN CARTRIDGES (Neo-Recormon®) 10,000units and 20,000units.

Dosage:

TREATMENT OF RENAL ANAEMIA IN DIALYSIS AND PRE-DIALYSIS PATIENTS

The SC route is unlicensed in children under 2 years.

SC injection, initially 50-100units/kg three times a week until target haemoglobin reached, then adjust until maintenance dose achieved.

IV injection, initially 100-150units/kg three times a week until target haemoglobin reached, then adjust until maintenance dose achieved.

For both routes maximum total weekly dose is 720units/kg.

ANAEMIA OF PREMATURITY

SC injection, 200units/kg on alternate days.

Administration: SC injection, reconstitute or dilute to obtain a final concentration not exceeding 2000units in 1ml with water for injection.

IV injection, reconstitute or dilute to obtain a final concentration not exceeding 1000units in 1ml with water for injection; inject over 2 minutes.

Notes:

a) Target haemoglobin is between 9-11g/100ml. Aim to increase haemoglobin at a rate not exceeding 2g/100ml/month.

b) Deficiencies of folic acid, cobalamin (vitamin B_{12}) and iron, and aluminium toxicity may reduce the effectiveness of epoetin.

c) The clinical efficacy of epoetin alpha and beta is similar, they can be used interchangeably.

d) Hypertension, haemodialysis access thrombosis and convulsions are reported as side effects of epoetin.

e) Epoetin beta pen cartridges and multidose vials are not suitable for use in neonates due to the benzyl alcohol content.

f) Epoetin beta pen cartridges are stable, if stored as directed, for 6 weeks.

EPOPROSTENOL (PROSTACYCLIN)

Preparations: INJECTION 500microgram.

Dosage: **PULMONARY HYPERTENSION, PLATELET AGGREGATION INHIBITOR, DIGITAL ISCHAEMIA**

These are unlicensed indications.

IV infusion, 2nanogram/kg/minute, increasing to 40nanogram/kg/minute if necessary. Doses of up to 120nanogram/kg/minute have occasionally been necessary.

Administration: Reconstitute each vial with 10ml of the glycine buffer. Return the resulting epoprostenol solution into the residue of the 50ml vial of glycine buffer, and mix well to give a solution of **10microgram in 1ml.** This solution should then be filtered using the 0.2micron filter provided. The 10microgram in 1ml solution can be further diluted with sodium chloride 0.9% Do not dilute below 1.7microgram in 1ml. (In general 10ml of the epoprostenol 10microgram in 1ml solution is added to 40ml of sodium chloride 0.9% to give 2 microgram in 1ml). The 10microgram in 1ml solution can be infused neat via central line. The manufacturers recommend changing the infusion every 12 hours due to instability, however in practice the loss in potency following 12 hours is not clinically significant as the dose is titrated to the response. The use of infusions for **up to 24 hours is therefore recommended.**

Notes:

a) 5nanogram equals 0.005microgram.

b) As epoprostenol is very unstable, **only** the glycine buffer, which has a very alkaline pH is suitable for reconstitution and sodium chloride 0.9% must be used for further dilution.

c) Vasodilation can produce flushing, headache and profound hypotension during infusion.

d) Platelet aggregation inhibition can result in unwanted bleeding therefore anticoagulant monitoring is required especially if concomitant heparin is infused.

e) Additional 0.2micron filters may be obtained from the Pharmacy Department if necessary.

ERGOCALCIFEROL (CALCIFEROL, VITAMIN D2)

Preparations: LIQUID 3000 units in 1ml (**Manufactured special**).
INJECTION 300,000units in 1ml (**Manufactured special, Non-formulary**).

Dosage: **PREVENTION OF RICKETS**
Orally,

Premature babies	900 units (0.3ml) once a day.
All other ages	600 units (0.2ml) once a day.

TREATMENT OF RICKETS
Orally,

0 - 12months	1,500 units/day.
1 - 4 years	1,500-3,000 units/day.
5 - 13 years	3,000-6,000 units/day.

Reduce dose within a few weeks, as there is a significant risk of hypercalcaemia if treatment is continued long term. The resolution of induced hypercalcaemia may be delayed. Monitor serum calcium and phosphate levels.

TREATMENT OF VITAMIN D RESISTANT RICKETS OR HYPOPARATHYROIDISM
Doses of 20,000-100,000 units *orally*, per day may be required. Consider using **calcitriol** or **alfacalcidol** if treatment fails.

PROPHYLAXIS IN CHOLESTATIC JAUNDICE
Intramuscularly,
30,000units (0.1ml) once a month.

Notes:

a) 300 units is equivalent to 7.5microgram.
b) Abidec multivitamin drops and ketovite liquid contain 400 units of ergocalciferol in 0.6ml and 5ml respectively.
c) For a comparison of vitamin D preparations see section 9.6.4 of Adult Formulary.
d) Liquid is sucrose free.

ERYTHROMYCIN

Preparations: TABLETS erythromycin stearate 250mg and 500mg. LIQUIDS erythromycin ethylsuccinate 125mg in 5ml and 250mg in 5ml. INJECTION erythromycin lactobionate 1g.

Dosage: **TREATMENT OF INFECTION**

All ages,

Orally or IV injection,	12.5mg/kg	4 times a day

OR

Orally

Up to 2 years	62.5-125mg	4 times a day
2 - 8 years	125-250mg	4 times a day
Over 8 years	250-500mg	4 times a day

Doses can be doubled in severe infection. Maximum dose 4g/**day**.

Total oral daily dose may be given in 2 divided doses, although gastrointestinal side effects may occur.

GASTRIC STASIS

This is an unlicensed indication.

Orally or IV injection, all ages, 3mg/kg 4 times a day.

Administration: Reconstitue each 1g vial with 20ml water for injection to give 1g in 20ml (i.e. 50mg in 1ml). Dilute to 5mg in 1ml with sodium chloride 0.9% **(do not use glucose 5%)** and give slowly over 20-60 minutes to avoid thrombophlebitis (see note d).

In cases of severe fluid restriction concentrations of up to 10mg in 1ml have been used without problems, however the risk of thrombophlebitis is increased.

Notes:

a) **CSM Warning:** Avoid concomitant administration with astemizole, terfenadine and cisapride due to increased risk of arrhythmias.

b) Use with caution in impaired liver function and **severe** renal failure. The estolate salt is best avoided in patients with liver failure.

c) Erythromycin inhibits the hepatic metabolism of carbamazepine and theophylline, therefore blood levels should be monitored. Warfarin, digoxin, midazolam, phenytoin and ciclosporin may also be potentiated.

d) If for clinical reasons sodium chloride 0.9% is not suitable **neutralised** glucose 5% can be used as a diluent. This is prepared by adding 5ml of 8.4% sodium bicarbonate injection to 1L of glucose 5%.

e) Erythromycin injection does not contain sodium.

f) Erythromycin liquids stocked are sugar free.

ESMOLOL

Preparations: INJECTION 2.5g in 10ml and 100mg in 10ml.

Dosage: ***ANTIARRHYTHMIC***

This indication is unlicensed for use in children.

SEEK EXPERT ADVICE BEFORE PRESCRIBING

IV injection, loading dose of 500microgram/kg over 1 minute then maintenance *infusion* of 50microgram/kg/minute. Reduce rate to 25microgram/kg/minute if heart rate or blood pressure is low.

If inadequate response after 5 minute intervals, repeat loading dose and increase maintenance infusion by 50microgram/kg/minute increments. Doses above 200microgram/kg/minute have not been shown to have a significantly increased benefit. (Doses above 300microgram/kg/minute not recommended).

After adequate control achieved initiate oral therapy with digoxin or alternative, see tachycardia guidelines page 239. Decrease infusion rate by 50% one hour after first oral dose and stop infusion one hour after second oral dose, as long as patient is stable.

Administration: Dilute to 10mg in 1ml or less with sodium chloride 0.9% or glucose 5% and administer via a large vein. In fluid restricted patients dilute to 20mg in 1ml and administer via a central line. Esmolol causes venous irritation, avoid extravasation.

Notes:

a) Esmolol is very short acting (half life is approximately 9 minutes) and is only indicated for short term treatment.

b) Esmolol blood levels may be increased by warfarin and morphine - whilst esmolol may increase digoxin levels by 10-20% and prolong neuromuscular blockade duration.

c) Esmolol is contraindicated if patient is on concomitant verapamil.

ETHAMBUTOL

Preparations: TABLETS 100mg and 400mg.

LIQUID (**Extemporaneously prepared**).

Dosage: ***TUBERCULOSIS THERAPY***

SEEK EXPERT ADVICE BEFORE PRESCRIBING

Treatment: *Orally,* all ages, 15mg/kg once a day. Maximum dose is 1.5g/day. Give for the first 2 months of treatment only. Only include if there is a high risk of resistant infection.

IN RENAL FAILURE

Creatinine clearance (ml/minute/1.73m^2)	Dosage
10-50	50% of normal dose
<10	25% of normal dose

Ethambutol is only slightly dialysed.

Maintain levels between 2-5mg/L.

Notes:

    a)   Ethambutol may cause visual impairment due to optic neuritis and routine ophthalmological examinations should be carried out, particularly in young children, every 6 months. The condition is difficult to diagnose in children under 6 years of age and is more likely to occur in renal failure.

    b)   Ethambutol may be omitted in previously untreated patients who are HIV negative, on negative risk assessment and not a contact of a suspected drug resistant case.

ETHOSUXIMIDE

Preparations: CAPSULES 250mg. LIQUID 250mg in 5ml (Both purchased on request).

Dosage: **EPILEPSY**

Initially, *orally*,

15mg/kg/day increased gradually by 5mg/kg increments as necessary, to a maximum of 50mg/kg/day.

OR

Under 6 years   250mg a day,
Over 6 years   500mg a day,
Increase dose by 125-250mg a day at 4 to 7 day intervals.

Notes:

    a)   A full blood count is recommended before and 4-6 weeks after starting treatment. Counsel patients or their carers to report any fever, sore throat, mouth ulcers, bruising or any other symptoms of blood disorders.

    b)   Blood levels:
        i)   Approximate time to steady state: 1-2 weeks.
        ii)   Therapeutic range: 40-100mg/L.
        iii)   Take trough sample, immediately prior to next oral dose.

    c)   Blood levels of ethosuximide may be reduced by carbamazepine, phenytoin, phenobarbitone or primidone and increased by isoniazid and sodium valproate.

    d)   Ethosuximide may increase blood levels of phenytoin.

    e)   Use with caution in renal and hepatic impairment.

    f)   The liquid (Zarontin®) is raspberry flavoured and contains 3g of sucrose in 5ml and is alcohol free.

FANSIDAR

Preparations: TABLETS containing 25mg pyrimethamine and 500mg sulfadoxine.

Dosage: **TREATMENT OF MALARIA (RADICAL CURE)**

Under 4 years (5-10kg)	0.5 tablet	As a single dose
4 - 6 years (11-20kg)	1 tablet	As a single dose
7 - 9 years (21-30kg)	1.5 tablets	As a single dose
10 - 14 years (31-45kg)	2 tablets	As a single dose
Over 14 years (>45kg)	2-3 tablets	As a single dose

A single dose is given following oral or IV quinine in the treatment of cerebral malaria or malignant tertian malaria due to chloroquine resistant strains.

Notes:

a)   **Caution:** Fansidar is not recommended in premature babies and infants under 2 months of age as it contains a sulphonamide.

b)   Fansidar may cause a higher incidence of blood dyscrasias if administered concomitantly with co-trimoxazole, trimethoprim, methotrexate or anticonvulsants.

c)

> Advice on TREATMENT can be obtained from the microbiology department or the duty doctor at:
> **The Hospital for Tropical Disease**
> (0171-387 4411 (All hours)

FENTANYL - (CD)

Preparations: INJECTION 50microgram in 1ml (2ml, 10ml).

Dosage: **OPIATE ANALGESIA/RESPIRATORY DEPRESSANT FOR CHILDREN WITH ASSISTED VENTILATION**

IV injection, 5-15microgram/kg with supplemental doses of 1-3microgram/kg as necessary.

IV infusion, initially 1-3microgram/kg/hr although may require 4-8microgram/kg/hr.

OPIATE ANALGESIA FOR CHILDREN WITH SPONTANEOUS RESPIRATION

ONLY USE IF A VENTILATOR IS AVAILABLE, OR IF GIVEN BY AN ANAESTHETIST.

IV injection, 1-3microgram/kg with supplemental doses of 1microgram/kg as necessary.

Administration: Dilute if required with glucose 5% or sodium chloride 0.9%.

Notes:

a)   Short acting but potentially cumulative. Dependency may also be seen sooner than with a longer acting opiate.

b)   In intensive care it is an alternative opiate when a patient has an unstable cardiovascular system.

c)   Use with caution in infants under 1 year, because of their increased susceptibility to respiratory depression.

FLECAINIDE ACETATE

Preparations:	TABLETS 100mg. INJECTION 150mg in 15ml.
	LIQUID 50mg in 5ml (**Named patient**).
Dosage:	***SUPRAVENTRICULAR, RE-ENTRY & VENTRICULAR TACHYCARDIA***

SEEK EXPERT ADVICE BEFORE PRESCRIBING

These indications are unlicensed for use in children.

IV injection, 2mg/kg/dose. Continue if required by *IV infusion*, 1.5mg/kg/hour for the first hour and then 100-125microgram/kg/hour subsequently. Infusion should be stopped when arrhythmia is controlled.

The IV route should only be used with ECG monitoring and facilities must be available for cardiopulmonary resuscitation.

Orally, initially, 2mg/kg 2-3 times a day. Adjust dose according to levels.

IN RENAL FAILURE
Reduce dose by 50% if creatinine clearance is less than 35ml/minute/1.73m^2 and monitor plasma levels.

Administration:	IV injection over at least 10-30 minutes. Dilute if required with glucose 5% **not** sodium chloride 0.9%.
Notes:	

a) Following preliminary findings in adults, use of flecainide for ventricular arrhythmias has been restricted to life-threatening ventricular tachycardias. However this restriction does not apply to supraventricular tachycardias with a structurally normal heart and normal ventricular function. Treatment should only be initiated by the cardiologists where first line treatment has failed.

b) Flecainide has a negative inotropic effect and can itself precipitate serious arrhythmias.

c) Caution, reduce dose in severe liver failure.

d) Cimetidine may reduce the metabolism of flecainide resulting in increased blood levels. Phenytoin, phenobarbitone and carbamazepine may reduce blood levels.

e) Flecainide may increase blood levels of digoxin.

f) Flecainide dose should be reduced by 50% with concomitant amiodarone.

g) Blood levels:
   i) Approx. time to steady state: 2 days.
   ii) Therapeutic range: 200-400microgram/L.
   iii) Take trough sample i.e. immediately prior to the next dose.

h) Do **NOT** store liquid in a fridge as precipitation occurs. The liquid has a local anaesthetic effect and should be given at least 30 minutes before or after food.

FLUCLOXACILLIN

Preparations: CAPSULES 250mg and 500mg. LIQUIDS 125mg in 5ml and 250mg in 5ml. INJECTION 250mg and 500mg.

Dosage: **TREATMENT OF INFECTION**

Orally,

Neonates, dose as for parenteral (see below)

1 month - 1 year	62.5mg	4 times a day
1 - 5 years	125mg	4 times a day
Over 5 years	250mg	4 times a day

IV or IM injection,

Premature neonates,	< 7 days	25mg/kg twice a day
Premature neonates	7-14 days	25mg/kg 3 times a day
Premature neonates and Full term neonates	> 14 days	25mg/kg 4 times a day
Infants and children		12.5-25mg/kg 4 times a day

In severe infection the above doses can be doubled.
Maximum dose is 8g/**day**.

IN RENAL FAILURE

If creatinine clearance is less than 10ml/minute/1.73m^2, increase the dosage interval to every 8 hours. Flucloxacillin is not significantly dialysed.

Administration: On reconstitution 250mg displaces 0.2ml.

IM injection, add 1.3ml water for injection to 250mg vial to give 250mg in 1.5ml and 1.6ml to 500mg vial to give 500mg in 2ml.

IV injection, dilute reconstituted dose to 5-10ml with water for injection, sodium chloride 0.9% or glucose 5% and give over 3-5 minutes.

Notes:

a) In confirmed penicillin allergy, cephalosporins may be an alternative treatment although approximately 10% of these patients will also be allergic to cephalosporins. Where severe allergy symptoms have occurred previously or the extent of the allergy is unknown an alternative antibiotic should be given. Contact the microbiology department for further information.

b) **CSM warning:** Cholestatic jaundice may occur up to several weeks after treatment stopped. Risk is increased with prolonged courses.

c) Whenever possible an alternative to oral flucloxacillin, such as erythromycin, should be prescribed for young children as flucloxacillin liquid is unpalatable.

d) Each 1g of flucloxacillin injection (Beecham and Berk) contains 2.26mmol of sodium.

e) Flucloxacillin liquids contain approximately 2.87g of sucrose in 5ml.

f) See also antibiotic treatment guidelines page 259.

FLUCONAZOLE

Preparations: CAPSULES 50mg, 200mg. INJECTION 2mg in 1ml, 25ml and 100ml. LIQUIDS 50mg in 5ml and 200mg in 5ml.

Dosage: **MUCOSAL CANDIDIASIS**
Orally, IV infusion,

Neonates	<2weeks	3mg/kg every 72 hours
Neonates	2-4 weeks	3mg/kg/every 48 hours
Children	>4weeks	3mg/kg once a day.

SYSTEMIC CANDIDIASIS, CRYPTOCOCCAL MENINGITIS
Orally, IV infusion,

Neonates	<2weeks	6-12mg/kg every 72 hours
Neonates	2-4 weeks	6-12mg/kg/every 48 hours
Children	>4weeks	6-12mg/kg once a day.

PROPHYLAXIS WHILST NEUTROPENIC
Orally, IV infusion,

Neonates	<2weeks	3-12mg/kg every 72 hours
Neonates	2-4 weeks	3-12mg/kg/every 48 hours
Children	>4weeks	3-12mg/kg once a day.

IN RENAL FAILURE
Children with impaired renal function should receive the normal dose on days 1 and 2 and then dose adjusted as per table below.

Creatinine clearance (ml/min/1.73m^2)	Dosage interval (hours)
21-40	48 (**or** half normal daily dose)
10-20	72 (**or** one-third normal daily dose)
Haemodialysis	Give normal dose after each dialysis session.

Intermittent peritoneal dialysis, give normal dose on days 1 and 2 and then give half the normal dose once a day after dialysis session.

Administration: Infuse undiluted over 10-20 minutes. Dilute if required with sodium chloride 0.9% or glucose 5%.

Notes:

a) **CSM Warning:** Avoid concomitant administration with astemizole, terfenadine and cisapride due to increased risk of arrhythmias.
b) Fluconazole may potentiate the effects of warfarin and also increase blood levels of phenytoin, theophylline, ciclosporin, tacrolimus and zidovudine.
c) Infusion vial contains 0.15mmol sodium in 1ml.
d) Fluconazole liquid contains 2.8g of sucrose in 5ml.

FLUCYTOSINE

Preparations:	INJECTION 2.5g in 250ml.
Dosage:	**SEVERE FUNGAL INFECTIONS**

This indication is unlicensed for use in neonates.

IV injection,

0 - 4 weeks	25mg/kg	4 times a day
Over 4 weeks	50mg/kg	4 times a day

IN RENAL FAILURE

Creatinine clearance (ml/min/1.73m²)	Dosage interval (hours)
20-40	12
10-20	24
Less than 10	Initial dose of 50mg/kg then according to blood concentration (maximum 80mg/L).

Flucytosine is cleared by haemodialysis.

Administration: Infuse over 20-40 minutes using a giving set incorporating a 15 micron filter. Dilute further if required with sodium chloride 0.9% or glucose 5%.

Notes:

a) **Caution:** monitor blood count and liver function before and during treatment.

b) Blood levels:
   i) Approx. time to steady state: 1 day.
   ii) Therapeutic range: 40-60mg/L. Do not exceed 80mg/L.
   iii) Take peak sample, 1-2 hours after dose if necessary.
   Send sample to department of microbiology.

c) Resistance may develop rapidly, so flucytosine should not be used alone for fungal or yeast infections other than localised candidiasis (e.g. urinary tract or peritoneal infection). Amphotericin acts synergistically with flucytosine.

d) The infusion contains 34.5mmol of sodium in 250ml.

FLUDROCORTISONE

Preparations:	TABLETS 100microgram. LIQUID (**Extemporaneously prepared**).
Dosage:	**ADRENOCORTICAL INSUFFICIENCY**

Orally, adjust according to response, but start with approximately 2-5microgram/kg/day.

OR

up to 10 years (including neonates)	50microgram/day
over 10 years	100microgram/day

Notes:

a) Fludrocortisone is a potent mineralocorticoid, dose and electrolytes should be monitored to avoid hypertension, fluid overload and electrolyte disturbances.

b) For relative potencies see Hydrocortisone (page 123, note b).

FLUMAZENIL

Preparations: INJECTION 500microgram in 5ml (**Restricted use**).
Dosage: ***REVERSAL OF BENZODIAZEPINE-INDUCED SEDATION***

This indication is unlicensed for use in children.

IV injection, 10microgram/kg repeat at 1 minute intervals to a maximum of 40microgram/kg(2mg). If necessary this may be followed by an infusion of 2-10microgram/kg/hour.

Administration: IV infusion, dilute with sodium chloride 0.9% or glucose 5%.

Notes:

a) The half-life of flumazenil is very short (50-60 minutes) and is shorter than midazolam or diazepam therefore an infusion may be necessary if drowsiness returns after single doses.

b) As flumazenil is metabolised in the liver, careful titration of the dose is necessary in hepatic failure.

c) Flumazenil is not recommended in epileptics who have received prolonged benzodiazepine therapy as it may induce a withdrawal syndrome.

d) Flumazenil is expensive and is **NOT** indicated for routine reversal of benzodiazepine pre-medications.

e) Although flumazenil may antagonise the obvious effects of sedation, higher cognitive functions may still be impaired.

f) At Guy's flumazenil is stocked in the anaesthetic, bronchoscopy and dental departments and on paediatric wards where midazolam is stocked. It is stocked in the anaesthetic and X-ray departments at St. Thomas'. At Lewisham contact the resident pharmacist.

FLUOXETINE

Preparations: CAPSULES 20mg. LIQUID 20mg in 5ml.
Dosage: ***ATTENTION DEFICIT HYPERACTIVITY DISORDER*, OBSESSIVE COMPULSIVE DISORDER***

SEEK EXPERT ADVICE BEFORE PRESCRIBING

*This indication is unlicensed. These indications are unlicensed for use in children.

Orally, initially, 0.5mg/kg once a day. Increase dose according to response. Maximum 60mg/**day**.

OR

initially,

6 - 8 year	10mg once a day
8 years and over	20mg once a day

Notes:

a) Patients should be monitored weekly for side effects whilst dose is being established.

b) Use with caution in epilepsy, seizure threshold may be lowered. Fluoxetine may increase carbamazepine and phenytoin levels.

c) Fluoxetine has a long duration of action and this should be taken into account when adjusting dosage. It may take up to 5 weeks to clear after discontinuing.

FLUTICASONE

Preparations:	AEROSOL INHALER 25microgram/metered inhalation, 50microgram/metered inhalation **(Non-formulary)**, 125microgram/metered inhalation*, 250microgram/metered inhalation*, 120 dose units. * Not licensed for use in children.
Dosage:	**ASTHMA THERAPY**

ON CONSULTANT ADVICE ONLY

This indication is unlicensed for use in children under 4 years.
Inhaled, doses (see note a).

Under 1 year	25-50microgram	twice a day
1 - 4 years	50-100microgram	twice a day
4 - 12 years	100-250microgram	twice a day
Over 12 years	250-500microgram	twice a day

Doses should be doubled (maximum 1mg twice a day), for at least 4 weeks, after an acute attack.

Notes:

a) Fluticasone is not a first line inhaled corticosteroid and although it is twice the potency of beclomethasone and budesonide when converting to fluticasone from the latter keep inhaled dose the same until control is achieved and then reduce dose.

b) Children under 10 years are usually incapable of using inhalers.

c) A Volumatic® spacer can be used with fluticasone inhalers.

d) Rinse mouth and wash face (if using mask) after use.

e) See also guidelines on management of chronic asthma page 241.

FOLIC ACID

Preparations:	TABLETS 5mg. LIQUID 2.5mg in 5ml. INJECTION 15mg in 1ml.
Dosage:	**FOLIC ACID SUPPLEMENTATION, PROPHYLAXIS IN DIALYSIS**

Orally,

Premature neonates	100-200microgram	once a day
Infants and children	250microgram/kg	once a day

OR,

4 weeks - 12 months	250microgram/kg	once a day
1 - 4 years	2.5mg	once a day
5 - 12 years	5mg	once a day
Over 12 years	5-10mg	once a day

TO TREAT MEGALOBLASTIC ANAEMIA

Orally,

Up to 1 year	500microgram/kg	once a day	) for up to
Over 1 year	5mg	once a day	) 4 months

Doses up to 15mg may be necessary in malabsorption states.

MAINTENANCE THERAPY

The above treatment doses - at daily to weekly intervals.

Notes:

a) Folic acid is well absorbed orally even in malabsorptive states, therefore parenteral therapy is only necessary when the oral route cannot be used.

b) Before treating megaloblastic anaemia with folic acid, **vitamin B12 deficiency** must be excluded, as neuropathy may be precipitated.

c) Folic acid liquid (Lexpec®) is sucrose free.

FRUSEMIDE (FUROSEMIDE)

Preparations:	TABLETS 20mg, 40mg and 500mg.
	LIQUID 1mg in 1ml and 10mg in 1ml.
	INJECTION 10mg in 1ml (2ml, 5ml and 25ml).
Dosage:	*DIURESIS*
	Orally,
	Neonates - 1 year 1mg/kg 3 times a day up to 4mg/kg/dose
	1 year - 12 years 1-4mg/kg once or twice a day
	Cardiac patients may require the above dose 3 to 4 times a day.
	Maximum dose is **12mg/kg/day**.
	IM injection, (all ages) 1-2mg/kg/dose.
	IV injection, (all ages) 0.5-1mg/kg/dose, every 6 to 12 hours.
	May increase to 5mg/kg/dose in resistant cases.
	IV infusion, 0.1-2mg/kg/hour.
Administration:	Give IV injection at a rate of 0.1mg/kg/min.
	Can be given by continuous infusion in sodium chloride 0.9% (do not use glucose 5% - see note d).

Notes:

a) Nephrocalcinosis has been reported in preterm neonates.

b) A marked fall in blood pressure may occur if an ACE-inhibitor is added to treatment with frusemide.

c) Do **not** mix frusemide injection with adrenaline, dopamine or dobutamine.

d) If for clinical reasons sodium chloride 0.9% is not suitable neutralised glucose 5% can be used as a diluent. This is prepared by adding 5ml of 8.4% sodium bicarbonate injection to 1L of glucose 5%.

e) Injection can be given orally.

f) Frusemide 1mg in 1ml liquid (Lasix®) is sugar free and contains sorbitol. Frusemide 10mg in 1ml is cherry flavoured and sugar free.

GABAPENTIN

Preparations: CAPSULES 100mg, 300mg; 400mg (**Non-formulary**).

Dosage: *EPILEPSY*

This indication is unlicensed for use in children.

Orally, initially, (see note a),

Day 1	5mg/kg	once a day
Day 2	5mg/kg	twice a day
Day 3	5mg/kg	three times a day

Then increase to maintenance dose of up to 8mg/kg three times a day, (maximum **45mg/kg/day** or 2.4g/day in adults). Anecdotally doses as high as 60mg/kg/day have been used. Maximum time between maintenance doses should not exceed 12 hours.

IN RENAL FAILURE

Creatinine clearance (ml/minute/1.73m^2)	Maintenance dose	Interval
30-60	8mg/kg	twice a day
15-30	8mg/kg	once a day
<15	8mg/kg	alternate days

Haemodialysis: 8-12mg/kg loading dose then 6-8mg/kg after each 4 hour dialysis period.

Notes:

a) Although the manufacturer's recommend daily increments in initial adult doses, some children may not tolerate such rapid increases and up to weekly increases may be more appropriate.

b) Avoid concomitant administration with antacids as they reduce the absorption of gabapentin.

c) Gabapentin is bitter; however capsules may be opened and mixed with a strong tasting liquid i.e. blackcurrant, immediately before administration. An aliquot may be given for doses less than the capsule strength.

GANCICLOVIR

Preparations: INJECTION 500mg. CAPSULES 250mg.

Dosage: **LIFE OR SIGHT THREATENING CMV INFECTION IN IMMUNOCOMPROMISED PATIENTS**

Ganciclovir is unlicensed for the treatment of congenital or neonatal CMV infections.

Treatment IV injection, 5mg/kg every 12 hours for 14-21 days.

Maintenance for patients at risk of relapse.

IV injection, 6mg/kg/day given for 5 days of each week

OR 5mg/kg/day for 7 days per week.

IN RENAL FAILURE

Creatinine clearance (ml/minute/1.73m^2)	Dose reduction (mg/kg)	Dosing Interval (hours)
>80	normal dose	normal
50-80	50% of normal dose	normal
10-50	25-50% of normal dose	halve frequency
<10 and peritoneal and haemodialysis	25% of normal dose	halve frequency

Ganciclovir is removed by haemodialysis therefore doses should be given following dialysis.

Clearance of ganciclovir during peritoneal dialysis is unknown therefore dose as for creatinine clearance less than 10ml/minute/1.73m^2 ensuring dose is given after dialysis session.

Administration: Reconstitution by the pharmacy manufacturing department is advised. Reconstitute (see note d) each vial with 10ml of water for injection to produce a 50mg in 1ml solution and dilute to at least 10mg in 1ml with sodium chloride 0.9% or glucose 5%. Infuse over 1 hour.

Notes:

a) Neutropenia occurs in 40% of patients and ganciclovir should not be administered if neutrophil count is less than 500 cells/mm^3. Thrombocytopenia occurs in 20% of patients.

b) The risk of neutropenia is greatly increased with concomitant administration of zidovudine and the two are not normally given together especially during initial ganciclovir therapy. White blood cell counts should be taken every 2 days for the first 2 weeks.

c) Toxicity is additive if flucytosine, amphotericin or co-trimoxazole are administered concomitantly.

d) When reconstituting the vial the use of polythene gloves and safety glasses is recommended as the resulting solution is very irritant (pH11) and ganciclovir is a potential carcinogen. If solution comes in contact with skin or mucosa, wash immediately with soap and water.

e) Ganciclovir can cause aspermatogenesis, mutagenicity, teratogenicity and carcinogenicity and should be considered as a potential carcinogen and teratogen.

f) The oral absorption of ganciclovir is extremely poor and therefore the intravenous route is recommended for treatment.

g) Sodium content is 2mmol per 500mg vial.

GAVISCON

Preparations:	INFANT SACHETS, LIQUID and TABLETS.
Dosage:	**GASTRIC REFLUX, DYSPEPSIA**

Orally,

Sachets

See note b).

Full term neonates and infants under 4.5kg, one sachet mixed with each feed.

Infants over 4.5kg and young children, two sachets mixed with each feed **or** half a glass of water, after each meal.

Liquid, tablets

1-12 years, 1 tablet or 5-10ml after meals and at bedtime.

Notes:

a) Carobel is preferred in neonates and infants less than 6 months. Gaviscon is not recommended in premature neonates.

b) One sachet is equal to one dose of a dual sachet.

c) Infant Gaviscon® provides 0.8mmol of sodium in 100ml when one sachet is mixed with 115ml (4 fluid oz) of feed/water.

d) Each sachet contains 0.92mmol of sodium, 225mg of sodium alginate, 87.5mg of magnesium alginate, 112.5mg of aluminium hydroxide with colloidal silica and mannitol. Each sachet contains 0.92mmol of sodium, 225mg of sodium alginate, 87.5mg of magnesium alginate, 112.5mg of aluminium hydroxide with colloidal silica and mannitol.

e) Each tablet contains 2mmol of sodium, 500mg alginic acid, 100mg of aluminium hydroxide, 25mg of magnesium trisilicate and 170mg of sodium bicarbonate.

f) Each 5ml of liquid contains 3mmol of sodium, 250mg of sodium alginate, 133.5mg of sodium bicarbonate and 80mg of calcium carbonate. The pharmacy departments currently stock the aniseed flavour.

g) Gaviscon infant sachets are sucrose and lactose free, the liquid and tablets are sugar free.

GENTAMICIN

Preparations: INJECTIONS 20mg in 2ml and 80mg in 2ml.
INTRATHECAL INJECTION 5mg in 1ml.

Dosage: **TREATMENT OF INFECTION (STANDARD REGIMEN)**
IV injection,
For neonates less than 7 days postnatal age

Gestational age	Dose	Dosage interval
<25 weeks	3.5mg/kg	36 hourly
26-30 weeks	3.0mg/kg	24 hourly
30-35 weeks	2.5mg/kg	18 hourly
>35 weeks	2.5mg/kg	12 hourly

For neonates more than 7 days postnatal age

Corrected gestational age (see note c)	Dose	Dosage interval
<27 weeks	3.0mg/kg	36 hourly
27-30 weeks	2.5mg/kg	24 hourly
30-34 weeks	2.5mg/kg	18 hourly
34-38 weeks	2.5mg/kg	12 hourly
>38 weeks	2.5mg/kg	8 hourly

Infants and children up to 12 years, *IV or IM injection*, 2.5mg/kg every 8 hours. Doses above 80mg should be according to levels.

TREATMENT OF INFECTION ON PICU (ONCE DAILY REGIMEN)

IV infusion, infants and children, 5mg/kg every 24 hours (see notes a and e).

In overweight or grossly oedematous patients ideal body weight must be used for calculating the dose.

Neonates: give 5mg/kg and await plasma level result before further dosing. For premature neonates use standard regimen.

IN RENAL FAILURE (STANDARD REGIMEN)

Creatinine clearance (ml/minute/1.73m^2)	Dose	Dosage Interval (hours)
30-70	2mg/kg	12
10-30	2mg/kg	24
<10	2mg/kg	48 or after haemodialysis

The above doses may be used in infants and children as a guide. Monitor levels and adjust dose accordingly.

Peritoneal dialysis;

Gentamicin is removed by peritoneal dialysis. If systemic therapy only is required give 2mg/kg after dialysis period.

APD/IPD: 5mg/L in every bag for 5 days. Monitor levels (as for once daily regimen) if cycles are rapid or treatment is prolonged. Systemic levels are not wanted.

IN RENAL FAILURE ON PICU (ONCE DAILY REGIMEN)

Give 5mg/kg and await plasma level result before further dosing.

INTRATHECAL, INTRAVENTRICULAR DOSE

> **INTRATHECAL PREPARATIONS ONLY AVAILABLE FROM PHARMACY.**
> **SEEK EXPERT ADVICE BEFORE PRESCRIBING**

1-5mg daily (see note b). CSF levels not to exceed 10mg/L. In addition, an IV/IM injection of 2mg/kg 8 hourly (3mg/kg by IV or IM injection 12 hourly if under 2 weeks old) should be administered.

CYSTIC FIBROSIS

IV or IM injection: Due to the increased rate of excretion of aminoglycosides in cystic fibrosis, the dose given needs to be increased (unless renal function is compromised) to 8-10mg/kg/day in divided doses. Adjust dose according to levels.

Nebulised: 40-80mg diluted to 3-4ml with sodium chloride 0.9% 2-3 times a day, after physiotherapy, depending on patient's age and clinical condition (see note g).

PROPHYLAXIS OF BACTERIAL ENDOCARDITIS

See guidelines page 265.

Administration: IV injection over 3 minutes (longer in neonates), either directly into a vein or into an IV giving set, **OR** by IM injection. Do **NOT** give by continuous infusion.

IV infusion over 30 minutes. Dilute if required with 0.9% sodium chloride.

Notes:

a) The ONCE DAILY REGIMEN is for use on PICU only until this dosing regime has been further evaluated.

b) Only intrathecal preparations of gentamicin should be used I.T. Do **NOT** use intravenous preparations as they often contain bacteriostats.

c) Corrected gestational age = gestational age + postnatal age.

d) Increased risk of ototoxicity with concomitant frusemide. Increased risk of nephrotoxicity with concomitant amphotericin, cisplatin or ciclosporin.

e) Blood levels *(STANDARD REGIMEN)*:
   i)   Approx. time to steady state: 3-4 doses.
   ii) Therapeutic level: trough   <2mg/L
                             peak   6-10mg/L
   iii) Take trough sample, immediately prior to next dose **and** peak sample, 1 hour after IV or IM dose.
   Blood levels on PICU *(ONCE DAILY REGIMEN)*:
   i)   Take level 18 hours post dose.
   ii) Therapeutic level: trough   <1mg/L
                             peak   NOT REQUIRED
   iii) Redose patient at 24 hours if trough level achieved. If trough is >1mg/L, recheck level 6-12 hours later and redose, appropriately adjusting the frequency of subsequent dose.

f) Do NOT store gentamicin blood samples if on concomitant beta-lactam antibiotics e.g. cefotaxime.

g) To reduce environmental contamination, gentamicin should be nebulised using a scavenging system or 'elephant' tubing vented via an external window or with a filter attached. Contact PICU ventilator technician on bleep 1360 for filter and advice on setting up tubing.

GLUCAGON

Preparations:	INJECTION 1mg.
Dosage:	**DIAGNOSTIC USE AND TREATMENT OF HYPOGLYCAEMIA**

IV, IM or SC injection,

0 - 4 weeks	20microgram/kg.
1 month - 4 years	500microgram.
Over 5 years	500microgram-1mg.

If not effective within 15 minutes for treatment of hypoglycaemia give IV glucose.

GROWTH HORMONE STIMULATION TEST

This is an unlicensed indication.

> **USE ENDOCRINE PROTOCOL**

IM injection, 15microgram/kg, maximum 1mg, as a single dose.

TREATMENT OF CARDIOGENIC SHOCK DUE TO BETA BLOCKER POISONING

This is an unlicensed indication.

> **IF IN ANY DOUBT CONTACT THE MEDICAL TOXICOLOGY UNIT**
> ☎ 0171-635-9191 ☎

IV injection, 50-150microgram/kg. Repeat if necessary.
If an infusion is required or glucagon is not available isoprenaline is an alternative.

Administration:	Reconstitute each vial with 1ml of diluent provided. Dilute if required with sodium chloride 0.9% or glucose 5%. For doses higher than 2mg reconstitute with water for injection not diluent. In treatment of beta blocker poisoning avoid phenol diluent.
Notes:	

a) If particles are observed in the solution, discard immediately.
b) Glucagon can **NOT** be added to infusion fluids containing calcium ions as this causes precipitation of the glucagon.

GLUCOSE

Preparations:	INFUSIONS 5%, 10%, 15%, 20% and 50% (500ml).
	INJECTION 50% (50ml).
	PRE-FILLED SYRINGE 50% (50ml).
Dosage:	**HYPOGLYCAEMIA**

Preterm and term neonates, *slow IV injection*, 200mg/kg (2ml/kg of glucose 10%), followed by an infusion of 6mg/kg/minute adjusting as necessary to maintain normoglycaemia.
Over 1 month, *IV injection*, 500mg-1g/kg (5-10ml/kg of glucose 10%).

HYPERKALAEMIA
IV injection, 500mg-1g/kg (2.5-5ml/kg of glucose 20%) and 0.5 units/kg of soluble insulin.

GLUCOSE TOLERANCE TEST
Orally, 1.75g/kg, up to 75g. See note c). This should then be made into a flavoured drink with concentration no greater than 25g in 100ml.

Administration: Slow IV injection over 5 minutes, not greater than 25% concentration, or as an infusion not greater than 30%, via central access. 50% glucose should only be administered in emergency situations. Concentrations greater than 10% should not be administered peripherally, see note d).

Notes:

a) To avoid rebound hypoglycaemia after injections of 50% glucose, use an infusion of 10% glucose after initial injection.
b) 50% glucose from the pre-filled syringe may be given orally for hypoglycaemia.
c) Lucozade® (from food stores), Fortical® (from dietitian), dextrose powder or 50% glucose can be used for the glucose tolerance test. Lucozade® comes in two strengths depending on the pack size. The 76kcal/100ml strength (739ml, 1L, 1.5L) contains 1.75g of glucose in 8.3ml and the 73kcal/100ml strength (300ml, 500ml) contains 1.75g of glucose in 8.9ml.
d) Concentrations of glucose greater than 10% are irritant to peripheral veins and greater than 30% are irritant to central veins.

GLYCEROL

Preparations:	SUPPOSITORIES: Infant 1g, child 2g and adult 4g.
Dosage:	**CONSTIPATION**

Rectally, insert appropriate suppository moistened with water, as necessary.

Notes:

Many small children who experience pain or fear during defecation find rectal administration very distressing, alternatives should be considered.

GLYCERYL TRINITRATE

Preparations: INJECTION 1mg in 1ml (5ml; 50ml) (Nitronal®). PATCHES 5mg.

Dosage: **VASODILATION**

This indication is unlicensed for use in children.

IV infusion, all ages, initially 0.1microgram/kg/minute, increasing to a maximum of 10microgram/kg/minute. Tolerance may occur with prolonged infusion.

Transdermally, initially,

Below 5kg	2.5mg (see note c)
5-10kg	5mg
Above 10kg	10mg

Patches should be changed daily. See note d). Tolerance may occur with prolonged use.

Administration: Dilute if required with sodium chloride 0.9%, glucose 5% or glucose/saline. As nitrates are adsorbed onto PVC, administration should be via a syringe pump (with plastipak or gillette sabre syringe) or via a rigid burette set with non-PVC tubing (Lectrocath or Gloucester tubing).

Notes:

a) Hypotension is more likely if patient is hypovolaemic, therefore central venous pressure should be monitored.

b) The formulation of glyceryl trintrate intravenous preparations varies, however Nitronal® contains **NO** alcohol or propylene glycol but does contain polyethylene glycol 400.

c) The 5mg Deponit® patches can be cut in half to provide a 2.5mg dose.

d) The site of the patch should be rotated each time it is changed to avoid skin sensitisation.

GLYCOPYRRONIUM BROMIDE

Preparations: AMPOULES 600microgram in 3ml. TABLETS 1mg and 2mg (**Named patient**).

Dosage: **PREMEDICATION AND INTRA-OPERATIVE USE**

IM or IV injection, 4-8microgram/kg. Maximum dose 200microgram. Dose may be repeated.

ANTAGONISM OF NEOSTIGMINE MUSCARINIC EFFECTS

IV injection, 10microgram/kg with 50microgram/kg neostigmine. Both can be mixed in the same syringe. See note below.

CONTROL OF UPPER AIRWAY SECRETIONS

Orally, 40-100microgram/kg 3 to 4 times a day.

Notes:

a) A 1ml premixed ampoule containing glycopyrronium 500microgram and neostigmine 2.5mg (Robinul-Neostigmine®) is available.

b) The tablets are scored and can be dispersed in water.

GRANISETRON

Preparations:	TABLETS 1mg. LIQUID 1mg in 5ml.
	INJECTION 1mg in 1ml and 3mg in 3ml.
Dosage:	**CYTOSTATIC INDUCED EMESIS**

Orally, over 1 month, 20microgram/kg, up to 1mg, twice a day. Initial dose to be administered approximately 1 hour **prior** to starting cytostatic therapy.

IV injection, over 1 month, 40microgram/kg, up to 3mg, immediately **prior** to starting cytostatic therapy. An additional dose may be given within a 24 hour period (at least 10 minutes after initial dose).

POST-OPERATIVE NAUSEA AND VOMITING

This indication is unlicensed for use in children.

IV injection, over 1 month, 40microgram/kg, up to 1mg, before, during or after induction of anaesthesia.

An additional dose may be given within a 24 hour period (at least 10 minutes after initial dose). Maximum 2mg/**day**.

Administration: Slow IV injection, over 5 minutes. Dilute if required with sodium chloride 0.9% or glucose 5%.

Notes:

a) Granisetron and other $5HT_3$ antagonists are very effective at controlling early emesis (24-48 hours) however they are not very effective at controlling late emesis. Dexamethasone should be considered see antiemetic guidelines page 277.

b) Granisetron is not first line treatment for post-operative nausea and vomiting and should only be used where first line therapy has failed or is contra-indicated.

c) Granisetron liquid (Kytril®) is sucrose free and contains 20%w/v sorbitol.

GRISEOFULVIN

Preparations:	LIQUID 125mg in 5ml. TABLETS 500mg.
Dosage:	**TREATMENT OF DERMATOPHYTE INFECTIONS OF SKIN, HAIR AND NAILS**

Orally, over 1 month, 10mg/kg once a day, after food. May be given in divided doses if not tolerated as a single dose. Treatment is usually continued for 4-6 weeks for hair and skin and 6 to 12 months for nails. Continue for at least 2 weeks after signs of infection have disappeared (see note d).

Notes:

a) Griseofulvin is contraindicated in severe liver disease and porphyria. It may also aggravate systemic lupus erythematosus.

b) Photosensitivity reactions may occur. Sunblock creams are required during periods of intense artificial or natural sunlight e.g. during summer.

c) Griseofulvin reduces the effect of warfarin and may also reduce ciclosporin blood levels. Phenobarbitone and primidone reduce the effectiveness of griseofulvin.

d) Tinea capitis may respond slowly. If still infected after 8 weeks seek advice from dermatologist.

e) Griseofulvin liquid is chocolate flavoured and contains 2.5g of sucrose in 5ml.

HAEMOPHILUS INFLUENZAE TYPE B (Hib) VACCINE

Preparations: INJECTION, 0.5ml of vaccine containing capsular antigens of Haemophilus Influenzae type B conjugated to proteins.

Dosage: **PRIMARY IMMUNISATION OR UNIMMUNISED AT LESS THAN 13 MONTHS OLD**

See immunisation guidelines page 296.

IM injection, 3 doses of 0.5ml with an interval of one month between each dose for infants from 2 months of age (see note a). Primary immunisation is usually given at the same time as Diptheria/Tetanus/Pertussis (see note b) and oral Polio vaccine.

UNIMMUNISED 13 MONTHS AND OVER

IM injection, a single dose of 0.5ml (see note c and d).

Administration: IM injection into the anterolateral thigh.

Notes:

a) Sufficient evidence now shows that there is no loss of immunogenicity or increased reactogenicity with different sequences of Hib vaccine.

b) A combined adsorbed diptheria, tetanus, pertussis with H.influenzae type b (Act-HiB DTP® or Trivax Hib®) is stocked in the pharmacy departments.

c) The dose may be given at the same time as the MMR vaccine.

d) Children over 4 years of age or adults do not usually require routine vaccination against Hib as the risk of invasive infection falls markedly after the first 4 years of life. However it may be given to those who are considered at increased risk e.g. immunocompromised, asplenic or with sickle cell disease.

HALOPERIDOL

Preparations: CAPSULES 500microgram. TABLETS 1.5mg, 5mg, 10mg and 20mg. LIQUID 2mg in 1ml. INJECTION 5mg in 1ml and 20mg in 2ml.

Dosage: **PSYCHOTIC DISORDERS, BEHAVIOURAL DISORDERS WITH SEVERE AGGRESSION/VIOLENCE, GILLES DE LA TOURETTE SYNDROME**

SEEK EXPERT ADVICE BEFORE PRESCRIBING

Over 4 weeks, *orally*, 12.5-25microgram/kg twice a day. Maximum 10mg/**day**, although adolescents may require up to 30mg or exceptionally up to 60mg/day for psychotic disorders.

PREMEDICATION

This is an unlicensed indication.

Orally, IM injection, 50-150microgram/kg.

Notes:

a) Extrapyramidal side effects occur at higher doses and are more common in children than adults.

b) Haloperidol is less sedating and has fewer antimuscarinic or hypotensive effects than chlorpromazine and is therefore the preferred treatment.

c) Haloperidol liquid (Rosemont®) is sucrose free.

HEPARIN SODIUM

Preparations: INJECTION 1,000 units in 1ml, 5,000 units in 1ml, 5,000 units in 0.2ml, 50 units in 5ml (Heplok®), 200 units in 2ml (Hepflush®) and 1,000 units in 1ml, (10ml and 20ml, Pump-hep®).

Dosage: ***ANTICOAGULANT THERAPY***
See notes below.
All ages, *IV injection*, of 75units/kg then *IV infusion,* starting at 20 units/kg/hour.
Adjust dose/rate according to APTT (Activated Partial Thromboplastin Time) ratio to maintain between 1.5 and 2.5 using the table below as a guide.

APTT RATIO	DOSE/RATE CHANGE	RECHECK APTT IN
>5	reduce by 35%❶	4 hours
4.1 - 5	reduce by 20%	4 hours
3.1 - 4	reduce by 10%	4 hours
2.6 - 3	reduce by 5%	4 hours
1.5 - 2.5	no change	24 hours
1.2 - 1.4	increase by 15%❷	4 hours
<1.2	increase by 30%❷	4 hours

❶ Stop infusion for 1 hour before recommencing at reduced infusion rate.
❷ Give *IV bolus* 50units/kg, before recommencing at increased infusion rate.

PROPHYLACTIC DOSE
This indication is unlicensed for use in children.
All ages, *SC injection*, 100units/kg up to 5000units, every 12 hours.

Administration: To prepare infusion take (500 x Wt (kg)) units of heparin and make up to 50ml with sodium chloride 0.9% to give a solution where 1ml/hour = 10units/kg/hour.
e.g. 20kg child: 500 x 20 = 10,000 units of heparin made up to 50ml with sodium chloride.

Notes:
a) **CSM Warning:** monitor platelet count in patients receiving heparin for longer than 5 days due to risk of immune mediated thrombocytopaenia.
b) A baseline full blood count, INR and APTT should be performed prior to commencing heparin infusion.
c) High doses of penicillins may prolong bleeding time and therefore increase the effects of heparin when used concurrently.
d) Antidote is **protamine** (see page 184).
e) For maintaining peripheral catheter patency, sodium chloride 0.9% is as effective as heparinised saline 50 units in 5ml.

HEPATITIS B IMMUNOGLOBULIN

Preparations: INJECTION 200 units and 500 units.

Dosage: ***PASSIVE IMMUNISATION***

IM injection, neonates 200units ideally within 12 hours but up to 24-48 hours of delivery.

Under 5 years	200 units
5 - 9 years	300 units
10 years and over	500 units

Hepatitis B vaccine should be administered concurrently, at a different site. See also immunisation guidelines page 296.

Administration: IM into the anterolateral thigh.

Notes:

a) Hepatitis B immunoglobulin should only be given under certain criteria. For use in neonates see hepatitis B vaccine page 121. For use in accidental inoculation see immunisation guidelines page 296.

b) **Caution:** There is a theoretical risk that new variant CJD may be transmitted in this product.

c) For supplies at Guy's and St Thomas': Contact the clinical pharmacist or resident (if out of hours) and Lewisham: available from Haematology Department.

HEPATITIS B VACCINE

Preparations: INJECTION 10microgram in 0.5ml (Engerix B® paediatric),
5microgram in 0.5ml (HB-Vax® II paediatric).
20microgram in 1ml (Engerix B® adult).
10microgram in 1ml (HB-Vax® II adult).
40microgram in 1ml (HB-Vax® II 40).

See immunisation guidelines page 296.

STANDARD IMMUNISATION REGIMEN,

Neonates and children under 10 years, *IM injection*, 0.5ml.

Children over 10 years, *IM injection*, 1ml.

Repeat dose, 1 and 6 months after first dose. Test for antibodies at 1-2 months after final dose and if no seroconversion has occurred retest and give a further dose.

ACCELERATED REGIMEN

The accelerated regimen should be used for all babies born to hepatitis B positive mothers and where accidental innoculation has occured. First dose should be given as above and then repeated at 1, 2 and 12 months after first dose. Test for antibodies 2-4 months after final dose and if no seroconversion has occured retest and give a further dose.

DIALYSIS REGIMEN

Dialysis or immunocompromised patients require larger doses.

IM injection,

Under 10 years	0.5ml	} of 40 microgram in 1ml
Over 10 years	1ml	} HB-Vax II® 40.

Repeat dose at 1 and 6 months after first dose. Test for antibodies 1-2 months after final dose and if no seroconversion has occured retest and give a further dose.

Administration:	Give IM into the deltoid muscle if over 10 years or into the anterolateral thigh in infants and children under 10 years.
	If immunoglobulin is to be administered at same time, inject at different sites.
Notes:	

a) Infants born to mothers who are HBsAg and HBeAg positive **or** HBsAg positive without c markers **or** with acute hepatitis B during pregnancy should receive vaccine **and** immunoglobulin (HBIG). Infants born to mothers who are HBsAg and anti-HBe positive require vaccine only.

b) Hepatitis B vaccine must not be injected IV or intradermally. In patients with severe bleeding tendencies e.g. haemophiliacs, SC injection may be considered.

c) Hepatitis B vaccine brands are interchangeable as long as the same dose (**in volumes**) is used.

HISTAMINE

Preparations:	INJECTION 0.1mg in 1ml (**Extemporaneously prepared**).
Dosage:	*TEST FOR FAMILIAL DYSAUTONOMIA*

SEEK EXPERT ADVICE BEFORE PRESCRIBING

Intradermal injection of 0.2-0.5ml.

Notes:

a) Injection produces a wheal but no pain or axon flare in a positive test.

b) This test is often performed in conjunction with the instillation of methacholine chloride 2.5% eye drops, see page 146.

HYDRALAZINE HYDROCHLORIDE

Preparations:	TABLETS 25mg and 50mg. INJECTION 20mg.
	LIQUID (**Extemporaneously prepared**).
Dosage:	*HYPERTENSION*

This indication is unlicensed for use in children.

Slow IV injection, all ages, 300-500microgram/kg/dose, maximum 4 hourly, (i.e. maximum 3mg/kg in 24 hours).

IV infusion, (preferred route in cardiac patients), all ages, 25-50microgram/kg/hour. Maximum 3mg/kg in 24 hours.

Orally, all ages, initially 250-500microgram/kg 2-3 times a day.

IN RENAL FAILURE

Dose may need to be reduced in patients with a creatinine clearance less than 30ml/minute/1.73m^2.

Administration:	Slow IV injection, reconstitute each vial with 1ml of water for injection and use immediately. Administer over at least 5 minutes. IV infusion, further dilute with sodium chloride 0.9%.
Notes:	

a) Treatment for longer than 6 months, particularly with high doses may be associated with a lupus-like syndrome which may require steroid therapy. This is more common in slow acetylators.

b) Injection solution can be given orally.

c) Hydralazine (Apresoline®) tablets contain gluten and sucrose.

HYDROCORTISONE

Preparations:	TABLETS 10mg and 20mg. PELLETS (lozenges) 2.5mg. INJECTION 100mg. LIQUID (**Extemporaneously prepared**).
Dosage:	*ASTHMA, ACUTE ADRENAL INSUFFICIENCY AND EMERGENCIES*

IV injection or *IM injection*, 4-8mg/kg, additional doses of 2-4mg/kg every 6 hours depending on the condition being treated and the patient's response.

Change to oral **prednisolone** as soon as possible.

OR

Up to 1 year	25mg	3-4 times a day
1 - 5 years	50mg	3-4 times a day
5 - 12 years	100mg	3-4 times a day
Over to 12 years	100-500mg	3-4 times a day

REPLACEMENT THERAPY MAINTENANCE

Orally, all ages, initially, 20mg/m^2/**day**. The correct dose is determined by a profile of plasma cortisol levels.

CONGENITAL ADRENAL HYPERPLASIA

SEEK EXPERT ADVICE BEFORE PRESCRIBING

Orally, neonates, 20-25mg/m^2 body surface area/**day** (equivalent to 5mg/day) in 3 divided doses. Fludrocortisone may be required and high doses may cause growth suppression. Dose can be reduced over next 2 years.

REFRACTORY HYPOTENSION

IV injection, premature (VLBW) neonates, 2.5mg/kg every 4 hours for 2 **doses** then every 6 hours. Once normotension has been maintained for 24 hours wean the hydrocortisone by halving the doses every 48 hours. If hypotension recurs resume therapy at previous dose

Administration:	Over at least 1-5 minutes. Dilute if required with sodium chloride 0.9%, glucose 5% or glucose/saline.
Notes:	
	a) Injection can be given orally.
	b) For relative potencies see table 1.

TABLE 1. RELATIVE POTENCIES AND APPROXIMATE EQUIVALENT DOSES

Drug	Relative Glucocorticoid (Anti-inflammatory) Potency	Relative Mineralo-corticoid Potency	Approximate Biological Half-life	Equivalent Anti-inflammatory dose❶
Dexamethasone	25	0	36-72 hours	4mg
Betamethasone (NF)	25	0	36-72 hours	4mg
Methylprednisolone	5	0.5	12-36 hours	20mg
Triamcinolone (NF)	5	0	12-36 hours	20mg
Prednisolone	4	0.8	12-36 hours	25mg
Hydrocortisone	1	1	8-12 hours	100mg
Fludrocortisone	--	125	8-12 hours	--

❶ Applies only to oral or intravenous administration; relative potencies may differ greatly when injected intramuscularly or into joint spaces.

HYDROXOCOBALAMIN

Preparations: INJECTION 1mg in 1ml.
Dosage: ***INBORN ERRORS OF METABOLISM***
This is an unlicensed indication.

SEEK EXPERT ADVICE BEFORE PRESCRIBING

Neonates and infants, *IM injection*, initially, 1mg once day for 5 days then assess. Adjust dose according to response. Maintenance dose may be as high as 1mg 1-2 times each week.

CONFIRMED VITAMIN B12 DEFICIENCY
Adults and children (all ages), *IM injection*, initially 250microgram-1mg 3 times weekly for 2 weeks, then 250microgram weekly until blood count is normal. Maintenance *IM injection*, 1mg every 2-3 months.

Notes:

Injection solution can be given orally, but the effect will not be prolonged and it will not be absorbed in pernicious anaemia, post gastrectomy or other malabsorption syndromes. Cyanocobalamin liquid and tablets are also available.

HYOSCINE BUTYLBROMIDE (SCOPOLAMINE BUTYLBROMIDE)

Preparations: TABLETS 10mg. INJECTION 20mg in 1ml.
Dosage: ***RENAL OR BILIARY COLIC***
This indication is unlicensed for use in children.
IM or IV injection,

Under 6 years	5mg up to 3 times a day
Over 6 years	5-10mg up to 3 times a day

GASTROINTESTINAL SPASM
Orally,

6 - 12 years	10mg 3 times a day.
Over 12 years	20mg 4 times a day.

Administration: IV injection over at least 1 minute. Dilute if required with glucose 5% or sodium chloride 0.9%.
Notes:

Injection can be given orally.

HYOSCINE HYDROBROMIDE (SCOPOLAMINE HYDROBROMIDE)

Preparations:	INJECTION 400microgram in 1ml. PATCHES 1mg.
Dosage:	**PREMEDICATION**

Orally, SC or IM injection,

1 - 4 years	10microgram/kg/dose
5 - 12 years	10microgram/kg/dose to a maximum of 400microgram

Over 12 years 400microgram/dose

HYPERSALIVATION

This is an unlicensed indication.

Transdermally

Under 3 years	¼ patch every 72 hours
3 - 9 years	½ patch every 72 hours
10 years and over	1 patch every 72 hours

Notes:

Injection can be given orally.

IBUPROFEN

Preparations:	TABLETS 200mg and 400mg. LIQUID 100mg in 5ml.
	INJECTION 100mg (**Named patient**).
Dosage:	***ANALGESIA FOR MILD TO MODERATE PAIN, ANTIPYRETIC***

These indications are unlicensed for use in children under 1 year or 7kg.

Orally, 4-10mg/kg every 6 to 8 hours,

OR

1 - 2 years	2.5ml (50mg)	3-4 times a day.
3 - 7 years	5ml (100mg)	3-4 times a day.
8 - 12 years	10ml (200mg)	3-4 times a day.

JUVENILE ARTHRITIS

Orally, 10-15mg/kg 3 times a day.

CLOSURE OF PATENT DUCTUS ARTERIOSUS
(see note c).

Neonates, *IV injection,* at 24 hour intervals (only if renal function has returned to normal - monitor weight, urine output and U+E's):

1st dose	10mg/kg
2nd dose	5mg/kg
3rd dose	5mg/kg

Above course may be repeated if the duct reopens or has not successfully closed 48 hours after the first course.

Administration:	Reconstitute vial with 3ml of water for injection to provide a 33mg in 1ml solution. Roll gently, do not shake, to avoid frothing. Dilute further with sodium chloride 0.9%. Administer over 15 minutes.
Notes:	

a) Ibuprofen is contraindicated in patients with a history of hypersensitivity (including asthma, angioedema, urticaria or rhinitis) to aspirin or any other non-steroidal anti-inflammatory drug or with a coagulation defect.

b) Caution, use in renal, cardiac or hepatic failure may cause a deterioration in renal function; the dose should be kept as low as possible and renal function monitored.

c) Currently, ibuprofen injection is being assessed for closure of patent ductus arteriosus within the neonatal units of the Trust. Assessment forms must be completed for each patient.

d) Ibuprofen liquid (Nurofen®) is orange flavoured and sugar free.

e) See recommended analgesics page 255.

IMIPRAMINE

Preparations: TABLETS 10mg and 25mg. LIQUID 25mg in 5ml.
Dosage: ***ATTENTION DEFICIT HYPERACTIVITY DISORDER***

This is an unlicensed indication.

SEEK EXPERT ADVICE BEFORE PRESCRIBING

Orally, initially, 10mg at night for 1 week, then 25mg at night. Increase if necessary, usual maintenance dose between **0.5-1.5mg/kg/day**. Doses over 1.5mg/kg/day should be given in 2 divided doses to decrease risk of cardiotoxic effects.

Notes:

a)   Baseline ECG must be performed and further monitoring is advisable at higher doses i.e. between 1.5 and 2.5mg/kg/day.

b)   Imipramine is contraindicated in patients with arrhythmias, particularly heart block and severe liver disease should be used with caution in patients with a history of epilepsy, thyroid disease or hepatic impairment.

c)   Avoid concomitant administration with astemizole and terfenadine, antiarrhythmics including sotalol and anaesthetic agents due to increased risk of arrhythmias. Methylphenidate may also inhibit the metabolism of imipramine.

d)   Imipramine liquid (Tofranil®) contains 0.63g of sucrose in 5ml and 50%w/v sorbitol.

INDOMETACIN

Preparations: CAPSULES 25mg. LIQUID 25mg in 5ml. INJECTION 1mg.
Dosage: ***RENAL FANCONI SYNDROME, CYSTINOSIS***

These indications are unlicensed.

Orally, all ages, initially, 300microgram/kg 3 times a day up to **3mg/kg/day**.

CLOSURE OF PATENT DUCTUS ARTERIOSUS

Neonates, *IV injection* at 12-24 hour intervals (only if renal function has returned to normal):

Age at time of first dose	1st dose (microgram/kg)	2nd dose (microgram/kg)	3rd dose (microgram/kg)
< 48 hours	200	100	100
2-7 days	200	200	200
> 7 days	200	250	250

OR *IV injection* 100microgram/kg every 24 hours for 6 doses.

Administration: Reconstitute vial with 1-2ml of water for injection. Administer over 20 minutes (see note b). Dilute if required with sodium chloride 0.9%. Precipitation may occur below pH6, **DO NOT** use glucose solutions.

Notes:

a) Indometacin is contraindicated in patients with a history of hypersensitivity (including asthma, angioedema, urticaria and rhinitis) to aspirin or any other non steroidal drug or with a coagulation defect.
b) Indometacin causes a reduction in cerebral blood flow. A 20 minute infusion results in a smaller reduction than a bolus.
c) Indometacin reduces glomerular filtration, therefore, in neonates with a PDA reduce fluid intake. Plasma creatinine, digoxin and aminoglycoside levels will rise.
d) Indometacin may antagonise thiazide diuretics and frusemide, and can potentiate warfarin.
e) Indometacin liquid (Indocid®) is sucrose free.

INFLUENZA VACCINE

Preparation: PRE-FILLED SYRINGE containing 0.5ml of strains A and B.
Dose: **PROPHYLAXIS OF INFLUENZA**
IM, deep SC injection,
6 months - 4 years 0.25ml, repeat at 4-6 weeks if receiving vaccination for first time
4 - 12 years 0.5ml, repeat at 4-6 weeks if receiving vaccination for first time
13 years and over 0.5ml single dose
In infants less than 6 months seroconversion cannot be assured.

Notes:

a) Vaccination is recommended in the following conditions: chronic respiratory disease (including asthma), chronic heart disease, chronic renal failure, diabetes mellitus and immunosuppression due to disease or treatment.
b) Do not administer within 3 days of DTP, due to increased risk of febrile illness.
c) Neurological disorders such as encephalomyelitis and neuritis have been reported but are rare.
d) Influenza vaccine is contraindicated in those hypersensitive to eggs.

INSULIN

Preparations:

SHORT ACTING	**Human Actrapid** (soluble) 10ml vials and pen cartridges for Novopen.	OR	**Humulin S** (soluble) pen cartridges for B-D pen.		
MEDIUM ACTING	**Humulin I** (isophane) pen cartridges for B-D pen.	OR	**Human Insulatard** (isophane) 10ml vials and pen cartridges for Novopen, and pre-loaded pen	OR	**Human Monotard** (insulin zinc suspension) 10ml vial.
BIPHASIC FIXED MIXTURES	**Human Mixtard 30** (soluble + isophane) 10ml vial and 1.5ml pen cartridges and pre-loaded pen.	OR	**Humulin M3** (soluble and isophane) 1.5ml and 3ml pen cartridges and pre-loaded pen. **Humulin M5** (soluble and isophane) 10ml vial.		
LONG ACTING	**Humulin-Zn** (insulin zinc suspension 10ml vials.				

Dosage:

INSULIN DEPENDENT DIABETES MELLITUS
All preparations contain 100 units in 1ml (store in fridge).
See page 268 for details of insulin administration in children.

MAINTENANCE THERAPY
Most children are maintained on twice a day *subcutaneous* human preparations, usually a mixture of short and medium acting preparations. Some children may benefit from more intensive therapy regimes (dosing up to four times a day).

DIABETIC KETOACIDOSIS
A soluble insulin (Human Actrapid) *IV infusion*, by syringe pump, rate determined by frequent blood glucose estimations. See guidelines on page 275.

PERI-OPERATIVE MANAGEMENT AND PATIENTS WHO ARE "NIL BY MOUTH"
See guidelines on page 272.

⊥

INTRAVENOUS IMMUNOGLOBULIN (HUMAN)

Preparations: INJECTION Sandoglobulin® containing 1g with 33ml diluent, 3g with 100ml diluent, 6g with 200ml diluent and 12g with 400ml diluent.

Dosage: **PROPHYLAXIS OF LATE ONSET SEPSIS**

This is an unlicensed indication. There is conflicting evidence of the efficacy of use of immunoglobulin for this indication.
Preterm neonate (<32 week gestation and <1500g).
IV infusion, 500mg/kg up to 750mg/kg. Two doses are given 7 days apart.

REPLACEMENT THERAPY FOR CONGENITAL AGAMMAGLOBULINAEMIA AND HYPOGAMMOGLOBULINAEMIA

IV infusion, initially, 0.4 to 0.8g/kg, then 0.2 - 0.6g/kg every 2-4 weeks, according to severity of clinical signs and symptoms. Trough levels should be measured in order to adjust the dose and dosage interval.

IDIOPATHIC THROMBOCYTOPENIC PURPURA

SEEK EXPERT ADVICE BEFORE PRESCRIBING

THIS IS NOT FIRST LINE TREATMENT
IV infusion, 0.4g/kg/day for 5 days or 2g/kg as a single infusion. Maintenance doses 0.4g/kg given to maintain platelet count.

KAWASAKI SYNDROME

IV infusion, 0.4g/kg/day for 4-5 days or 2g/kg as a single infusion; with aspirin, see page 30.

Administration: The vials should be reconstituted immediately before use. Dissolve the contents of the vial in the diluent (sodium chloride 0.9%), resultant solution concentration is 3% i.e. 30mg of immunoglobulin in 1ml. In fluid restricted patients, use half the volume of diluent, resultant solution concentration is 6%. Avoid frothing and **do not shake the solution**. The immunoglobulin may take up to 20 minutes to dissolve. Ensure solution is clear before administering.
For IV infusion,
Neonates: infuse dose over 4 hours.
Infants and children: initial starting rate is 0.01-0.02ml/kg/minute for 30 minutes. If well tolerated increase rate to 0.08ml/kg/minute.
Infuse 2g/kg dose over 12 hours.
Observe patient for signs of anaphylaxis.
May be further diluted with sodium chloride 0.9% if required.

Notes:

a) Intravenous immunoglobulin has been associated with anaphylactoid reactions. These are most likely during the first infusion. Patient should be monitored for a further 20 minutes after infusion completed. Cardiopulmonary resuscitation facilities should be available.

b) Sandoglobulin® is prepared by cold alcohol fractionation of human plasma and is stabilised with 5g sucrose for every 3g of protein (immunoglobulin). Dose is based on protein (immunoglobulin) content. The sucrose content is only relevant for diabetic or hyperglycaemic patients and should not be included in dosage calculations.

⊥

INULIN (POLYFRUCTOSAN)

Preparations: INJECTION 5g in 20ml. (**Named patient**).
Dosage: **MEASUREMENT OF GLOMERULAR FILTRATION RATE (GFR) USING IV INJECTION METHOD**

IV injection, all ages, 75mg/kg, up to 5g, as a slow IV injection over 1-2minutes. See notes below.

Administration:

> Available from pharmacy in prefilled syringes. Must be ordered at least 24 hours in advance of test. Contact pharmacy manufacturing on ☎Guy's ext. 3712, Lewisham ext. 3201, St Thomas' ext. 3051☎

Notes:

a) **Caution:** Bronchospasm and anaphylaxis have been reported. Caution required in asthmatic patients. Resuscitation facilities must be available.

b) Inulin is almost entirely cleared by glomerular filtration without secretion or reabsorption in the renal tubule.

c) Dose **administered** should be recorded on the inulin test form sent to the Children Nationwide Kidney Research Laboratory, ext 4502, 12th floor, Guy's Tower.

d) Blood samples should be taken at 5 minutes, 1 hour, 2 hours, 3 hours and 4 hours post injection. Accurate time of injection and sampling must be recorded.

e) Height (cm) and weight (kg) must be recorded on inulin test form for calculation of surface area as GFR is expressed as ml/minute/1.73m^2.

IODINE

Preparations: AQUEOUS LIQUID containing iodine 130mg in 1ml.
Dosage: **THYROTOXICOSIS (PRE-OPERATIVE)**

Children (all ages), *orally*, 0.1-0.3ml 3 times a day for 6 days. Treatment is started the day before the MIBG scan.
Administration: Dilute well with milk or water.

IPRATROPIUM

Preparations:	NEBULISER SOLUTION 250microgram in 1ml and 500microgram in 2ml.
	INHALERS 20microgram and 40 microgram per metered dose (200 dose units).
	BREATH ACTIVATED INHALER® 20microgram per metered dose (200 dose unit).

Dosage: **ASTHMA THERAPY**

Nebulised,

This route is unlicensed for use in children under 3 years.

4 weeks -1 year	62.5microgram	every 6-8 hours
1 - 4 years	125-250microgram	every 6-8 hours
5 - 12 years	250-500microgram	every 6-8 hours

Optimal volume for nebulisation is 4ml, unless smaller reservoir is used. Dilute dose where appropriate with sodium chloride 0.9%. Nebulisers may be administered more frequently in hospital with close monitoring.

Inhalation,

Up to 6 years	20microgram (1 puff) 3 times a day
6 - 12 years	20-40microgram (1-2 puffs) 3 times a day
Over 12 years	20-40microgram (1-2 puffs) 3-4 times a day. Up to 80microgram (4 puffs) at a time.

Notes:

a) As paradoxical bronchospasm can occur, first dose should be inhaled under medical supervision.
b) Children under 10 years are usually incapable of using inhalers.
c) The ipratropium aerosol inhaler loosely fits into the Nebuhaler® and fits into the Volumatic® spacers.
d) Ipratropium and salbutamol solutions are compatible and may be nebulised concomitantly.
e) See also guidelines on the management of acute and chronic asthma page 241 and 244.

⊥

IRON (ORAL SUPPLEMENTATION)

Preparations: FERROUS SULPHATE TABLETS 200mg (65mg elemental iron).
SYTRON® ELIXIR (sodium iron edetate) 55mg elemental iron in 10ml.
NIFEREX® ELIXIR 100mg elemental iron in 5ml.

Dosage: *IRON DEFICIENCY*
Dosage should be calculated using the amount of ELEMENTAL IRON (E.I.) in the preparation.
Infants and premature neonates:
Orally, 4-6mg/kg E.I. per day in 2 to 3 divided doses,
OR
Sytron® initially 1ml/kg once a day, larger volumes may be given in 2-3 divided doses.
Niferex® 2 drops/kg 3 times a day (2 drops contains approximately 1mg E.I.)
Children:
Orally, 1 - 5 years 40-50mg E.I. (approximately 7.5ml Sytron® or 2.5ml Niferex®) per day.
6 - 12 years 80-100mg E.I. (approximately 15ml Sytron® or 5ml Niferex®) per day. Sytron® should be given in 2-3 divided doses.

IRON PROPHYLAXIS
Premature neonates over 4-6 weeks or on discharge from unit, *orally,* 1ml (of Sytron®) once a day until weaned.

Notes:

a) Acute iron toxicity after accidental ingestion may occur with as little as 30mg/kg of E.I. and may be fatal in young children. Urgent treatment with oral or parenteral desferrioxamine is required, see page 79.

> **IF IN ANY DOUBT CONTACT THE MEDICAL TOXICOLOGY UNIT**
> ☎ 0171-635-9191 ☎

b) Niferex® 30ml size is on the government "black list" for all indications except for prophylaxis and treatment of iron deficiency in infants born prematurely. Prescrptions should be endorsed "SLS".

c) Niferex® and Sytron® are sucrose free and do not stain dental enamel. Sytron® is cherry flavoured and Niferex® is caramel flavoured.

ISOLEUCINE see Metabolic dietitian

⊥

ISONIAZID

Preparations:	TABLETS 100mg. LIQUID 50mg in 5ml (**Manufactured special**). INJECTION 50mg in 2ml.
Dosage:	*TUBERCULOSIS THERAPY (UNSUPERVISED REGIMEN)*

SEEK EXPERT ADVICE BEFORE PRESCRIBING

TREATMENT
Orally, IM or Slow IV injection injection,
Neonates, 3-5mg/kg once a day.
Over 1 month, 5-10mg/kg once a day. Maximum dose 300mg/**day**.
Exceptionally, a higher dose of 20mg/kg once a day (maximum 500mg/**day**), may be required in tuberculous meningitis.

PROPHYLAXIS
Orally, IM or Slow IV injection injection,
Over 1 month, 5-10mg/kg once a day. Maximum dose 300mg/**day**.

IN RENAL FAILURE
Dosage adjustments are not usually necessary until creatinine clearance is less than 10ml/minute/1.73m^2. Maximum dose 200mg/**day** (see note b).
Isoniazid is removed by haemodialysis and peritoneal dialysis.

Administration: Slow IV injection over 2-5 minutes; dilute if required with water for injection, use immediately.

Notes:

a) Main route of excretion is hepatic, reduce the dose and use with caution in liver failure. See note below.
b) Therapeutic drug monitoring:
   i) Isoniazid blood levels are not routinely monitored however in severe renal failure and liver impairment monitoring may be useful to reduce the risk of side effects.
   ii) Trough level should be below 1mg/L in liver impairment and severe renal failure.
   iii) Take a trough sample, immediately prior to next dose.
c) Hepatitis has been reported with isoniazid. Base line liver function tests should be performed before commencing treatment. Frequent checks in the first 2 months are then required in those with pre-existing liver disease. Further routine checks are not required if there is no evidence of liver disease or dysfunction. Patients/carer should be warned to seek medical advice immediately if there are any signs of liver disorder e.g. persistent nausea, vomiting, malaise, fever or jaundice.
d) Pre-existing risk factors such as malnutrition, chronic renal failure, HIV infection, diabetes and slow acetylator status increase the risk of developing peripheral neuritis. If considered necessary, **pyridoxine** should be given concurrently (see page 186).
e) The metabolism of phenytoin, diazepam and carbamazepine may be reduced by isoniazid. Corticosteroid effects of prednisolone may also be enhanced.
f) The absorption of isoniazid may be inhibited by concomitant administration of antacids.
g) Isoniazid liquid (Martindale) is sugar free.

134

ISOPRENALINE

Preparations:	INJECTIONS 200microgram in 10ml, 2mg in 2ml and 5mg in 5ml.
Dosage:	**ASYSTOLE**

Neonates and older children, *IV injection,* 5microgram/kg.

BRADYCARDIA
IV infusion, 0.02microgram/kg/minute, increasing to a maximum of 0.5microgram/kg/minute if necessary.

INOTROPE FOR COMPLETE HEART BLOCK
IV infusion, 0.1-1microgram/kg/minute.

Administration: Dilute if required with glucose 5% or sodium chloride 0.9%.

Notes:

a) Isoprenaline may precipitate ventricular extrasystole and arrhythmias and should only be used with ECG monitoring and cardiopulmonary resuscitation facilities available.

ISOSORBIDE

Preparations:	LIQUID 50%w/v (50g in 100ml) (**Extemporaneously prepared**).
Dosage:	**OSMOTIC DIURETIC IN HYDROCEPHALUS**

SEEK EXPERT ADVICE BEFORE PRESCRIBING

Orally, all ages, initially, 0.5g/kg every 6 hours increasing to 1-2g/kg every 6 hours.

Notes:

a) **Note** this is the dose for **ISOSORBIDE - not** to be confused with isosorbide dinitrate or mononitrate.
b) Monitor plasma osmolarity and sodium levels. Isosorbide should not be used if there is diarrhoea or vomiting, particularly in young children.

ITRACONAZOLE

Preparations:	CAPSULES 100mg. LIQUID 10mg in 1ml.
Dosage:	

CONSULT MICROBIOLOGY BEFORE PRESCRIBING

SYSTEMIC FUNGAL INFECTIONS
This indication is unlicensed for use in children.
Orally, all ages, 3-5mg/kg once a day. Up to 10mg/kg once a day in severe infections.

Notes:

a) Itraconazole is predominantly hepatically metabolised; no dosage adjustment is required in renal failure.
b) Liver function tests should be performed if pre-existing liver disease or treatment is to be continuous for more than 1 month. Patient/carer should be warned to seek medical advice immediately if there are any signs of liver disorder e.g. persistent nausea, vomiting, malaise, fever or jaundice.
c) **CSM Warning:** Avoid concomitant administration with astemizole, terfenadine and cisapride due to increased risk of arrhythmias.
d) Phenytoin and rifampicin decrease blood levels of itraconazole.
e) Itraconazole increases ciclosporin, midazolam, digoxin and possibly tacrolimus levels and potentiates warfarin.
f) Itraconazole liquid (Sporanox®) is cherry flavoured and sugar free.

KETAMINE (CD restrictions apply at Guy's).

Preparations:	INJECTION 200mg in 20ml, 500mg in 10ml, 500mg in 5ml.
Dosage:	***INTERMITTENT INJECTION***

INDUCTION OF ANAESTHESIA

All ages (under 15 years), *IV injection,* 1-2mg/kg given slowly over 1 minute. Maximum initial dose 4.5mg/kg.

MAINTENANCE OF ANAESTHESIA

IV or IM injection, give additional dose of 50% of full induction dose.

CONTINUOUS INFUSION

INDUCTION OF ANAESTHESIA

IV injection, 0.5-2mg/kg given slowly over 1 minute.

MAINTENANCE OF ANAESTHESIA

IV infusion, 10-45 microgram/kg/minute.

The dosage used may require reduction if a long acting neuromuscular blocking agent is used.

Notes:

a) The incidence of psychological reactions during recovery e.g. hallucinations, is higher in children over 15 years. The use of a benzodiazepine e.g. midazolam, diazepam, lorazepam as an adjunct to ketamine is effective in reducing the incidence of emergence reactions. Minimised verbal and tactile stimulation during the recovery phase may also reduce emergence reactions.

b) Although ketamine has been used outside of the operating theatre, it should be remembered that it is a general anaesthetic, requiring appropriate skills and equipment such as those usually found within an intensive care environment. Ketamine should not be administered on a general ward or department.

KETOVITE®

Preparations:	TABLETS containing ascorbic acid 16.6mg, riboflavine 1mg, thiamine 1mg, pyridoxine 330microgram, nicotinamide 3.3mg, calcium pantothenate 1.16mg, alphatocopheryl acetate 5mg, inositol 50mg, biotin 170microgram, folic acid 250microgram, acetomenaphthone 500microgram.

LIQUID containing in 5ml vitamin A 2500 units (750microgram), ergocalciferol 400 units, choline chloride 150mg, cyanocobalamin 12.5microgram.

Dosage:	***MULTIVITAMIN SUPPLEMENT***

Orally, all ages, 5ml of liquid **and** 3 tablets per day.

Notes:

a) Tablets **and** liquid must **both** be given for complete vitamin supplementation.

b) These preparations do not contain sucrose, lactose, starch, sodium or artificial colouring.

LABETALOL

Preparations:	TABLETS 100mg and 200mg; 400mg (**Non-formulary**). INJECTION 100mg in 20ml.
Dosage:	These indications are unlicensed for use in children. ***HYPERTENSIVE CRISIS*** All ages, *IV infusion*, 1mg/kg/hour titrating according to response to maximum of 3mg/kg/hour.
	HYPERTENSION All ages, *orally,* 1-2mg/kg 3 to 4 times a day.
Administration:	For continuous IV infusion, dilute in sodium chloride 0.9% or glucose 5%. Can be given undiluted in fluid restricted patients.
Notes:	

a) In hypertensive encephalopathy, rapid uncontrolled reduction in blood pressure to normotensive level can result in water shed cerebral infarction, blindness or death. Aim to reduce blood pressure to normal over 24-48 hours. If patient is fitting then a rapid initial decrease in blood pressure is required but not to normal levels.

b) No dosage reduction is required in renal impairment and it is not significantly cleared by dialysis.

c) **Caution:** Hepatotoxicity has been reported after both short and long term therapy. Avoid in hepatic impairment.

d) Injection can be given orally with squash or juice.

LACTULOSE

Preparations:	SOLUTION containing lactulose 3.35g in 5ml.
Dosage:	***CONSTIPATION*** *Orally*, initially,

under 1 year	2.5ml twice a day
1 - 5 years	5ml twice a day
5 - 10 years	10ml twice a day
Over 10 years	15ml twice a day

Then adjust dose to individual requirements.

Notes:

a) Lactulose is an osmotic laxative and has a 48 hour onset of action therefore prescribe regularly for at least 2 days.

b) Lactulose solution is sucrose free and 5ml provides approximately 20kJoules (5cals).

c) May be diluted with water or fruit juice.

LAMOTRIGINE

Preparations: DISPERSIBLE TABLETS 5mg, 25mg and 100mg.

Dosage: *EPILEPSY*

This indication is only licensed as adjunctive therapy in children over 2 years and as monotherapy in children over 12 years.

Orally,

	AGE	INITIAL DAILY DOSE (Week 1 +2)	SUBSEQUENT DAILY DOSE (Week 3 + 4)	MAINTENANCE DAILY DOSE (Week 5+)
ADJUNCTIVE WITH SODIUM VALPROATE (± other AED's)	<12 years	0.2mg/kg	0.5mg/kg	Increase by 0.5-1mg/kg every 1-2 weeks to 1-5mg/kg
	≥12 years	12.5mg	25mg	Increase by 25-50mg every 1-2 weeks to 100-200mg
ADJUNCTIVE with enzyme inducing AED's (see note b) Except SODIUM VALPROATE (± other AED's)	<12 years	2mg/kg	5mg/kg	Increase by 2-3mg/kg every 1-2 weeks to 5-15mg/kg
	≥12 years	50mg	100mg	Increase by 100mg every 1-2 weeks to 200-400mg, up to 700mg
MONOTHERAPY	≥12 years	25mg	50mg	Increase by 50-100mg every 1-2 weeks to 100-200mg, up to 500mg

The total daily dose should be given in one or two divided doses when patient is **on** sodium valproate or if monotherapy.

Total daily dose should be given in two divided doses when used as adjunctive therapy and patient is **not on** valproate.

Notes:

a) **Caution:** Severe rashes have been reported in children. Increased risk associated with concomitant valproate, increased initial doses and rapid dose escalation. Discontinue lamotrigine at first sign of a rash unless it is clearly not drug related. Withdrawal should be considered if fever, influenza-like symptoms, drowsiness, worsening of seizure control or other symptoms associated with hypersensitivity develop.

b) Phenytoin, phenobarbitone, primidone and carbamazepine increase the clearance of lamotrigine.

c) Sodium valproate reduces the clearance of lamotrigine.

d) Lamotrigine may raise plasma concentration of an active carbamazepine metabolite carbamazepine epoxide. If side effects occur these usually resolve with a reduction in carbamazepine dose.

e) In patients taking concomitant antiepileptic drugs where the pharmacokinetic interaction is not known, use the dosage regimen for concomitant sodium valproate for initial therapy, thereafter, the dose should be increased until response is optimised.

f) Lamotrigine dispersible tablets (Lamictal®) are blackcurrant flavoured.

LENOGRASTRIM (G-CSF)

Preparations:	INJECTION 105microgram (13.4 million units).
	263 microgram (33.6 million units).
Dosage:	*CYTOTOXIC INDUCED NEUTROPENIA*

> SEEK EXPERT ADVICE BEFORE PRESCRIBING

This indication is unlicensed for use in children under 2 years.
SC injection, 5microgram/kg (19.2 million units/m^2) once a day starting the day after completion of chemotherapy and continuing until neutrophil count is stable in acceptable range.
SEVERE CONGENITAL AND RELATED NEUTROPENIAS
These are unlicensed indications.
SC injection, initially, 5microgram/kg once a day, increase at weekly intervals to 20microgram/kg until neutrophil count stabilised. Reduce to minimum effective maintenance dose.

Administration: SC injection, reconstitute vial with 1ml water for injection. Dilute if required with sodium chloride 0.9% to not less than 2.7microgram (336,000units) in 1ml.

LEUCINE see Metabolic dietitian

LEVAMISOLE

Preparations:	TABLETS 50mg (**Named patient**).
Dosage:	*NEPHROTIC SYNDROME*

> SEEK EXPERT ADVICE BEFORE PRESCRIBING

Orally, 2.5mg/kg 3 times a week or alternate days.

Notes:

Neutropenia, agranulocytosis and vasculitis have been reported, patient/carer should be advised to report any 'flu' like symptoms such as sore throat, fever, chills or rash.

LIGNOCAINE (LIDOCAINE)

Preparations: INJECTION 0.5% in 10ml; 1% in 2ml, 5ml and 10ml; 2% in 5ml.
INFUSION 0.4% in glucose 5% 500ml.
PREFILLED SYRINGES 100mg in 5ml.

Dosage: **VENTRICULAR TACHYCARDIA**
This indication is unlicensed for use in children.
All ages, *IV injection,* initially 500microgram-1mg/kg over 1 minute (0.05-0.1ml/kg of 1%). Repeat at 5 minute intervals to a maximum of 3mg/kg, followed by an, *IV infusion* of 1mg/kg/hour. Maximum rate of infusion 3mg/kg/hour.
STATUS EPILEPTICUS
This is an unlicensed indication.

SEEK EXPERT ADVICE BEFORE PRESCRIBING

IV infusion, 4mg/kg/hour, increasing if necessary to maximum of 10-12mg/kg/hour, see note b). If seizure-free dose is above 4mg/kg/hour, decrease by 1-2mg/kg/hour every 6 to 8 hours until 4mg/kg/hour achieved. Decrements should then not exceed 1mg/kg/hour every 24-48 hours. Increase dose if seizures recur.

Notes:

a)   See page 234 for cardiopulmonary resuscitation guidelines.
b)   Lignocaine infusions can cause respiratory depression, convulsions, hypotension and bradycardia therefore they must be administered with concurrent ECG monitoring and with cardiopulmonary resuscitation facilities available.
c)   Dose should be reduced in liver or renal impairment.

LOPERAMIDE

Preparations: CAPSULES 2mg. LIQUID 2mg in 10ml.
Dosage: **CHRONIC DIARRHOEA**
This indication is unlicensed for use in children.
Orally,

Under 1 year	0.1mg/kg	2 times a day
1 - 2 years	0.25-0.5mg	2-3 times a day
2 - 5 years	1mg	3-4 times a day
6 - 12 years	2mg	3-4 times a day

Doses up to 1.25mg/kg/day may be required.

Over 12 years	2mg	2-4 times a day up to 16mg/**day**

Notes:

a)   Loperamide is **not** recommended for the treatment of acute diarrhoea. First line therapy is prevention of fluid and electrolyte depletion (see page 163).
b)   Do not use if inflammatory bowel disease suspected due to risk of precipitating toxic bowel disease.
c)   Loperamide should be used with caution in the very young because of the risk of respiratory depression.
d)   Loperamide is contraindicated in children with chronic diarrhoea due to overflow as a result of chronic constipation.
e)   Loperamide liquid (Imodium®) is raspberry/redcurrant flavoured, sucrose free and contains a negligible amount of alcohol.

LORAZEPAM

Preparations: TABLETS 1mg. INJECTION 4mg in 1ml.

Dosage: **PREMEDICATION, PRE OPERATIVE ANXIETY, SEDATION WITH AMNESIA**

The use for premedication is unlicensed in children under 5 years and the use for anxiety or sedation is unlicensed for use in children.

Over 1 month, *orally*, 50microgram/kg (to the nearest 500microgram) given the night before and/or at least 1 hour before the procedure.

STATUS EPILEPTICUS

The rectal and the sublingual routes are unlicensed.

IV injection, *rectally*, *sub-lingually* 50microgram/kg. Repeat if necessary. Maximum single dose of 4mg. Maximum of 8mg or 100microgram/kg in 12 hours.

Administration.   IV injection, into large vein over 1-2 minutes, dilute if required with an equal volume of water for injection or sodium chloride 0.9%.

Notes:

a) Hypotension and apnoea may occur with intravenous lorazepam; resuscitation facilities should be available.

b) Should be used with caution in severe liver disease as may induce coma.

c) The injection solution can be given rectally or sublingually.

MAGNESIUM GLYCEROPHOSPHATE

Preparations: TABLETS each containing 95mg (4mmol) of magnesium (**Manufactured special**).
LIQUID (**Extemporaneously prepared**).

Dosage: *MAGNESIUM SUPPLEMENT*
Orally, all ages, according to plasma magnesium levels. If below 0.4mmol/L give 0.2mmol/kg 3 times a day.

Notes:
The tablets can be dispersed in water immediately before administration.

MAGNESIUM SULPHATE

Preparations: INJECTION 50% (500mg in 1ml), 2ml, 10ml, contains 2mmol of magnesium in 1ml.

Dosage: *MAGNESIUM SUPPLEMENT IN DEFICIENCY*
All ages, *slow IV injection,* 100mg/kg (maximum 10ml) as a single dose, repeated every 12 hours as necessary.

CONVULSIONS ASSOCIATED WITH LOW MAGNESIUM LEVELS
This is an unlicensed indication.
All ages, *slow IV injection,* 20-40mg/kg (0.1-0.2ml/kg of a 20% solution) repeated every 4-6 hours if necessary.

SEVERE PERSISTENT PULMONARY HYPERTENSION
This is an unlicensed indication.
Neonates, *IV infusion,* loading dose 200mg/kg over 20-30 minutes, then continuous infusion of 20-50mg/kg/hr. Monitor blood pressure, renal function, electrolytes and blood glucose.

Administration: Dilute to concentration of 10% (100mg in 1ml) with glucose 5% or glucose/saline. If fluid restricted, maximum concentration is 20% (200mg in 1ml).
Rate of administration should not exceed 10mg/kg/minute.
May be part of total parenteral nutrition regimen, see page 279

Notes:
Magnesium glycerophosphate is the oral preparation for magnesium supplementation as it is better absorbed. Oral magnesium sulphate is a purgative.

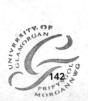

MALATHION

Preparations: AQUEOUS LOTION 0.5% (Derbac-M®).
               ALCOHOLIC LOTION 0.5% (Suleo-M®).

Dosage: ***PEDICULOSIS***
Use only under medical supervision in babies under six months.
Rub liquid gently into dry hair until all hair is thoroughly moistened. Comb and allow to dry naturally, away from heat or sunshine. Leave for 12 hours and remove by washing. Comb hair while still wet. Repeat after 7 days only if live lice are found again. Do not use for more than 3 consecutive weeks.

CRAB LICE IN THE EYE LASHES

UNDER OPHTHALMOLOGY SUPERVISION

This is an unlicensed indication.
Apply **aqueous** lotion to eye lashes and eyebrows using a cotton bud. Allow to dry naturally. Wash face thoroughly after 12 hours. Repeat after 7 days if necessary.

SCABIES
Use only under medical supervision in babies under six months.
Apply **aqueous** lotion to the whole body from the neck downwards. In children under 2 years, the scalp, face and ears, avoiding the eyes and mouth, should be treated as well. Leave for 24 hours. Wash off thoroughly. Can be repeated after 1-2 days.

Notes:

PEDICULOSIS
a) Avoid contact with the eyes. Rarely, skin irritation has been reported.
b) Alcoholic based preparation is preferred since it dries quickly after application. Aqueous preparation should be used in cases of skin sensitivity, abrasions of the scalp, in asthmatic patients and young children.
c) Rotation of preparations is now outmoded. A mosaic pattern of use should be employed, i.e. an alternative preparation used if after repeat administration of the initial preparation there are still live lice.
d) Household contacts should **NOT** routinely be treated, only treat if infestation has occurred. Prophylactic use of an insecticide is not recommended.

SCABIES
a) Refer to guidelines on page 295.
b) If hands are washed with soap and water during treatment period reapply lotion.
c) It is often advisable, to repeat application after 1-2 days, to cover any areas that may have been missed.
d) Only the aqueous solution should be used in the treatment of scabies.
e) Household contacts should be treated for scabies.

MANNITOL

Preparations: INJECTION 10% (1g in 10ml) and 20% (2g in 10ml) 500ml.
Dosage: **CEREBRAL OEDEMA**

IV infusion, all ages, 250-500mg/kg over 30-60 minutes.
May be repeated if required provided the serum osmolality is not greater than 325mOsm/L.

Notes:

The 20% solution is supersaturated, warming will dissolve any crystals that form.

MEASLES, MUMPS AND RUBELLA VACCINE (MMRII®)

Preparations: LIVE, ATTENUATED VACCINE.
Dosage: **VACCINATION**

See immunisation guidelines page 296.
First dose, 12-18 months old, 0.5ml by *deep subcutaneous* or *IM injection*, into outer aspect of arm.
Second dose, not less than 3 months after first dose, usually at the same time as the pre-school DT and polio boosters (i.e. 4-5 years), 0.5ml by *deep subcutaneous* or *IM injection*, into outer aspect of arm.

Administration: Reconstitute each vial with all of the diluent provided.
Notes:

a) The Department of Health can find no established causal link between MMR vaccine and bowel disease or autism and recommend the continued use of MMR vaccine.

b) MMRII® vaccine is a live vaccine and is contra-indicated in immunosuppressed patients (see immunisation guidelines page 296). It is also contraindicated in patients who have received another live vaccine within 3 weeks, immunoglobulin within 3 months or who have an acute febrile illness.

c) MMRII® is also contraindicated in children with allergies to neomycin or kanamycin.

d) There is increasing evidence that MMR vaccine can be given safely to children even when they have had an anaphylactic reaction to food containing egg.

e) Vaccination is not recommended in infants less than 12 months of age as they may fail to respond to the measles component of the vaccine due to presence of maternal antibodies. If vaccination is **absolutely necessary** repeat vaccination after 15 months of age.

MELATONIN

Preparations: CAPSULES 2mg, 5mg and 10mg (**Named patient**).
Dosage: *SLEEP DISTURBANCE*

SEEK EXPERT ADVICE BEFORE PRESCRIBING

Orally, all ages, initially, 2mg 30-60 minutes before bedtime.
Increase dose according to response.
Doses above 10mg are not considered to be of greater efficacy and may increase side effects.

Notes:

Melatonin may have a proconvulsive effect and should be avoided in epilepsy and used with caution in neurologically impaired children.

MEROPENEM

Preparations: INJECTION 250mg, 500mg and 1g.
Dosage: *TREATMENT OF INFECTION*

This indication is unlicensed for use in children under 3 months.
IV injection, all ages, 10-20mg/kg every 8 hours.
Maximum 3g/**day**.
Increase dose up to 40mg/kg every 8 hours in severe infection including meningitis, cystic fibrosis. Maximum 6g/**day**.

IN RENAL FAILURE

Creatinine clearance (ml/minute/1.73m^2)	Dose	Dosage Interval (hours)
25-50	100%	12
10-25	50%	12
<10	50%	24

Haemodialysis: administer the normal dose after dialysis session.
Continuous haemofiltration or haemodiafiltration: administer 50% of dose every 12 hours. In life threatening infections increase interval to every 8 hours.

Administration: On reconstitution 250mg displaces 0.22ml.
Reconstitute with water for injection by adding:
4.78ml   to 250mg vial to give   50mg in 1ml
9.56ml   to 500mg vial to give   50mg in 1ml
19.12ml   to 1g vial to give   50mg in 1ml
IV injection, give over at least 5 minutes, dilute if required with glucose 5% or sodium chloride 0.9% and give immediately.
IV infusion, dilute as above and give over 15-30 minutes.

Notes:

a) Meropenem is a beta-lactam antibiotic. There is partial cross allergenicity between penicillins and cephalosporins. In confirmed allergy an alternative antibiotic should be prescribed. Contact the Microbiology department for further advice.
b) Each 1g of powder contains 3.9mmol of sodium.

MESNA

Preparation:	INJECTIONS 400mg in 4ml and 1g in 10ml.
	TABLETS 400mg and 600mg.
Dosage:	***PREVENTION OF UROTHELIAL TOXICITY BY CYCLOPHOSPHAMIDE***

IV injection, dose of mesna is 40% of the cyclophosphamide dose given at the same time and then repeated 3 times at 3 hourly intervals (i.e. 0, 3, 6, 9 hours)

Total dose is 160% w/w of cyclophosphamide dose.

Orally, dose of mesna is 40% of the cyclosphosphamide dose given 2 hours prior to and repeated 2 and 6 hours after dose. More doses may need to be given and more frequently.

Administration:	IV infusion can be given over 15 minutes, dilute if required with sodium chloride 0.9%.
Notes:	

Injection can be given orally diluted with orange juice or cola.

METHACHOLINE

Preparations:	EYE DROPS 2.5% (**Extemporaneously prepared**).
Dosage:	***TEST FOR FAMILIAL DYSAUTONOMIA***

> **SEEK EXPERT ADVICE BEFORE PRESCRIBING**

Instil drops into conjunctival sac of **ONE** eye.

Notes:

Miosis should occur in the treated eye; this does not occur in unaffected patients.

METHIONINE

Preparations:	TABLETS 250mg.
Dosage:	***PARACETAMOL OVERDOSE***

> **IF IN ANY DOUBT CONTACT THE MEDICAL TOXICOLOGY UNIT ☎ 0171-635-9191 ☎.**

Orally, methionine is highly effective in preventing toxicity and is easier to administer than acetylcysteine. It can be used if the child presents within 8 hours of ingestion, is conscious, not vomiting and has not been given activated charcoal.

Under 6 years,   1g every 4 hours for 4 doses (total of 4g)
6 years and over,   2.5g every 4 hours for 4 doses (total of 10g)

Notes:

a) If the child presents after 8 hours from ingestion of paracetamol or cannot be given an oral preparation give acetylcysteine (page 13). Discuss with the Medical Toxicology Unit.

b) Do not use in patients with metabolic acidosis.

METHOTREXATE

Preparations: TABLETS 2.5mg.

Dosage: ***SEVERE UNCONTROLLED PSORIASIS***

This indication is unlicensed for use in children.

SEEK EXPERT ADVICE BEFORE PRESCRIBING

Orally, initially, 200-400microgram/kg **once a week**.

IN RENAL FAILURE
Reduce dose if creatinine clearance is between 20-50ml/minute/1.73m^2. Seek expert advice. Avoid if creatinine clearance is less than 20ml/minute/1.73m^2.

Notes:

a) **CSM warning:** Monitor liver and renal function and perform a full blood count before starting therapy, weekly whilst stabilising and then every 2-3 months during therapy. Patient/carer should be warned to report the onset of sore throats, mouth ulcers, bruising and other indicators of blood dyscrasias.

b) Aspirin and NSAIDs may reduce excretion of methotrexate and therefore increase toxicity, AVOID concomitant administration.

c) Phenytoin, trimethoprim and co-trimoxazole, and antimalarials increase the antifolate effect of methotrexate. Penicillins, acitretin, probenecid and ciclosporin increase the risk of toxicity.

METHYLCELLULOSE

Preparations: TABLETS 500mg. GEL 200mg in 5ml (**Manufactured special**).

Dosage: ***CONSTIPATION***

This indication is unlicensed for use in children.
Orally, 50mg/kg twice a day
OR

1 - 7 years	10ml or 500mg twice a day
7 - 14 years	20ml or 1g twice a day
Over 14 years	1.5 to 3g twice a day

Notes:

a) Methylcellulose is a bulk forming laxative; the full effect may take some days to develop therefore prescribe regularly.

b) Avoid in intestinal obstruction, faecal impaction and colonic atony.

c) Dose should be taken with copious amounts of water and **NOT** taken at bedtime.

d) Methylcellulose tablets contain lactose.

METHYLPHENIDATE - (CD)

Preparations: TABLETS 10mg.

Dosage: ***ATTENTION DEFICIT HYPERACTIVITY DISORDER***

Orally, over 6 years, 5mg once or twice a day, 30 minutes before breakfast and lunch. Increase by 5-10mg a day every week. Usual maintenance dose 1mg/kg/day. If required, doses may be increased by 5mg a day every 3 days, side effects permitting. Maximum of 60mg/day.

Notes:

a) Patients/carers should be counselled to report any side effects particularly whilst dose is being established.

b) Methylphenidate decreases appetite and lead to reversible growth retardation if weight gain not maintained. Baseline assessment of weight and height should be performed and subsequently monitored 3 monthly.

c) If anorexia is a problem, give dose after breakfast and lunch.

d) A baseline blood pressure should be performed. As methylphenidate may, rarely, cause leucopenia or thrombocytopenia, a baseline full blood count should, also be performed and monitored three monthly.

e) Doses may be given in more divided doses if rebound hyperactivity occurs in the latter part of the day but because methylphenidate may cause insomnia, the last dose should not usually be given later than 4pm.

f) Use with caution in patients with a diagnosis or family history of tics, Tourette's syndrome or epilepsy.

g) Regimen should regularly be reviewed and drug holidays considered if prolonged poor weight gain.

h) Methylphenidate may inhibit the metabolism of tricyclic antidepressants, phenytoin and possibly phenobarbitone and primidone.

METHYLPREDNISOLONE

Preparations: INJECTION 40mg, 500mg, 1g.

Dosage: *GRAFT REJECTION*

IV injection, $600mg/m^2$ body surface area, once a day for 3 days. (Maximum dose 1g/day). Can be given alternate days for 3 doses.

Administration: Reconstitue 40mg vial with 1ml of water for injection to give 40mg in 1ml. Reconstitute 500mg and 1g vials with 7.8ml and 15.6ml, respectively, with water for injection to give 62.5mg in 1ml. Dilute if required with sodium chloride 0.9%, glucose 5% or glucose/saline and give over 20-30 minutes. Do not give more rapidly because of the risk of cardiovascular collapse.

Notes:

a) Severe hypertension may occur after IV injection, especially if dose is given too rapidly.

b) Methylprednisolone is no longer recommended for septic shock.

c) High dose methylprednisolone, as above, increases blood ciclosporin levels.

d) Each 1g of methylprednisolone injection contains 7mmol of sodium.

METOCLOPRAMIDE

Preparations:	TABLETS 10mg. LIQUID 5mg in 5ml. INJECTION 10mg in 2ml.
Dosage:	***NAUSEA AND VOMITING***

The licensed use of metoclopramide in children is for severe intractable vomiting of known cause, vomiting associated with radiotherapy/chemotherapy, as an aid to gastrointestinal intubation and as a premedicant prior to surgery.

Orally, IM or slow IV injection,

Up to 1 year (<10kg)	100microgram/kg	3 times a day
1 - 3 years (10-14kg)	1mg	2-3 times a day
3 - 5 years (15-19kg)	2mg	2-3 times a day
5 - 9 years (20-29kg)	2.5mg	3 times a day
9 - 14 years (>30kg)	5mg	3 times a day
Over 15 years (>30kg)	5-10mg	3 times a day

Total daily dose should not exceed 500microgram/kg.

Administration:	Slow IV injection over 1-2 minutes. Dilute if required with sodium chloride 0.9% or glucose 5%.
Notes:	

a) Extrapyramidal disturbances may be experienced and are more common in the young. They can be treated with an anticholinergic, e.g. procyclidine (see page 181).
b) Injection can be given orally.
c) Metoclopramide liquid (Maxolon®) is lemon/lime flavoured and sucrose free.

METOLAZONE

Preparations:	TABLETS 5mg.
Dosage:	***DIURESIS***

This indication is unlicensed for use in children.

Orally, 0.1-0.2mg/kg once or twice a day. Maximum 80mg/**day**.

Notes:

a) Metolazone has a synergistic effect with frusemide and the combination will sometimes produce diuresis in patients with seriously impaired renal function.
b) Suspension can not be prepared but the tablets may be crushed and mixed with water immediately before use.

METOPROLOL

Preparations:	TABLETS 50mg and 100mg.
	LIQUID (**Extemporaneously prepared**).
Dosage:	***HYPERTENSION***

This indication is unlicensed for use in children.

Orally, initially 1mg/kg twice a day. Increase to maximum of 8mg/kg/**day**. Daily dose can be given in up to 4 divided doses.

METRONIDAZOLE

Preparations: TABLETS 200mg and 400mg. LIQUID 200mg in 5ml.
SUPPOSITORIES 500mg and 1g. INJECTION 500mg in 100ml.

Dosage: TREATMENT OF ANAEROBIC INFECTION, PROPHYLAXIS FOR SURGERY

Orally or IV injection,

AGE	LOADING DOSE	DOSE
Neonates	15mg/kg loading dose followed 24 hours later by	7.5mg/kg every 12 hours
Over 1 month	---	7.5mg/kg every 8 hours

Rectally,

AGE	DOSE	
Less than 1 year	125mg	
1 - 5 years	250mg	three times
5 - 10 years	500mg	a day
Over 10 years	1g	

After 3 days of rectal therapy, change to oral therapy or reduce
frequency to twice a day.

GIARDIASIS
Orally,

AGE	DOSE	
Less than 1 year	40mg/kg	
1 - 3 years	500mg	once a day
3 - 7 years	600-800mg	for
7 - 10 years	1g	3 days
Over 10 years	2g	

IN RENAL FAILURE AND LIVER FAILURE
Metronidazole is rapidly removed by dialysis and therefore dose
should be administered immediately following period of
haemodialysis. No dosing adjustments are necessary for
intermittent peritoneal dialysis or continuous ambulatory
peritoneal dialysis.
Reduce dose in severe liver disease. Avoid in hepatic
encephalopathy. If required, reduce daily dose to 1/3 and give
once a day.

Administration: IV injection over 20 minutes. Dilute if required with sodium
chloride 0.9% or glucose 5%.

Notes:

   a)   Metronidazole is well absorbed orally and rectally. The IV preparation
is very expensive and should only be used where the oral/rectal routes
are not possible or for initiating treatment of serious conditions.

   b)   The effects of oral anticoagulants may be potentiated by concurrent
metronidazole, however heparin is not affected.

   c)   Barbiturates may enhance the metabolism of metronidazole.

   d)   Metronidazole 500mg injections contain 13.6mmol (Flagyl®) and
14.53mmol (Metrolyl®) of sodium.

   e)   Metronidazole liquid (Flagyl®) contains 0.63g of sucrose in 5ml.

MICONAZOLE

Preparations:	ORAL GEL 2% (80g). CREAM 2% (30g) (Lewisham and St Thomas' only).
Dosage:	**ORAL CANDIDIASIS**

Oropharangeally,

Less than 2 years	2.5ml twice a day
2 - 6 years	5ml twice a day
6 - 12 years	5ml four times a day
Over 12 years	5-10ml four times a day

Gel should be retained in mouth for as long as possible before swallowing. Use for at least 2 days after the infection has cleared. For a localised infection the gel can be applied directly to the affected area. Administer after meals or feeds.

DERMATOPHYTE AND CANDIDA SKIN INFECTIONS

Apply cream to the affected area two to three times a day. To prevent relapse, continue for 10 days after lesions have healed.

Notes:

Miconazole oral gel (Daktarin®) is orange flavoured and sucrose free but does contain alcohol.

MIDAZOLAM

Preparations:	INJECTION 10mg in 5ml, 10mg in 2ml.
Dosage:	**SEDATION, PREMEDICATION**

This indication is unlicensed for use in children.
Slow IV injection, all ages, 100-200microgram/kg (see note a).
Orally, all ages, 500microgram/kg.

SEDATION FOR ARTIFICIAL VENTILATION

All ages, *slow IV injection*, 200microgram/kg then an initial *IV infusion,* 30microgram/kg/hour. Dosage should be increased according to response.

INDUCTION OF ANAESTHESIA

Over 7 years, *slow IV injection,* 150microgram/kg. Up to 3 supplementary doses of 50microgram/kg can be given at 2 minute intervals.

STATUS EPILEPTICUS

This is an unlicensed indication.
See note f).

Slow IV injection	all ages	100-200microgram/kg
IV infusion	all ages	30-300microgram/kg/hour
Intranasally	all ages	200microgram/kg, maximum 10mg
Sublingually	all ages	500microgram/kg, maximum 10mg

Administration:	For IV infusion, dilute if required with sodium chloride 0.9% or 5% glucose.

Notes:

a) When used with opiates, potentiation of respiratory or cardiovascular depression may occur. Intravenous midazolam has caused respiratory depression, sometimes with severe hypotension.
b) Erythromycin inhibits the metabolism of midazolam resulting in profound sedation. This effect is also seen with cimetidine, itraconazole, ketoconazole and possibly fluconazole.
c) Flumazenil, page 107, is the specific antidote for midazolam induced respiratory depression.
d) Treatment beyond one to two weeks, especially at large doses, has been associated with an acute benzodiazepine withdrawal syndrome. Infusions should be gradually reduced over several days. Diazepam is treatment of choice for withdrawal symptoms.
e) Injection is painful and may cause thrombophlebitis.
f) Injection solution may be used intranasally, sublingually or orally however it is extremely bitter and may be irritant to mucosa.
g) For oral administration, the injection solution should be diluted, immediately before use, with neat blackcurrant squash.
h) See also sedation guidelines page 247.

MINOXIDIL

Preparations: TABLETS 5mg and 10mg. LIQUID (**Extemporaneously prepared**).
Dosage: ***SEVERE HYPERTENSION***

> **SEEK EXPERT ADVICE BEFORE PRESCRIBING**

Under 12 years, *orally*, initially 200microgram/kg/day in 1-2 divided doses. Increase by 100-200microgram/kg/day every 3 days, to a maximum of 1mg/kg/day.
Over 12 years, *orally*, initially 5mg once a day, increasing by 5mg a day every 3 days. Maximum dose 100mg/day.

Notes:

a) Minoxidil may cause sodium and water retention and tachycardia, therefore it is generally prescribed along with a diuretic and a beta-blocker.
b) Dose should be taken after dialysis where appropriate.
c) Hypertrichosis occurs in most patients. This is generally reversible 1-3 months after treatment is stopped.

MONTELUKAST

Preparations: CHEWABLE TABLETS 5mg. TABLETS 10mg.
Dosage: ***ASTHMA THERAPY IN ASPIRIN SENSITIVE ASTHMA***

> **ON CONSULTANT ADVICE ONLY**

This indication is unlicensed for use in children under 6 years.
Orally, 4 years - 14 years 5mg at night.
Over 14 years 10mg at night.

Notes:

a) **Note:** Montelukast is not for immediate relief of acute asthma attacks and existing corticosteroid therapy should not be withdrawn or reduced.
b) Phenobarbitone, phenytoin and rifampicin may reduce the levels of montelukast.
c) **Caution:** Leukotriene receptor antagonists (montelukast) may be associated with the emergence of Churg-Strauss Syndrome.
d) Montelukast chewable tablets are cherry flavoured and contain aspartame (0.842mg phenylalanine/5mg of montelukast).

MORPHINE SULPHATE - (CD)

Preparations: INJECTION 1mg in 2ml (**Manufactured special**), 10mg in 1ml, 15mg in 1ml, 60mg in 2ml. LIQUID 10mg in 5ml. CONCENTRATED LIQUID 100mg in 5ml. IMMEDIATE RELEASE TABLETS 10mg and 20mg. SLOW RELEASE TABLETS (MST) 10mg, 30mg, 60mg and 100mg. CONTROLLED RELEASED GRANULES 20mg and 30mg (**Restricted use**).

Dosage: ***PREMEDICATION AND ANALGESIA FOR MODERATE TO SEVERE PAIN***
These indications are unlicensed for use in children via the parenteral route.
See notes below.
Orally, over 1 month, 200-500microgram/kg/dose not more frequently than every 4 hours. Maximum of 2.5mg/kg/day.
OR

1 - 5 years	2.5-5mg	every 4 hours
6 - 12 years	5-10mg	every 4 hours
Over 12 years	10-20mg	every 4 hours

Slow or controlled release products are given as the total daily dose in 2 divided doses (see note d). The dose is usually, *orally*, 200-800microgram/kg every 12 hours.
SC infusion, via an indwelling butterfly needle. Over 1 month, loading dose 100-200microgram/kg, then 20microgram/kg/hr. Only suitable for 48-72 hours at any one site.
IV injection, over at least 5 - 10 minutes.

Neonates,	50-100microgram/kg/dose
Over 1 month,	100-200microgram/kg/dose

IV infusion,

Preterm neonates,	loading dose 25-50microgram/kg then 5microgram/kg/hr.
Neonates,	loading dose 50-100microgram/kg then 5-10 microgram/kg/hr.
Over 1 month,	loading dose 100-200microgram/kg then 10-30micrograms/kg/hr.

Under 6 months the initial infusion rate is 10microgram/kg/hour and over 6 months 20microgram/kg/hour. In non-ventilated patients maximum dose is 60microgram/kg/hour. Ventialted patients may need to exceed these doses to achieve adequate sedation and pain management.

IN RENAL FAILURE

Creatinine clearance (ml/minute/1.73m^2)	Dosage adjustment
10-50	75% of dose
< 10	50% of dose

Notes:

a) Neonates and infants under 1 year show an increased susceptibility to respiratory depression however this should not exclude them from adequate analgesia. The above doses reflect the increased sensitivity and decreased metabolism seen in neonates and infants. All non-ventilated patients should be assessed regularly for pain, sedation and respiration.

b) Naloxone, page 156, is the specific antidote for morphine induced respiratory depression.

c) Dosage titration should be made by increasing or decreasing the previous dose by 30-50%.

d) Conversion to MST should only be made after the total daily dose required has been established. The first dose of MST is given prior to discontinuing previous treatment.

e) See section 4.7.2 of Adult Formulary for equivalent opioid doses

f) Liquid contains 1.6g sucrose and 10% v/v alcohol in 5ml. The concentrated liquid is sucrose and alcohol free.

g) See also premedication guidelines page 250 and pain management guidelines page 251.

MULTIVITAMIN DROPS

Preparations: ABIDEC® DROPS: 0.6ml contains vitamin A 4000 units (1.2mg), ergocalciferol 400 units, vitamin C 50mg, thiamine 1mg, riboflavine 400microgram, nicotinamide 5mg, pyridoxine 500microgram.

Dosage: **MULTIVITAMIN SUPPLEMENT**

Orally,
Premature babies, 0.6ml once a day.
Infants, 0.3ml once a day.
Children over 1 year, 0.6ml once a day.

Notes:

a) Abidec drops contain 45mg of sucrose in 0.6ml.

b) In cystic fibrosis doses are doubled.

MUSTINE HYDROCHLORIDE
(CHLORMETHINE HYDROCHLORIDE)

Preparations: INJECTION 10mg.
Dosage: **NEPHROTIC SYNDROME**

SEEK EXPERT ADVICE BEFORE PRESCRIBING

IV injection, 100microgram/**kg** once a day for 4 days.
In overweight or grossly oedematous patients ideal body weight must be used for calculating the dose.
Repeat the course after 4 weeks or when neutrophils >1000.

Administration: Mustine is a cytotoxic drug; therefore it will be reconstituted in the oncology pharmacy department.

☎Guy's ext. 5418, Lewisham ext. 3201, St Thomas' ext. 3851☎

Administer as an injection, over approximately 2 minutes, through the side port of a fast running (approximately 150-200ml/hour) infusion of sodium chloride 0.9% or glucose 5%.

Notes:

a) **CAUTION: MUSTINE IS A VESICANT.** Extravasation during injection and any contact with skin, eyes or mucosa should be avoided.

b) If extravasation occurs stop infusion immediately, aspirate as much fluid as possible and leave needle in situ. Apply an ice pack and contact a member of the Plastics team immediately.

c) If eyes contaminated, flush with copious amounts of water or 1.26% sodium bicarbonate (in polyfusor) for at least 10 minutes. Seek urgent medical advice. If skin contaminated, wash in copious amounts of water, and seek urgent medical advice.

d) Whenever possible, mustine should be prescribed as a weekday course as it is only stable for 6 hours, if refrigerated, after reconstitution.

e) Ensure patient is hydrated before and after mustine dose. If patient is vomiting institute intravenous fluid therapy.

f) Mustine is highly emetogenic (see antiemetic guidelines page 277).

g) Mustine may cause thrombophlebitis especially if concomitant infusion rate is too slow. Superficial thrombophlebitis can be treated with a heparinoid cream e.g. Lasonil®.

MYCOPHENOLATE MOFETIL

Preparations: CAPSULES 250mg.

Dosage: **PREVENTION OF RENAL ALLOGRAFT REJECTION**

This indication is unlicensed for use in children.

SEEK EXPERT ADVICE BEFORE PRESCRIBING

Orally, 600mg/m^2 (maximum 1g) twice a day.

PREVENTION OF LIVER TRANSPLANT REJECTION

This indication is unlicensed for use in children.

SEEK EXPERT ADVICE BEFORE PRESCRIBING

Orally, 10-20mg/kg twice a day.

Notes:

a) Monitor full blood count at least every week during the first month, twice monthly during the second and third months and then monthly through the first year.

b) Mycophenolate absorption is reduced by antacids and anion exchange resins (e.g. cholestyramine).

c) Elevated plasma concentrations of aciclovir and mycophenolate occur with concomitant administration.

d) Prophylaxis against cytomegalovirus infection or reactivation should be considered. Discuss with Medical Virologist on call.

NALOXONE

Preparations:	INJECTION 400microgram in 1ml.
	PRE-FILLED SYRINGE 400microgram in 1ml.
Dosage:	***REVERSAL OF OPIOID INDUCED RESPIRATORY DEPRESSION***

(See notes below).

Neonates: *IV injection,* 10microgram/kg, repeated every 2-3 minutes as necessary. Doses up to 100microgram/kg have been used. In neonates with respiration depressed by maternal opioids, it is generally preferred to give an *IM injection* of 200microgram (60microgram/kg) for a prolonged effect.

Children: *IV injection,* 10microgram/kg. If respiratory improvement is not achieved, a larger dose of 100microgram/kg (maximum 2mg) may be administered. If there is still no response, other causes may be responsible.

Administration:	Dilute if required with sodium chloride 0.9% or glucose 5%.
Notes:	

a) **CAUTION:** The half-life of an opioid may be longer than that of naloxone. A second dose of naloxone may be required to prevent respiratory depression recurring.

b) It should not be used in neonates born to opioid addicted mothers. Check before administering.

c) Naloxone can be given by IM or SC injection, however the IV route is preferred **except** for neonates with respiration depressed by maternal opioids. Given by IM injection, onset of action of naloxone is approximately 3-4 minutes and duration is 18 hours. The onset is approximately 2 minutes if given IV, but duration is only 3-4 hours.

d) Naloxone also reverses analgesic action of opioids. Pain management must be considered when naloxone is used especially if post surgery or trauma.

NAPROXEN

Preparations:	TABLETS 250mg and 500mg. LIQUID 125mg in 5ml.
	SUPPOSITORIES 500mg (**Non-formulary**).
Dosage:	*JUVENILE RHEUMATOID ARTHRITIS, NON-STEROIDAL ANTI-INFLAMMATORY ANALGESIC**

*This indication is unlicensed for use in children. Naproxen is unlicensed for use in children under 5 years.

Orally, 5mg/kg twice a day.

IN RENAL FAILURE

Use with caution, avoiding if creatinine clearance is less than 20ml/minute/1.73m^2, unless dialysis patient.

Notes:	

a) Naproxen is contraindicated in patients with a history of hypersensitivity (including asthma, angioedema, urticaria or rhinitis) to aspirin or any other non-steroidal anti-inflammatory drug or with a coagulation defect.

b) Caution, use in renal, cardiac or hepatic failure may cause a deterioration in renal function; the dose should be kept as low as possible and renal function monitored.

c) Naproxen liquid (Naprosyn®) is pineapple/orange flavoured and contains 1.3g of sucrose and 1.7mmol of sodium in 5ml.

d) See recommended analgesics page 255.

NASEPTIN

Preparations:	CREAM containing chlorhexidine hydrochloride 0.1% and neomycin sulphate 0.5%.
Dosage:	***ERADICATION OF NASAL STAPHYLOCOCCI***
	Apply to inside of each nostril 4 times a day for 10 days.
	PROPHYLAXIS
	Apply to the insides of the nostrils twice a day.
Notes:	

a) Prolonged use of neomycin can lead to skin sensitisation, ototoxicity and nephrotoxicity.
b) **Note:** Naseptin® cream contains arachis (peanut) oil and should not be administered in patients who have known or suspected hypersensitivity reactions to peanuts.

NEOSTIGMINE

Preparations:	TABLETS 15mg. INJECTION 2.5mg in 1ml.
	LIQUID **(Extemporaneously prepared)**.
Dosage:	***MYASTHENIA GRAVIS***

Neonates
Orally, initially, 1-2mg followed by 1-5mg every 4 hours.
IM injection, initially, 100microgram followed by 50-250microgram *IV, IM or SC injection* every 4 hours (see note a). Neostigmine should be given at least 30 minutes before feed is due.

Over 1 month
Orally, initially,
Under 6 years   7.5mg then at suitable intervals during the day.
6 - 12 years   15mg then at suitable intervals during the day.
Adjust according to response, range usually 15-90mg per day.
Neostigmine usually produces a therapeutic effect for 4 hours.
Maximum dose is 300mg/**day** although most patients can only tolerate a dose of 180mg/**day**.
IV, IM or SC injection, 200-500microgram as required.

REVERSAL OF NON-DEPOLARISING MUSCLE RELAXANTS
Slow IV injection 50-70microgram/kg in combination with a slow IV injection of atropine 10microgram/kg over 1 minute.

Administration:	Oral neostigmine should be administered at least 30 minutes before food.
Notes:	

a) 1microgram IV is equivalent to 2-3microgram given by IM or SC injection or to 30microgram orally.
b) When used in a conscious child e.g. in myasthenia gravis, neostigmine may cause severe gastro-intestinal pain. Simultaneous administration of atropine may prevent the muscarinic side effects.
c) In neonates with myasthenia gravis, treatment beyond 8 weeks is only required in the rare condition of congenital and familial infantile myasthenia.

NIFEDIPINE

Preparations:	CAPSULES 10mg. MODIFIED RELEASE (MR) TABLETS (Adalat Retard®) 10mg and 20mg. SLOW RELEASE TABLETS (Adalat LA®) 30mg and 60mg. LIQUID 2% (20mg in 1ml) (**Named patient**).
Dosage:	These indications are unlicensed for use in children.

HYPERTENSIVE CRISIS

All ages, *orally*, 250-500microgram/kg (see note a).

HYPERTENSION

All ages, *orally*, 200-300microgram/kg 3 times a day **or** 5-10mg 3 times a day. Maximum 3mg/kg/day.
Modified release tablets, 10-20mg twice a day (see note b).
Slow release tablets, once a day.

Notes:

a) **For rapid effect**, bite the capsule releasing the contents into the mouth and then **swallow**. If less than 10mg is needed, syringe out the liquid contents of a capsule.
10mg Bayer capsules contain 10mg nifedipine in 0.34ml
10mg Norton capsules contain 10mg nifedipine in 0.45ml
Nifedipine is **very** light sensitive. Cover required dose of liquid from capsules in foil and administer immediately. Capsule contents may also be diluted with water to aid administration. Use immediately. Discard any remainder.

b) Tablets may be crushed to aid administration; however this alters the modified release characteristic of the tablet and so dose should be administered three times a day. Crushed tablets should also be administered within 30-60 seconds of crushing to avoid significant loss in potency of drug.

c) Nifedipine should be prescribed by generic name, strength, form and trade name to ensure continuity of the same preparation for the patient as NOT ALL PRODUCTS ARE BIOEQUIVALENT.

NIMODIPINE

Preparations:	INJECTION 10mg in 50ml. TABLETS 30mg.
Dosage:	These indications are unlicensed for use in children.

> **SEEK EXPERT ADVICE FROM NEUROLOGIST OR**
> **NEUROSURGEON BEFORE PRESCRIBING**

TREATMENT OF VASOSPASM FOLLOWING SUBARACHNOID HAEMORRHAGE
IV infusion, 15microgram/kg/hr increasing after 2 hours to 30microgram/kg/hr provided no severe decrease in blood pressure is observed. If blood pressure is unstable starting dose is 7.5microgram/kg/hr.
Treatment should start as soon as possible and continue for at least 5 days to a maximum of 14 days.

PREVENTION OF VASOSPASM FOLLOWING SUBARACHNOID HAEMORRHAGE
Orally, 0.9-1.2mg/kg every 4 hours
OR

1 - 4 years	15mg	every 4 hours
5 - 11 years	30mg	every 4 hours
12 - 16 years	45mg	every 4 hours
Over 16 years	60mg	every 4 hours

Administration:	Infuse neat via a central catheter. Nimodipine reacts with polyvinyl chloride (**PVC**) and should be avoided. **Use** polyethylene or polypropylene plastic infusion materials.
Notes:	

a) Tablets may be crushed or halved but are light sensitive therefore administer immediately and discard any remaining drug.
b) Infusion solution contains 20% ethanol and 17% polyethylene glycol-400.

NITRAZEPAM

Preparations:	TABLETS 5mg. LIQUID 2.5mg in 5ml (**Non-formulary**).
Dosage:	*EPILEPSY*
	This is an unlicensed indication.
	Orally, initially,

Up to 1 year	250-500microgram/kg	twice a day
1 - 4 years	2.5mg	twice a day
5 - 12 years	2.5-5mg	twice a day

Notes:

Nitrazepam liquid (Somnite®) is cherry flavoured and contains 2g of sucrose in 5ml.

NITROFURANTOIN

Preparations: CAPSULES (Macrodantin) 50mg and 100mg.
LIQUID 25mg in 5ml (**Named patient**).

Dosage: ***URINARY TRACT INFECTION***
Orally, over 3 months, 3mg/kg/day in 4 divided doses.
In severe infections the above dose can be doubled.

PROPHYLAXIS
Orally, over 3 months, 1mg/kg at night.

IN RENAL FAILURE
Use the above doses with caution. Nitrofurantoin should not be used if creatinine clearance is less than 60ml/minute/1.73m^2.

Notes:

a) Nitrofurantoin is not usually used in infants less than 3 months due to the theoretical risk of haemolytic anaemia.
b) Acute, subacute and chronic pulmonary reactions and peripheral neuropathy have been observed. If these occur treatment should be stopped immediately.
c) Nitrofurantoin may cause haemolysis in patients with glucose-6-phosphate dehydrogenase (G-6-PD) deficiency.
d) Nitrofurantoin and the quinolones are mutually antagonistic in vitro.

NORADRENALINE (NOREPINEPHRINE)

Preparations: INJECTION noradrenaline acid tartrate 8mg in 4ml (equivalent to noradrenaline base 4mg in 4ml).
INJECTION noradrenaline acid tartrate 400microgram in 2ml (equivalent to noradrenaline base 200microgram in 2ml) (**Manufactured special, Non-formulary**).

Dosage: ***VASOPRESSOR***
This indication is unlicensed for use in children.
IV infusion, 20-100nanogram/kg/minute
(0.02-0.1microgram/kg/minute) of noradrenaline **base**. Increase to a maximum of 1microgram/kg/minute of noradrenaline base.

Administration: IV infusion, dilute in glucose 5% or glucose/saline and administer, preferably, via a central line.

Notes:

a) Noradrenaline base 1mg is equivalent to noradrenaline acid tartrate 2mg.
b) Local extravasation into tissue may cause necrosis.
c) Noradrenaline is incompatible with sodium bicarbonate and alkaline solutions.

NORFLOXACIN

Preparations: TABLETS 400mg.
Dosage: *URINARY TRACT INFECTIONS*

> SEEK SPECIALIST ADVICE BEFORE PRESCRIBING

This indication is unlicensed for use in children and growing adolescents.
Orally, 5 years and over, 6mg/kg twice a day for 7-10 days (3 days in uncomplicated lower urinary tract infections).
IN RENAL FAILURE
If creatinine clearance is less than 30ml/minute/1.73m^2 reduce to once a day dose.

Notes:

a) **CSM Warning:** At the first sign of pain or inflammation, patients should discontinue treatment and rest the affected limb until tendon symptoms have resolved.
b) Theophylline levels, the anticoagulant effect of warfarin and the nephrotoxic effect and plasma levels of ciclosporin may be increased by norfloxacin.
c) Sucralfate, antacids and iron should not be administered concomitantly with norfloxacin.
d) Tablets may be crushed or halved but are light sensitive therefore administer immediately and discard any remaining drug.

NTBC(2-[2-nitro-4-trifluoro-methylbenzoyl]-1,3,-cyclohexanedione)

Preparations: CAPSULES 2mg, 5mg and 10mg (**Named patient**).
Dosage: *TREATMENT OF TYROSINAEMIA TYPE 1*

> SEEK EXPERT ADVICE FROM METABOLIC TEAM BEFORE PRESCRIBING

Orally, all ages, initially 1mg/kg/day in 1 to 2 divided doses.

Notes:

a) Aim to maintain plasma tyrosine levels below 600micromol/L.
b) NTBC treatment has been associated with some ophthalmological and haematological problems. All adverse effects must be reported as part of the protocol.

NYSTATIN

Preparations: LIQUID 100,000 units in 1ml. PASTILLES 100,000 units.
CREAM AND OINTMENT 100,000 units/g.
Dosage: *OROPHARYNGEAL CANDIDA*

Oropharangeally, 1ml of liquid dropped into the mouth and retained for one minute before swallowing, or 1 pastille dissolved in the mouth, 4 times a day, after meals or feeds.
PROPHYLAXIS IN THE NEWBORN
1ml of liquid once a day, after a feed.
TOPICAL CANDIDA
Apply cream or ointment 2-4 times a day. Continue for 7 days after lesions have healed.

Notes:

a) Nystatin liquid (Rosemont) is sugar free.
b) All children on peritoneal dialysis prescribed systemic broad spectrum antibiotics should receive concomitant nystatin.

OCTREOTIDE

Preparations: INJECTION 50microgram in 1ml and 500microgram in 1ml.
Dosage: *BLEEDING GASTRO-OESOPHAGEAL VARICES*

This is an unlicensed indication.
IV infusion, all ages, loading dose, 1microgram/kg then 1microgram/kg/hour for 2-5 days.
OR
IV infusion, all ages, 25microgram/hour for 2-5 days.

Administration: IV infusion, dilute to 500microgram in 40ml with sodium chloride 0.9% (25microgram/hour equals 2ml/hour).

Notes:

Octreotide should be withdrawn slowly to prevent rebleeding. Halve rate every 6 to 12 hours.

OMEPRAZOLE

Preparations: CAPSULES 10mg, 20mg. 40mg (**Non-formulary**).
Dosage: *SEVERE REFLUX OESOPHAGITIS*

This indication is unlicensed for use in children under 2 years.
Orally, initially, 0.7-1.4mg/kg once a day, up to 40mg/**day**. Doses should preferably be rounded to the nearest capsule size. Maximum dose 3mg/kg/**day** (120mg/**day**).
HELICOBACTER PYLORI ERADICATION

This indication is unlicensed for use in children.
The above doses should be used for 7 days in conjunction with standard treatment doses of amoxicillin see page 25 and metronidazole see page 150 also for 7 days.

Administration: Enteric coated granules may be emptied out of capsule and mixed with fruit juice or yoghurt. The granules must **not** be chewed as omperazole degrades rapidly in an acidic environment. If the granules cannot be administered e.g. unable to pass down nasogastric tube, then a suspension can be made. Make suspension by emptying granules from the capsule into 10ml of 8.4% sodium bicarbonate. Stand for approximately 10 minutes until solution becomes turbid. A small amount of carbon dioxide may be produced. Administer the suspension immediately.

Notes:

a) Omeprazole should only be used in the treatment of severe oesophagitis refractory to H_2 receptor antagonists. It is not recommended as first line therapy.
b) Omeprazole may increase levels of phenytoin, digoxin, diazepam and tacrolimus and increase the anticoagulant effect of warfarin.

ORAL CONTRACEPTIVES - see Adult Formulary section 7.3

ORAL REHYDRATION SOLUTION

Preparations:	DIORALYTE®; CITRUS, BLACKCURRANT OR UNFLAVOURED SACHETS containing sodium chloride 470mg, potassium chloride 300mg, disodium hydrogen citrate 530mg, glucose 3.56g per sachet. On reconstitution with 200ml of water (sterile or freshly boiled and cooled), solution contains Na 60mmol/L, K 20mmol/L, Cl 60mmol/L, citrate 10mmol/L and glucose 90mmol/L. Total osmolality is 240mmol/L.
Dosage:	***ORAL REHYDRATION***

Infants, 150ml/kg/day, **OR** 1-1.5 times the usual feed volume. Children and adults, 20-40ml/kg/day, **OR** 1 sachet after each loose motion.

Once rehydrated, reintroduce the normal diet. Breast feeding can continue to be offered between oral rehydration drinks.

Notes:

a) Treat mild to moderate diarrhoea with oral rehydration solutions, however if severe, intravenous therapy is indicated. Anti-diarrhoeals (e.g. codeine phosphate and loperamide) and antibiotics are not generally indicated as infections are usually viral and will resolve quickly.

b) The W.H.O. formulated oral rehydration salts (manufactured special) should be used for high output ileostomy losses and short bowel syndromes as it contains 90mmol/L of sodium.

c) Following reconstitution, Dioralyte® can be stored for up to 24 hours in a fridge.

d) Unflavoured Dioralyte® should only be added to feeds at the recommendation of the dietitian.

OXYBUTYNIN HYDROCHLORIDE

Preparations:	TABLETS 2.5mg and 5mg. LIQUID 2.5mg in 5ml.
Dosage:	***NEUROGENIC BLADDER DISORDERS, BLADDER SPASM, DAYTIME WETTING***

These indications are unlicensed for use in children under 5 years. The use in bladder spasm is unlicensed for use in children.

) *Orally,*

Under 5 years	initially 0.1mg/kg/**day**. Increase if necessary as tolerated.
5 - 12 years	2.5-5mg twice a **day**. Maximum 5mg 3 times a day.
Over 12 years	2.5-5mg 2-3 times a **day**. Maximum dose is 5mg 4 times a day.

Notes:

a) Ensure patient is able to empty bladder particularly if large doses prescribed.

b) The side effects of oxybutynin are mostly anticholinergic and include dry mouth, blurred vision, constipation and facial flushing.

c) Oxybutynin elixir (Ditropan®) contains 1.3g of sucrose in 5ml.

PANCREATIN PREPARATIONS

Preparations:

Preparations	Protease (units)	Lipase (units)	Amylase (units)
PANCREASE CAPSULES ❶ (enteric coated beads)	330	5,000	2,900
CREON 10000 CAPSULES (enteric coated beads)	600	10,000	8,000
CREON 25000 CAPSULES ❷ (enteric coated beads)	1000	25,000	18,000
NUTRIZYM GR CAPSULES (enteric coated beads) **(Non-formulary)**	650	10,000	10,000

❶ **Note** contents of Pancrease capsules are expressed in USP units on the container from the manufacturer. In the above table the contents are expressed as PhEur units.

❷ See note a).

Dosage:

PANCREASE, CREON, NUTRIZYM GR CAPSULES
Dose varies considerably according to the child's needs but initial doses are:
Orally,
Neonates, 1/4 capsule with feeds increasing in 1/4 capsule increments to 1 capsule.
Children, 1 capsule with snacks and 1-2 before each meal. The beads must not be chewed, but can be emptied out of the capsule and mixed with a small amount of liquid or soft food e.g. jam or apple juice. Do not add to hot food.
Increase slowly according to response. The total dose of pancreatin should not exceed 10,000 units of lipase/kg/day (see note a).
Development of new abdominal symptoms (or any change in existing abdominal symptoms) should be reviewed to exclude the possibility of colonic damage.

Notes:

a) Due to reported fibrotic strictures in the large bowel of cystic fibrosis children, aged between 3-13 years, the use of these high dose products should be avoided unless the benefits outweigh the risks.

b) Contact of the beads in the capsules with food of pH greater than 5.5 can dissolve the protective coat.

c) The use of a barrier cream (e.g. Metanium) will help prevent excoriation in neonates and infants.

d) High concentrations of pancreatin may burn the buccal mucosa and skin round the mouth and anus. If this occurs the dose should be reduced.

PANCURONIUM

Preparations:	INJECTION 4mg in 2ml.
Dosage:	*NEUROMUSCULAR BLOCKADE FOR VENTILATION AND SURGICAL PROCEDURES*

NEUROMUSCULAR CONDUCTION, USING A NERVE STIMULATOR, SHOULD BE MONITORED IN ALL PATIENTS IN WHOM REPEATED DOSES OR INFUSIONS ARE ADMINISTERED.

IV injection,
Neonates, initially, 30-40microgram/kg then 10-20microgram/kg.
Children, initially, 60-100microgram/kg then 10-20microgram/kg.
RENAL AND LIVER FAILURE
Use with caution in severe renal impairment or liver failure as duration is prolonged.

Administration: Dilute if required with sodium chloride 0.9% or glucose 5%.

Notes:

a) Pancuronium is only used in patients with assisted ventilation.
b) Dose is reduced in neonates as they have an increased sensitivity to non-depolarising muscle relaxants.
c) Although pancuronium lacks a histamine releasing effect, vagolytic and sympathomimetic effects can cause hypertension and tachycardia.

PARACETAMOL

Preparations: TABLETS 500mg. SOLUBLE TABLETS 500mg.
LIQUIDS 120mg in 5ml and 250mg in 5ml (Calpol® sugar free).
SUPPOSITORIES 60mg, 125mg and 500mg (**Manufactured special**).

Dosage: *ANTIPYRETIC AND ANALGESIA FOR MILD TO MODERATE PAIN.*

These indications are licensed in children over 3 months of age.
Over 2 months of age, licensed for post immunisation pyrexia.
Orally,
Under 3 months   10-15mg/kg   (5mg/kg if jaundiced)
Repeat dose every 4-6 hours as necessary.

MAXIMUM 60MG/KG IN 24 HOURS	
3 - 12 months	60-120mg
1 - 5 years	120-240mg
6 - 12 years	250-500mg

Repeat dose every 4-6 hours as necessary.

MAXIMUM 80MG/KG IN 24 HOURS

Rectally,
Under 3 months   30-60mg
Repeat dose every 4-6 hours as necessary.

MAXIMUM 60MG/KG IN 24 HOURS	
3 - 12 months	60-125mg
1 - 5 years	125-250mg
6 - 12 years	250-500mg

Repeat dose every 4-6 hours as necessary.

MAXIMUM 80MG/KG IN 24 HOURS

Notes:

a) Paracetamol is the drug of choice for mild analgesia in children under 12 years, as aspirin is contraindicated in this age group.
b) Soluble tablets contain 18.5mmol of sodium per 500mg.

PARALDEHYDE

Preparations: INJECTION 5ml.
Dosage: **STATUS EPILEPTICUS**

Rectally, 0.3ml/kg diluted with an equal volume of olive oil or 1 in 10 with sodium chloride 0.9% and given as a rectal enema.

OR

up to 3 months	0.5ml
3 - 6 months	1ml
6 - 12 months	1.5ml
1 - 2 years	2ml
3 - 5 years	3-4ml
6 - 12 years	5-6ml
over 12 years	5-10ml

Notes:

a)   Plastic syringes can be used if the dose is administered immediately, otherwise use a glass syringe.

b)   Do not use if it has a brownish colour or smells of acetic acid.

PENICILLAMINE

Preparations: TABLETS 125mg and 250mg.
Dosage: **CYSTINURIA**

Orally, all ages, 10mg/kg twice a day up to 30mg/kg/**day**. Adjust dose to maintain urinary cystine below 200mg/L.

WILSON'S DISEASE

Orally, all ages, initially 5mg/kg 1-2 times a day increasing at 2 week intervals, if tolerated, up to 10mg/kg twice a day.

JUVENILE RHEUMATOID ARTHRITIS

Orally, initially 2.5-5mg/kg once a day for 1 month, then increase at 4 week intervals to 15-20mg/kg/day.

Notes:

a)   Pyridoxine 10mg a day may be given concurrently in Wilson's Disease.

b)   Thrombocytopenia occurs commonly, neutropenia less often. A full blood count must be performed every week for the first 2 months of treatment, or after any dosage increase, and monthly thereafter. If platelet count is less than 120,000/mm^3 or WBC below 2500/mm^3 or if three successive falls are noted within normal range then stop drug, restarting at lower doses when recovery occurs. If thrombocytopenia or neutropenia recurs treatment should be withdrawn permanently.

c)   Counsel patients or their carers to report any fever, sore throat, mouth ulcers, bruising or any other symptoms of blood or skin disorders.

d)   Persistent heavy proteinuria should lead to withdrawal of the drug, however transient proteinuria is not an indication to stop the drug. Test urine every week for 2 months and then monthly.

PEPPERMINT WATER

| *Preparations:* | PEPPERMINT WATER STH. |
| | ALCOHOL FREE PEPPERMINT WATER (**Extemporaneously prepared**). |

Dosage: INFANT COLIC

3 - 6 months	2.5ml	20 minutes before feeds
6 months - 2 years	5ml	20 minutes before feeds
Over 2 years	10-40ml	before food

Maximum 4 doses in 24 hours for all age groups.

Notes:

a) Peppermint water STH contains chloroform and 6.25% w/v of alcohol and is not suitable for infants under 3 months.

b) Peppermint water STH contains 2.5% of concentrated peppermint water BP1973.

PERMETHRIN

Preparation: CREAM RINSE 1% w/w and DERMAL CREAM 5% (**Purchased on request**).

Dosage: PEDICULOSIS (HEAD LICE)

Use only under medical supervision in children under 6 months.

Apply **cream rinse 1%** to clean damp hair i.e. shampoo, rinse and towel dry hair. The scalp and hair should be saturated with the cream rinse. Leave for 10 minutes, then rinse and dry hair. **Repeat** after 7 days only if live lice are found again.

SCABIES

This indication is unlicensed for use in children under 2 months and should only be used under medical supervision in children under 2 years.

Apply **dermal cream 5%**

2 months to 1 year	up to 1/8 tube (3.8g)
1 - 5 years	up to 1/4 tube (7.5g)
5 - 12 years	up to 1/2 tube (15g)
Over 12 years	up to 1 tube (30g)

Apply over whole body including face, neck scalp and ears. Avoid immediate vicinity of the mouth and eyes.

The cream should be rubbed gently into the skin. Wash off after 8-24 hours. Repeat after 1-2 days if necessary.

Notes:

PEDICULOSIS

a) Rotation of preparations is now outmoded. A mosaic pattern of use should be employed, i.e. an alternative preparation used if after repeat application there are still live lice.

b) Household contacts should **NOT** routinely be treated, only treat if infestation has occurred. Prophylactic use of an insecticide is not recommended.

c) Cream rinse contains 20% isopropyl alcohol. Avoid contact with eyes.

SCABIES

a) Refer to guidelines page 295.

b) If hands are washed with soap and water during the treatment period reapply dermal cream.

c) It is often advisable, to repeat application after 1-2 days, to cover any areas that may have been missed.

PETHIDINE - (CD)

Preparations:	INJECTIONS 50mg in 1ml and 100mg in 2ml. TABLETS 50mg.
Dosage:	***ANALGESIA FOR MODERATE TO SEVERE PAIN***

Orally, SC or IV injection:

Neonates   500microgram - 1mg/kg/dose.

Over 1 month   500microgram - 2mg/kg/dose, usual dose is 1mg/kg.

Doses may be repeated every 4-6 hours.

IV infusion:

See note a)

Over 1 month, 1mg/kg loading dose then, initially 100-400microgram/kg/hr adjusting according to response. Ventilated patients may require higher doses.

Administration:	IV infusion, dilute with sodium chloride 0.9% or glucose 5%. IV injection, dilute with water for injection and give over 2-5 minutes.

Notes:

a) Neonates and infants under 1 year show an increased susceptibility to respiratory depression, however this should not exclude them from adequate analgesia. Non-ventilated patients should be assessed regularly for pain, sedation and respiration.

b) Avoid in patients with renal impairment as accumulation of metabolite, norpethidine, may induce seizures. Accumulation of this metabolite may also occur in sickle cell crisis and prolonged infusions.

c) Pethidine has antispasmodic properties.

d) Injection can be given orally.

e) See pain management guidelines page 251.

PHENOBARBITONE (PHENOBARBITAL)

Preparations:	TABLETS 15mg, 30mg and 60mg.
	INJECTION 60mg (sodium salt) in 1ml.
	LIQUID 15mg (base) in 5ml (**Extemporaneously prepared**).
Dosage:	*EPILEPSY*

SEEK EXPERT ADVICE BEFORE PRESCRIBING

Loading dose, *slow IV injection,*

Neonates, 20mg/kg

Infants and children, 15mg/kg

Maintenance dose, *slow IV injection or orally,*

All ages, 5mg/kg/**day** in 1-2 divided doses (see note d).

Increase by 2mg/kg/**day** as necessary. Maximum dose 10mg/kg/**day**.

IMPROVEMENT IN BILE FLOW

Orally, all ages, 5mg/kg/**day**, for 5 days prior to scintography scan and continued depending upon result.

In biliary atresia, all ages, 45mg once a day.

Administration:	Slow IV injection, dilute to 6mg in 1ml with water for injection and give at a maximum rate of 1mg/kg/minute.

Notes:

a) Therapeutic drug monitoring:
   i) Approx. time to steady state: 10-14 days. (Prolonged in neonates).
   ii) Therapeutic plasma levels: Epilepsy, 9-25mg/L.
   Febrile convulsions, 15-25mg/L.
   Some patients may tolerate levels up to 40mg/L.
   iii) Take trough sample, immediately prior to next dose.

b) Phenobarbitone reduces blood levels of carbamazepine, clonazepam, lamotrigine and sodium valproate and may reduce ethosuximide levels. The effect of phenobarbitone on phenytoin levels is unpredictable therefore blood levels should be checked if this drug combination is initiated. Reduced blood levels and/or increased elimination of chloramphenicol, theophylline, ciclosporin and warfarin also occur if phenobarbitone is given concomitantly.

c) Phenobarbitone liquid B.P. is sucrose free but contains 38% alcohol, and is very bitter. This preparation is not stocked and is **not** recommended for use in children. Phenobarbitone liquid contains phenobarbitone sodium and only 1.9% alcohol.
Injection contains 90% propylene glycol.

PHENOTHRIN

Preparation: LOTION 0.2% w/v in alcoholic base (**Purchased on request**).
Dosage: PEDICULOSIS (HEAD LICE):

Use only under medical supervision in children under 6 months.
Apply and rub gently into dry hair until entire scalp is moistened. Comb hair whilst still wet and then allow hair to dry naturally. DO NOT use heat to dry hair. Hair may be shampooed 2 hours after application.
Repeat after 7 days only if live lice are found again.

Notes:

a) Rotation of preparations is now outmoded. A mosaic pattern of use should be employed, i.e. an alternative preparation used if after repeat application there are still live lice.

b) Household contacts should **NOT** routinely be treated, only treat if infestation has occurred. Prophylactic use of an insecticide is not recommended.

c) Lotion contains 69.3% isopropyl alcohol. Avoid contact with eyes.

PHENOXYBENZAMINE HYDROCHLORIDE

Preparations: INJECTION 100mg in 2ml (**Hospital only**).
CAPSULES 5mg (**Named patient**) and 10mg.

Dosage:

SEEK EXPERT ADVICE BEFORE PRESCRIBING

PHAEOCHROMOCYTOMA
This indication is unlicensed for use in children.
Orally, 1-2mg/kg once a day.
IV infusion, 0.5-2mg/kg/day, titrating the dose according to response. Concomitant beta-adrenergic blockade may be required to prevent tachycardia and arrhythmias.

CARDIAC SURGERY
This is an unlicensed indication.
IV infusion, 1mg/kg, just prior to the institution of cardiopulmonary bypass.

POST CARDIAC SURGERY
This is an unlicensed indication.
IV infusion, initially 1mg/kg, then 0.5mg/kg every 8 to 12 hours.

Administration: IV infusion, dilute in sodium chloride 0.9% immediately before use and give over at least 2 hours or by continuous infusion.

Notes:

a) Continuous intra-arterial blood pressure monitoring is recommended during an IV infusion. If severe hypotension occurs and is not correctable with intravenous fluids then a noradrenaline infusion may be required.

b) Phenoxybenzamine is no longer recommended for urinary conditions as it has been shown to have carcinogenic effects in rats. For phaeochromocytoma it should only be used in children for whom alternative treatment is inappropriate.

c) The oral route is rarely used.

d) Avoid contact with skin/hands as risk of contact sensitisation. Phenoxybenzamine is also irritant to tissues, avoid extravasation.

PHENOXYMETHYLPENICILLIN (PENICILLIN V)

Preparations:	TABLETS 250mg. LIQUIDS 125mg in 5ml and 250mg in 5ml.
Dosage:	*TREATMENT OF INFECTION*

All ages, 6-12.5mg/kg 4 times a day,
OR

Up to 1 year	62.5mg	)
1 - 5 years	125mg	) 4 times a day
6 - 12 years	250mg	)
Over 12 years	500mg	)

PROPHYLAXIS

Up to 1 year	62.5mg	)
1 - 5 years	125mg	) twice a day
6 - 12 years	250mg	)
Over 12 years	500mg	)

Notes:

Penicillin V liquids (Kent) contain approximately 3g of sucrose in 5ml.

PHENTOLAMINE MESYLATE (PHENTOLAMINE MESILATE)

Preparations:	INJECTION 10mg in 1ml.
Dosage:	*PAROXYSMAL HYPERTENSION*

This indication is unlicensed.

IV infusion, 20-100microgram/kg loading dose then 5 to 50microgram/kg/min.

Administration:	IV infusion dilute in 5% glucose, sodium chloride 0.9% or glucose/saline.
Notes:	

a) Phentolamine should only be administered by an anaesthetist or in an intensive care unit.

b) Presence of sulphites in ampoule may lead to hypersensitivity with bronchospasm and shock, especially in asthmatic patients.

PHENYTOIN

Preparations:
CHEWABLE TABLETS (Infatabs®) 50mg.
LIQUID 30mg in 5ml and 90mg in 5ml (**Manufactured special**).
CAPSULES **phenytoin sodium** 25mg, 50mg, 100mg.
INJECTION 250mg **phenytoin sodium** in 5ml.

NOTE: PHENYTOIN 90MG IS EQUIVALENT TO PHENYTOIN SODIUM 100MG.
THEREFORE 45MG, 7.5ML OR 2.5ML RESPECTIVELY OF ABOVE SUSPENSIONS IS
EQUIVALENT TO A 50MG CAPSULE.

Dosage:
STATUS EPILEPTICUS
See note a).
Neonates (preterm and term), *slow IV injection*, 20mg/kg given over 20 minutes.
Infants and children, *slow IV injection*, 15mg/kg given over 20 minutes, followed by a further 10mg/kg given over 20 minutes if necessary.
A second dose may be necessary, after reviewing blood levels at 12 to 24 hours post dose, before initiating maintenance doses.

EPILEPSY
See note a).
Loading dose, *slow IV injection,*
Neonates, 20mg/kg
Infants and children, 15mg/kg
Maintenance dose, *slow IV injection* or *orally*, (see note d).
Neonates, 2-4mg/kg twice a day.
Metabolism increases over first 5-7 weeks then stabilises, dosage increases will be required over this time. Monitor levels regularly.
Infants and children, 2.5-7.5mg/kg twice a day
Usual maintenance dose is 5mg/kg twice a day. Measure blood levels after 2 weeks and adjust the dose accordingly. Dosage increments should not exceed 1mg/kg/day. For difficult to control fits, higher doses are often required, check blood levels regularly.

Administration:
Slow IV injection, at a maximum rate of 1mg/kg/minute. The ready-mixed injection solution (Epanutin®) does not need to be diluted. Dilute if required with sodium chloride 0.9% only to not more than 10mg in 1ml. Flush with sodium chloride 0.9% only after administration. Only give IV with concurrent ECG monitoring. Monitor B.P.

Notes:

a) Oral administration is not effective for loading the patient with phenytoin if they are in status or fitting.

b) Do not give by IM injection. If essential, IM dose should be 50% greater than established oral dose.

c) Administration of intravenous phenytoin to patients receiving thyroid hormones may induce supraventricular tachycardia.

d) Therapeutic drug monitoring:

   i) Approx. time to steady state: 1-2 weeks (highly variable)

   ii) Therapeutic plasma levels:

	Neonates	6-15mg/L.
	Infants and children	10-20mg/L. ❶

          ❶Caution above 16mg/L.

   iii) Take a trough sample, immediately prior to next dose.

e) The bioavailability of oral phenytoin is very good therefore the same daily dose of phenytoin can be given by IV injection if oral route becomes impossible. **However as** the infatabs and suspension are in the form of phenytoin and the injection is the sodium salt multiply oral dose by 1.1 to calculate equivalent IV dose.

f) **Enteral feeds** inhibit the absorption of phenytoin resulting in low plasma levels. **STOP** feed for at least 30 minutes prior to and post administration of oral phenytoin. Dose should be given with water to enhance absorption.

g) Phenytoin is highly protein bound; 90% bound to serum albumin. In states of low serum albumin or altered protein binding (e.g. renal failure) adjust the plasma level or measure free drug level (therapeutic range of free drug = 1- 2mg/L).

h) Phenytoin can affect the metabolism of many hepatically metabolised drugs due to enzyme induction. Also phenytoin blood levels may be increased or decreased by drugs which alter its absorption or metabolism. For further information contact your clinical pharmacist, drug information (Guy's ext. 3594, Lewisham ext. 3202, St Thomas' ext. 3069) or consult the Adult Formulary Chapter 4.8.

i) Counsel patient/carer to report the onset of fever, sore throats, mouth ulcers, bruising, rashes or any other indicators of skin or blood disorders.

j) Phenytoin liquid (Epanutin®) contains 1g of sucrose in 5ml. The chewable tablets Epanutin® contain 0.46g of sucrose per 50mg tablet.

PHOLCODINE

Preparations: LINCTUS 5mg in 5ml.

Dosage: *COUGH SUPPRESSANT*

Pholcodine is not usually recommended in children under 1 year.

3 months - 1 year	1mg	3 times a day
1 - 2 years	2.5mg	3-4 times a day
3 - 5 years	5mg	3-4 times a day
6 - 12 years	5mg	4-5 times a day
Over 12 years	5-10mg	4-6 times a day

Maximum 60mg in 24 hours.

Notes:

a) Pholcodine linctus (Pavacol D) is sucrose free and contains 1.2% w/v alcohol.

b) Can cause constipation.

PHOSPHATES

Preparations:

Phosphate-Sandoz®: SOLUBLE TABLETS each containing 16.1mmol phosphate, 20.4mmol sodium and 3.1mmol potassium.

Slow Phosphate®: SLOW RELEASE TABLETS each containing 3.13mmol phosphate, 3 16mmol sodium as sodium acid phosphate (**Manufactured special**).

Potassium acid phosphate 13.6%: INJECTION containing 10mmol potassium and 10mmol acid phosphate in 10ml (**Manufactured special**).

Neutral sodium phosphate: INJECTION (1ml) containing 1.5mmol sodium and 0.8mmol phosphate in 1ml (**Manufactured special**).

ORAL SOLUTION (20ml) containing 1mmol phosphate and 1.8mmol sodium in 1ml (**Manufactured special**).

Polyfusor phosphates: INFUSION containing 50mmol phosphate, 81mmol sodium and 9.5mmol potassium in 500ml.

Addiphos®: INJECTION containing 40mmol phosphate, 30mmol potassium and 30mmol sodium in 20ml.

Phosphate Enema: Sodium acid phosphate 12.8g sodium phosphate 10.24g in 128ml.

Dosage:

HYPERCALCAEMIA

See note c).

Orally, neonates, initially 1mmol/kg/day in 1-2 divided doses. Adjust dose according to serum phosphate levels.

Under 5 years	up to 3 tablets (Phosphate-Sandoz®)/day.
Over 5 years	up to 6 tablets/day.

HYPOPHOSPHATAEMIA, INCLUDING RICKETS AND OSTEOMALACIA

Orally, premature neonates, initially 1mmol/kg/day in 1-2 divided doses.

Under 5 years	2-3 tablets (Phosphate-Sandoz®)/day.
Over 5 years	4-6 tablets/day.

Adjust the dose according to response.

PARENTERAL PHOSPHATES

SEEK EXPERT ADVICE BEFORE PRESCRIBING

IV infusion, 0.15-0.33mmol/kg, up to 1mmol/kg/day of phosphate. This is repeated to maintain appropriate blood levels of phosphate.

CONSTIPATION

Rectally, see notes e and f).

Under 3 years	not recommended.
3 - 6 years	50ml as required.
Over 6 years	128ml as required.

Administration: IV infusion, dilute to 0.1mmol of phosphate in 1ml with sodium chloride 0.9% or glucose 5%. Administer at a rate of 0.05mmol/kg/hour.

In an emergency **and** in intensive care rate can be increased to 0.5mmol/kg/hour.

Notes:

a) **Use with great caution in renal failure.**
b) Phosphate infusion may cause hypotension, tachycardia, pulmonary oedema, fever, hypocalcaemia and tetany. It can also cause thrombophlebitis and calcification at infusion site.
c) Phosphate infusion is not the first line treatment for hypercalcaemia because of the risk of precipitation of calcium phosphate in tissues especially the kidneys. A high fluid throughput is essential and electrolyte load must be monitored. Seek expert advice.
d) **CAUTION:** monitor acid-base balance when infusing potassium acid phosphate as it may potentiate/cause acidosis.
e) Phosphate enema is not recommended in small children and renal impairment as absorption of phosphate results in serious electrolyte imbalance.
f) Many small children who experience pain or fear during defecation find rectally administered treatment very distressing and alternatives should be considered.
g) Neutral sodium phosphate injection can be given orally.
h) Phosphate-Sandoz® tablets contain 136mg of sucrose.

PHYTOMENADIONE

Preparations: TABLETS 10mg. INJECTION (Konakion MM®) 10mg in 1ml.
AMPOULES - oral and parenteral use (Konakion MM®) 2mg in 0.2ml.

Dosage: **PROPHYLAXIS AGAINST HAEMORRHAGIC DISEASE OF THE NEWBORN**
See notes below.
All well term babies,
Orally, 2mg dose at birth and on day 7.
Breast-fed babies require a further oral dose of 2mg at 4-6 weeks.
"At risk" and premature babies (<36 weeks gestation)
IM injection, a single dose at birth,
less than 2.5kg   0.4mg/kg
2.5kg or greater   1mg

NEONATAL HYPOPROTHROMBINAEMIA
IV injection, 1mg, repeated at 8 hourly intervals if necessary.

ANTIDOTE TO COUMARIN ANTICOAGULANTS WHERE CONTINUED ANTICOAGULATION IS REQUIRED.

SEEK EXPERT ADVICE BEFORE PRESCRIBING

Initially, *IV injection*, 25microgram/kg, maximum 1mg if no major bleeding and INR >8. Repeat if INR still too high after 24 hours. Restart warfarin when INR <5.

OTHER INDICATIONS

Orally, and infants,   1mg a day
Children,   5-10mg a day
IV or *IM injection,*
4 weeks - 12 months   1mg
1 - 4 years   3mg
5 - 12 years   5mg
Over 12 years   10mg
Repeat at intervals according to clotting time.

Administration:	IV injection, Konakion MM® injection solution may be diluted if required with glucose 5% or sodium chloride 0.9%. Give over 5-10 minutes.

Notes:

a) Injection (2mg in 0.2ml) is licensed to be given orally, intramuscularly or intravenously.

b) All well babies of 36 weeks and over should receive oral phytomenadione unless they are unable to absorb the oral dose or are at increased risk of haemorrhagic disease e.g. prematurity, birth asphyxia, bleeding problems, instrumental delivery, maternal liver disease or mother is on anticonvulsants or antituberculosis drugs.

c) The day 7 dose will be administered by the community midwife and the 4-6 week dose by either the general practitioner or baby health clinic at the 6 week health check. All mothers will be given a card at birth in which the dose and route of administration must be recorded by the person administering the dose.

d) Breast fed babies have a higher risk of haemorrhagic disease of the newborn.

e) Parenteral administration to premature babies weighing less than 2.5kg may increase the risk for the development of kernicterus.

f) IV injection may cause peripheral vascular collapse, cyanosis, sweating and flushing if given too rapidly.

g) In hepatic disease repeated IM injection may cause cutaneous or subcutaneous changes.

PIMOZIDE

Preparations:	TABLETS 2mg, 4mg; and 10mg (**Non-formulary**).
Dosage:	**SEEK EXPERT ADVICE BEFORE PRESCRIBING**

GILLES DE LA TOURETTE SYNDROME

This indication is unlicensed for use in children.

Orally, 1-2mg once a day, **OR** 200microgram/kg/day. Maximum dose 20mg/day.

SCHIZOPHRENIA

There is no recommended dose for children under 12 years as data from clinical use is limited.

Children over 12 years, initially 4mg/day. Adjust in increments of 2-4mg/day at weekly intervals. Maximum dose 20mg/day.

PARANOID STATES & PSYCHOSIS

There is no recommended dose for children under 12 years as data from clinical use is limited.

Children over 12 years, 4mg/day increasing to a maximum of 16mg/day.

Notes:

a) **CSM Warning:** Pimozide should be used with extreme caution in patients with cardiovascular disorders, liver disease, renal failure or epilepsy. An E.C.G. should be performed before initiating treatment and periodically where doses exceed 16mg/day.

b) Doses in excess of 20mg/day have been associated with rare sudden unexpected deaths.

c) Pimozide should **not** be given with other antipsychotic drugs, tricyclic antidepressants, other drugs which prolong the QT intervals, i.e. antimalarials (e.g. quinine), antiarrhythmics, antihistamines (e.g. terfenadine, astemizole), cisapride, or drugs which cause electrolyte imbalance e.g. diuretics.

POLIOMYELITIS VACCINE

Preparations: LIVE VACCINE (OPV) single dose and multidose.
INACTIVATED VACCINE (Salk) (**Named patient**).

Dosage: **PRIMARY IMMUNISATION**
Orally, course of three doses, each of 3 drops of multidose or entire contents of single dose at 2, 3 and 4 months of age.

BOOSTER DOSE
Orally, 3 drops of multidose or entire contents of single dose at 3-5 years and 15-18 years.

INACTIVATED VACCINE
IM or *deep SC injections,* a primary course of 3 doses each of 0.5ml, followed by booster doses of 0.5ml, at 3-5 years and 15-18 years.

Notes:

a) The inactivated vaccine should only be used where live vaccine is contraindicated e.g. In immunosuppressed patients or their household contacts or prior to renal transplantation. Supplies are available on a named patient basis via the pharmacy.

b) Polio vaccine is excreted in faeces and urine and vaccination should therefore be delayed until immediately prior to discharge from hospital. Parents/carers should be counselled with regard to strict personal hygiene. Unimmunised contacts (e.g. parents, grandparents, carers) should be immunised concomitantly.

c) Either live (oral) or inactivated vaccine may be used to complete a course started with the other as long as contraindications are adhered to.

d) See immunisation guidelines on page 296.

POTASSIUM CHLORIDE

Preparations: SLOW RELEASE TABLETS (Slow K®) potassium chloride 600mg, providing 8mmol each of potassium and chloride.
SOLUBLE TABLETS (Sando-K®) containing potassium bicarbonate and chloride,equivalent to 12mmol potassium and 8mmol chloride.
LIQUID (Kay-Cee-L®) containing 1mmol each of potassium and chloride in 1ml.
INJECTION containing 1.5g (20mmol) potassium and 20mmol chloride in 10ml.

Dosage: **POTASSIUM SUPPLEMENT**
All ages, *orally,* 2mmol/kg/day in 2-3 divided doses.
IV infusion, add 2mmol/kg/day to the infusion fluid, according to serum levels. See note b).

ACUTE DEPLETION
IV infusion, 1mmol/kg infused at a rate of 0.2mmol/kg/hr. Recheck potassium level after 3 hours. **Caution** is required in patients with renal failure.

Administration:	**Dilute injection before use**. Ensure thoroughly mixed before administration. Maximum concentration peripherally of potassium is 40mmol/L. Maximum infusion rate 0.5mmol/kg/hour of potassium. If patient is fluid restricted and being monitored by ECG, higher concentrations of potassium have been infused, however infusion rate **MUST NOT** exceed 0.5mmol/kg/hour of potassium.

Notes:

a) Potassium requirement in healthly individuals is 1- 2mmol/kg/day.
b) Intravenous fluids with added potassium are available on wards. Use the pre-mixed bags whenever practicable.
c) Injection can be given orally.
d) Slow release tablets (Slow K®) should **not** be crushed.
e) Potassium chloride liquid (Kay-Cee-L®) is cherry flavoured and sucrose free. Sando-K® effervescent tablets contain 0.5g of sucrose (approximately 4kcals) and 0.1mmol of sodium in each tablet.

PRAZOSIN

Preparations:	TABLETS 500microgram, 1mg and 2mg. LIQUID (**Extemporaneously prepared**).
Dosage:	*HYPERTENSION* This indication is unlicensed for use in children. *Orally*, initially, 10-15microgram/kg 2-4 times a day, increasing to a maximum of 500microgram/kg/day. *CONGESTIVE HEART FAILURE* This indication is unlicensed for use in children. *Orally*, initially, 5microgram/kg twice a day increasing to a maximum of 100microgram/kg/day.

Notes:

a) The patient's blood pressure should be monitored closely after the **first** dose since prazosin can cause a precipitous fall in blood pressure. It may be preferable to give first dose at bedtime.
b) Patients in chronic renal failure are more sensitive to the effects of prazosin.

PREDNISOLONE

Preparations: TABLETS 1mg and 5mg. ENTERIC COATED TABLETS 2.5mg and 5mg. SOLUBLE TABLETS 5mg. TABLETS 25mg are available if this strength is specified on the prescription.

Dosage:

CAUTION: SEVERE CHICKENPOX ASSOCIATED WITH SYSTEMIC CORTICOSTEROIDS SEE IMMUNISATION GUIDELINES ON PAGE 296.

GLUCOCORTICOSTEROID
Orally, 1-2mg/kg/day.

ASTHMA
Orally, 1-2mg/kg/day, maximum dose of 40mg, for 3-5 days and then stop. If treatment is required for 7 days or more, reduce dose gradually.

CROUP REQUIRING INTUBATION
Orally, 1mg/kg every 12 hours for 48 hours or until extubated.

IDIOPATHIC NEPHROTIC SYNDROME
Orally, initially, $60mg/m^2$/day (maximum 80mg/day) until proteinuria absent for 3 days then reduce to $40mg/m^2$ on alternate days for 4 weeks. For relapses give initial dose until protinuria absent for 3 days then reduce to $60mg/m^2$ alternate days and continue to reduce dose by 10mg every 3 doses.

RENAL GRAFT REJECTION
Orally, 3mg/kg/day for 3 days.

Notes:

a)   If therapy is long term, consider maintenance treatment on alternate days as steroids suppress growth in children.
b)   When long term treatment is to be discontinued, the dose should be reduced gradually over several weeks or months depending on the dosage and duration of the therapy.
c)   The absorption of enteric coated prednisolone is not always reliable in children.
d)   For relative potencies see Hydrocortisone (page 123, note b).

PRIMIDONE

Preparations:	TABLETS 250mg. LIQUID 250mg in 5ml.
Dosage:	*EPILEPSY*

Orally, 10-15mg/kg twice a day. If control is not achieved increase dose every 3 days. Maximum dose, under 9 years 1g/day, and over 9 years 1.5g/day.
OR

Under 2 years	125-250mg	twice a day
2 - 5 years	250-375mg	twice a day
6 - 9 years	375-500mg	twice a day
Over 9 years	500-750mg	twice a day

Notes:

a) Therapeutic drug monitoring of primidone is a poor indication of the appropriate dose as primidone is metabolised to phenobarbitone. See page 168 for phenobarbitone monitoring.

b) Some patients develop vertigo, vomiting and ataxia even at low doses.

c) Primidone reduces blood levels of carbamazepine, lamotrigine, ethosuximide, sodium valproate, chloramphenicol, cimetidine, ciclosporin, griseofulvin, corticosteroids and warfarin. Blood levels of isoniazid may be increased by concomitant administration of primidone. The effect of primidone on phenytoin levels is unpredictable therefore monitor blood levels.

d) Primidone liquid contains 1g of sucrose in 5ml.

PROCHLORPERAZINE

Preparations:	TABLETS 5mg. LIQUID 5mg in 5ml. SUPPOSITORIES 5mg and 25mg. INJECTION 12.5mg in 1ml.
Dosage:	*ANTIEMETIC*

This indication is unlicensed for use in children under 10kg or for the rectal or parenteral routes.
Orally, 100-250microgram/kg 2-3 times a day
OR

1 - 4 years (over 10kg)	1.25-2.5mg	2-3 times a day
5 - 12 years	2.5-5mg	2-3 times a day
Over 12 years	5-10mg	2-3 times a day

Rectally,

1 - 4 years (over 10kg)	2.5mg	Up to
5 - 12 years	5-10mg	3 times
Over 12 years	12.5-25mg	a day

IM injection,

1 - 4 years (over 10kg)	1.25-2.5mg	Up to
5 - 12 years	5-6.25mg	3 times
Over 12 years	12.5mg	a day

Notes:

a) There is an increased possibility of extrapyramidal side effects, especially in very ill children and children under 10kg. Prochlorperazine may, rarely, cause neuroleptic malignant syndrome.

b) The IV route is unlicensed and not recommended, however the above IM injection doses have been given as a slow IV injection, diluted 1 in 10 with sodium chloride 0.9%, over at least 10 minutes.

c) Prochlorperazine liquid (Stemetil®) contains 3.4g of sucrose in 5ml.

PROCYCLIDINE

Preparations: TABLETS 5mg. INJECTION 5mg in 1ml. LIQUID 5mg in 5ml.
Dosage: **ACUTE DYSTONIA**

> **IF IN ANY DOUBT CONTACT THE MEDICAL TOXICOLOGY UNIT**
> ☎ 0171-635-9191 ☎

This indication is unlicensed for use in children.
Orally,

7 - 14 years	1.25mg	3 times a day
Over 14 years	2.5mg	3 times a day

IM or IV injection (over at least 2 minutes),

Under 2 years	500microgram-2mg as a single dose
2 - 10 years	2-5mg as a single dose
Over 10 years	5-10mg as a single dose

Repeat if necessary after 20 minutes.

Notes:

Procyclidine liquid (Arpicolin®) is sugar free.

PROGUANIL

Preparations: TABLETS 100mg.
Dosage: **PROPHYLAXIS OF MALARIA**
Orally,

Up to 5 weeks	25mg (1/4 tablet)	once a day
6 weeks - 11 months	50mg (1/2 tablet)	once a day
1 - 5 years (10-19kg)	100mg (1 tablet)	once a day
6 - 11 years (20-39kg)	150mg (1 1/2 tablets)	once a day
12 years and over (40kg)	200mg (2 tablets)	once a day

Notes:

a) A tablet cutter can be used to cut tablets although they are scored and do break into fairly accurate quarters. Precise accuracy is not essential. The dose may be crushed and mixed with milk, jam or honey.

b) Proguanil should be started 1 week before arriving in endemic area and should be continued for 4 weeks after return.

c)
> Up to date advice on PROPHYLAXIS of malaria can be obtained from:
> **The Drug Information Centre**
> ☎Guy's ext 3594, Lewisham ext 3202, St Thomas' ext 3069☎
> or
> **The Malaria Reference Laboratory**
> ☎0171-387 4411 (TREATMENT) or 0171-636 8636 (PROPHYLAXIS)☎

PROMETHAZINE HYDROCHLORIDE

Preparations: TABLETS 10mg **(Non-Formulary)** and 25mg. LIQUID 5mg in 5ml.
INJECTION 50mg in 2ml.

Dosage: These indications are unlicensed for use in children under 2
years of age.

ALLERGIC DISORDERS

Orally, 125 microgram/kg 3 times a day and 500 microgram/kg
at night.
OR

4 weeks - 1 year	2.5mg	twice a day or 2.5-10mg as single dose. Maximum 10mg/**day**.
1 - 5 years	5mg	twice a day or 5-15mg as single dose. Maximum 15mg/**day**.
6 - 10 years	5-10mg	twice a day or 10-25mg as sinlge dose. Maximum 25mg/**day**.
Over 10 years	10-20mg	2-3 times a day or 25mg as single dose. Maximum 60mg/**day**.

SEDATION

Orally,

4 weeks - 1 year	5-10mg	at bedtime
1 - 5 years	10-20mg	at bedtime
6 - 10 years	20-25mg	at bedtime
Over 10 years	25-50mg	at bedtime

OR, for daytime sedation, give once or twice a day using the
lower dose.

PREMEDICATION

Deep IM injection or *slow IV injection* over at least 5 minutes,
500microgram/kg/dose.

Orally, 500microgram-1mg/kg/dose to a maximum of 50mg.

Notes:

a) **Caution:** in infants under 2 years because of the possible association
with 'cot deaths'.

b) Paradoxical hyperexcitability may be seen in some children.

c) Promethazine liquid (Rosemont) contains 1.7g of sucrose in 5ml.
Promethazine liquid (Phenergan®) is sugar free.

PROPANTHELINE

Preparations:	TABLETS 2.5mg **(Manufactured special)** and 15mg.
Dosage:	*ANTISPASMODIC, DAY TIME WETTING AND UNSTABLE BLADDER*

Use for day time wetting and unstable bladder are unlicensed indications and use as antispasmodic is unlicensed for use in children.

Orally, all ages, 300microgram/kg 3-4 times a day. Maximum dose 2mg/kg/day.

Notes:

The side effects are anticholinergic and include dry mouth, blurred vision and constipation.

PROPOFOL

Preparations:	INJECTION 200mg in 20ml and 500mg in 50ml.
	PREFILLED SYRINGE 500mg in 50ml.
Dosage:	

> THE CSM DOES NOT RECOMMEND THE USE IN CHILDREN FOR SEDATION AND HAS RECEIVED REPORTS OF CONVULSIONS FOLLOWING ANAESTHESIA.

ANAESTHESIA

Induction; over 3 years, *IV injection* 2.5mg/kg, adjust dose according to response. Larger doses are often required for children under 8 years. Lower dosage is recommended for children of ASA grades 3 and 4.

Maintenance; over 3 years, repeat injectiones as required or *IV infusion*, 9-15mg/kg/hour adjusting dose according to response.

SEDATION AND ICP CONTROL IN SEVERE HEAD INJURY

> SEEK EXPERT ADVICE BEFORE PRESCRIBING

These indications are unlicensed for use in children.

IV injection, 2-2.5mg/kg

IV infusion, 2-3mg/kg/hour adjust dose according to response. Infusion should not continue for more than 3 days. (see note a).

Administration:

Inject slowly or infuse, neat. If required propofol can be diluted in glucose 5% only. Dilutions must not exceed concentrations of 2mg in 1ml. Discard any diluted solution after 6 hours. Administer using PVC giving sets.

Notes:

a) Monitor blood lipid levels of all patients at risk of not clearing the fat contained in propofol injection emulsion.

b) Discolouration of the urine has been reported with prolonged infusions.

PROPRANOLOL

Preparations: TABLETS 10mg, 40mg, and 80mg. INJECTION 1mg in 1ml.
LIQUID 5mg in 5ml.

Dosage: **FALLOT'S TETRALOGY**
Orally, 1mg/kg 3-4 times a day.
IV injection, initially, 15-20microgram/kg, then increasing to a dose of 100-200microgram/kg, given slowly under ECG control. May be repeated 3-4 times each day.

DYSRHYTHMIAS, PHAEOCHROMOCYTOMA, THYROTOXICOSIS
Orally, 250-500microgram/kg 3-4 times a day. Start at low dose and increase to 1mg/kg 3 times a day or until response. Maximum 8mg/kg/**day**.
IV injection, 10-50microgram/kg slowly under ECG control. Repeat 3-4 times a day if necessary.

PORTAL HYPERTENSION
Orally, initially, 500microgram/kg twice a day. Adjust according to heart rate; aim to decrease rate by 25%.

MIGRAINE PROPHYLAXIS
Orally,

Under 12 years	10-20mg	2-3 times a day.
Over 12 years	20-40mg	2-3 times a day.

Notes:
a) Propranolol is contra-indicated in asthmatics due to increased bronchospasm.
b) Cardiac failure and heart block may be exacerbated by propranolol.
c) Administration of IV propranolol may be preceded by an IV dose of atropine sulphate.
d) Administration of IV, and possibly oral, propranolol is contraindicated in patients on concomitant verapamil.
e) Cimetidine potentiates the effects of propranolol and chlorpromazine concentrations are increased by propranolol.

PROTAMINE SULPHATE

Preparations: INJECTION 50mg in 5ml.
Dosage: **HEPARIN ANTIDOTE**
This indication is unlicensed for use in children.

Time since heparin given (minutes)	Protamine dose/100units of heparin
<30	1mg
30-60	0.5-0.75mg
60-120	0.375-0.5mg
>120	0.25-0.375mg

Maximum 50mg (5ml)/dose. Monitor APTT and INR.

Administration: *IV injection* over 10 minutes, dilute if required with sodium chloride 0.9%.

Notes:
a) May cause hypotension.
b) In excess, protamine has an anticoagulant effect.

PROTIRELIN (THYROTROPHIN RELEASING HORMONE)

Preparations: INJECTION 200microgram in 2ml (**Hospital only**).
Dosage: *TO ELUCIDATE BORDERLINE THYROTOXICOSIS OR HYPOTHYROIDISM BY EXAMINATION OF TSH RESPONSE*

Undiluted IV injection 1microgram/kg as a single dose. In some cases doses up to 20microgram/kg have been required.

Notes:
a) Take blood sample before the dose as a control, then again 20 minutes after injection, for peak TSH assay. If necessary take a further blood sample 60 minutes after the dose to detect a delayed TSH response.
b) IM injection should be avoided as no peak in blood levels occurs.
c) The response to thyrotrophin may be modified in patients taking thyroxine, antithyroid drugs, corticosteroids, theophylline, phenothiazines, metoclopramide, bromocriptine, salicylates, benzodiazepines, amiodarone, carbamazepine or spironolactone.

PYRAZINAMIDE

Preparations: TABLETS 500mg. LIQUID (**Extemporaneously prepared**).
Dosage: *TUBERCULOSIS THERAPY (UNSUPERVISED REGIMEN)*

SEEK EXPERT ADVICE BEFORE PRESCRIBING

This indication is unlicensed for use in children.
Orally, all ages, 35mg/kg/day, rounded to the nearest 125mg. Maximum dose is 2g/day. Give for first 2 months of treatment only. If not given, rifampicin and isoniazid should be administered for 9 months.

Notes:

Hepatitis has been reported with pyrazinamide. Base line liver function tests should be performed before commencing treatment. Frequent checks in the first 2 months are then required in those with pre-existing liver disease. Further routine checks are not required if there is no evidence of liver disease or dysfunction. Patients/carer should be warned to seek medical advice immediately if there are any signs of liver disorder e.g. persistent nausea, vomiting, malaise, fever or jaundice.

PYRIDOSTIGMINE BROMIDE

Preparations: TABLETS 60mg.
Dosage: **MYASTHENIA GRAVIS**
Orally, initially,
Neonates, 5-10mg every 4 hours, ½ - 1 hour before feeds.
Over 1 month, 1-1.5mg/kg 4-6 times a day.
Usual total daily dose 30-360mg.
Over 12 years, 30-120mg then at suitable intervals during the day. Maximum dose 1.2g however it is not advisable to exceed 720mg/**day**.

Notes:

Pyridostigmine is usually first line as it is longer acting and has a smoother onset of action than neostigmine. It is weaker than neostigmine and the decreased muscurinic action results in better gastrointestinal tolerability.

PYRIDOXINE

Preparations: TABLETS 10mg, 20mg and 50mg. INJECTION 50mg in 2ml.
LIQUID (**Extemporaneously prepared**).
Dosage: **CONVULSIONS**

Neonates, *orally,* 200mg a day as a therapeutic trial for up to 7 days.
IV injection (see notes a and b) 100mg as a therapeutic trial for up to 7 days. For maintenance, convert to oral therapy.
Children, *orally,* 20-100mg a day, but up to 1g may be required (see note c).

SUPPLEMENTATION ON DIALYSIS AND ISONIAZID PROPHYLAXIS
Neurological side effects of isoniazid are less common in children (see note d)
Orally, neonates and infants 5mg once a day and children 10mg once a day.

Administration: Slow IV injection over at least 5 minutes, dilute with sodium chloride 0.9%.

Notes:

     a)   Resuscitation facilities **must** be readily available when IV pyridoxine is administered due to the risk of cardiovascular collapse.
     b)   Initial IV therapeutic trial dose should be given, if possible, during concurrent EEG monitoring.
     c)   Ideal maintenance dose is not necessarily one that stops seizures but that allows best intellectual performance.
     d)   Risk factors for developing peripheral neuritis whilst on isoniazid are breast fed infants, malnutrition, diabetes and chronic renal failure.

QUININE

Preparations:	TABLETS quinine sulphate 200mg and 300mg.
	INJECTION quinine dihydrochloride 600mg in 2ml.
Dosage:	**_TREATMENT OF CHLOROQUINE RESISTANT MALARIA (P.FALCIPARUM)_**

See note e).

QUININE SULPHATE

Orally, 10mg/kg (of sulphate) 3 times a day, for 7 days.
Doses may need to be rounded to the nearest tablet size or given less frequently, to achieve a suitable total daily dose.

QUININE DIHYDROCHLORIDE

IV infusion, 20mg/kg (of dihydrochloride) as loading dose, maximum 1.4g (**See note a**). Then after 8-12 hours, 10mg/kg (of dihydrochloride) every 8 hours. Change to oral therapy as soon as practically possible. If IV treatment is required for more than 48 hours, reduce maintenance dose to 5-7mg/kg every 8 hours. A 7 day course of quinine should be completed.

Administration:	IV infusion; (administer over at least 4 hours) dilute to 2mg in 1ml with sodium chloride 0.9%. In fluid restricted patients dilute to a maximum concentration of 30mg in 1ml.
Notes:	

a) **Do not** give loading dose if patient has received quinine, quinidine or mefloquine during the previous 24 hours.
b) Monitor blood glucose levels as quinine and malaria may cause hypoglycaemia.
c) Monitor blood levels of quinine. To avoid toxicity, trough blood levels should remain below 8mg/L.
d) For IV injection or IM administration, **seek expert advice**, due to risk of hypoglycaemia or arrhythmias.
e) Fansidar should be given as a **radical cure** after quinine treatment. (See page 187).
f)

> Up-to-date information about the DISTRIBUTION OF CHLOROQUINE RESISTANCE
> can be obtained from:
> **Drug Information Centre**
> (Guy's ext 3594, Lewisham ext 3202, St Thomas' ext 3069)
> or
> **The Malaria Reference Laboratory**
> (0171-387 4411 (TREATMENT) or 0171-388 9600 (PROPHYLAXIS))

g) Quinine base 100mg is equivalent to quinine dihydrochloride 122mg or quinine sulphate 121mg.

RANITIDINE

Preparations:	TABLETS 150mg and 300mg. LIQUID 15mg in 1ml. INJECTION 50mg in 2ml. EFFERVESCENT TABLETS 150mg. **(Non-formulary)**.
Dosage:	*ULCER THERAPY, REFLUX OESOPHAGITIS*

The parenteral route is unlicensed for use in children.
IV injection, all ages, 1mg/kg 3-4 times a day.
The treatment of peptic ulcers is the only licensed indication for use in children.
Orally,

Less than 6 months	1mg/kg	3 times a day
6 months - 8 years	2mg/kg	twice a day
Over 8 years	up to 150mg	twice a day (300mg/day)

Doses as high as 4mg/kg twice a day, up to 300mg per **day**, can be used for treatment of peptic ulcer.

IN RENAL FAILURE

Creatinine clearance (ml/minute/1.73m^2)	Dosage
10-50	75% normal dose
<10	50% normal dose

Administration:	IV injection, dilute to 2.5mg in 1ml with sodium chloride 0.9% and administer over at least 2 minutes.

Notes:

a) Interactions due to blocking of cytochrome P450 mediated hepatic drug metabolism are less common with ranitidine compared with cimetidine.
b) Ranitidine effervescent tablets are sucrose and alcohol free but contain aspartame and 14.3mmol of sodium per 150mg tablet; the liquid is sucrose free but contains 7.5% w/v alcohol.

RIBOFLAVIN

Preparations:	POWDER **(Named patient)**.
Dosage:	*INHERITED METABOLIC DISEASE*

SEEK EXPERT ADVICE BEFORE PRESCRIBING

Orally, all ages, initially 10-20mg once a day. Maintenance, 5-10mg once a day. Doses up to 100mg/day have been used.

Notes:

a) Riboflavin is a co-enzyme in a number of different enzyme systems.
b) Large doses may interfere with some laboratory tests.
c) The powder is **not** stocked in the pharmacy department. The powder can be encapsulated in the manufacturing unit.

RIFAMPICIN

Preparations: CAPSULES 150mg and 300mg. LIQUID 100mg in 5ml.
INJECTION 600mg.

Dosage: **TUBERCULOSIS THERAPY (UNSUPERVISED REGIMEN)**

SEEK EXPERT ADVICE BEFORE PRESCRIBING

Orally or *IV infusion,*
Premature and newborn neonates, 10mg/kg once a day.
Over 1 month, 10mg/kg up to 20mg/kg once a day (maximum 600mg).

IN LIVER FAILURE
Avoid in liver failure or reduce dose to a maximum of 8mg/kg once a day.

PROPHYLAXIS OF MENINGITIS

Ciprofloxacin is first choice as prophylaxis for meningitis contacts at Guy's and St Thomas'.

Meninogococcal
Orally,

Less than 1 year	5mg/kg	twice a day	}
1 - 12 years	10mg/kg	twice a day	} for 2 days
Over 12 years	600mg	twice a day	}

Haemophilus influenzae type B
Orally,

Under 3 months	10mg/kg	once a day	}
3 months - 12 years	20mg/kg	once a day	} for 4 days
Over 12 years	600mg	once a day	}

PRURITUS DUE TO CHOLESTATIS
Orally, all ages, 5-10mg/kg once a day.

Administration: On reconstitution 600mg (Rifadin®)displaces 0.48ml. Add 4.52ml of the solvent provided to each vial to give 600mg in 5ml. Further dilute to a concentration of 1mg in 1ml with glucose 5%. Administer over 2-3 hours. Discard any remaining solution after 6 hours.

Notes:

a) Hepatitis has been reported with rifampicin. Base line liver function tests should be performed before commencing treatment. Frequent checks in the first 2 months are then required in those with pre-existing liver disease. Further routine checks are not required if there is no evidence of liver disease or dysfunction. Patients/carer should be warned to seek medical advice immediately if there are any signs of liver disorder e.g. persistent nausea, vomiting, malaise, fever or jaundice.

b) Occasional renal dysfunction and haematological abnormalities have been noted, particularly with intermittent, interrupted or prolonged treatment.

c) Rifampicin enhances the metabolism of many drugs thus reducing blood levels and efficacy. Some of the drugs affected are warfarin, ciclosporin, phenytoin, corticosteroids, theophylline, oral contraceptive pills and some antifungals and antiarrhythmics.

d) Rifampicin stains urine, sweat and tears (including soft contact lenses) red/orange.

e) Rifampicin liquid contains 2g of sucrose in 5ml and saccharin.

RISPERIDONE

Preparations: TABLETS 1mg and 3mg. 2mg and 4mg (**Purchased on request**).
LIQUID 1mg in 1ml.

Dosage: ***CHILDHOOD SCHIZOPHRENIA, BEHAVIOURAL DISORDERS***

SEEK EXPERT ADVICE BEFORE PRESCRIBING

These indications are unlicensed for use in children under 15 years.

	4 - 8 years	8 - 15 years	≥ 15 years	
Day 1	0.25mg	0.5mg	1mg	} TWICE
Day 2	0.5mg	1mg	2mg	} A
Day 3	0.75mg	1.5mg	3mg	} DAY

Increase dose according to response. Usual maintenance dose in adolescents and adults is 4-8mg/day. Maximum 16mg/day however doses above 10mg/**day** have not been shown to be more effective and side effects are more likely.

IN RENAL AND HEPATIC FAILURE

Initial starting dose should be reduced by 50%.

Notes:

a) Risperidone can cause postural hypotension. A baseline blood pressure should be performed. Blood pressure should be monitored whilst dose is being established and after any dosage increments.

b) Patient should be monitored at least weekly for side effects whilst dose is being established.

SALBUTAMOL

Preparations:	CONTROLLED RELEASE TABLETS 4mg (**Non-formulary**) and 8mg.
	LIQUID 2mg in 5ml.
	INJECTION 500microgram in 1ml and 5mg in 5ml (for continuous infusion).
	NEBULES (Preservative free) 2.5mg in 2.5ml and 5mg in 2.5ml.
	INHALER 100microgram/metered inhalation, 200 dose unit.
	BREATH ACTIVATED INHALER 100microgram/metered inhalation, 200 dose unit.
	VENTODISK® 200microgram and 400microgram/blister (**Non-formulary**).

Dosage:

ASTHMA THERAPY

Inhaled, initially, 100-200microgram up to 4 times a day. In some cases higher doses may be necessary - seek expert advice.

Nebulised,

Under 5 years	2.5mg	) every 4 hours as required
5 years and over	5mg	)

Nebulisers may be administered more frequently in hospital with close monitoring.

Orally, see note a).

All ages, 100microgram/kg 4 times a day,

OR

Liquid,

2 - 6 years	1-2mg	)
6 - 12 years	2mg	) 3-4 times a day.
Over 12 years	2-4mg	)

Controlled release tablets,

3 - 12 years	4mg	twice a day
Over 12 years	8mg	twice a day

PARENTERAL THERAPY FOR ASTHMA

This indication is unlicensed for use in children.

IV injection, 4-6microgram/kg.

IV infusion, 0.6-1microgram/kg/minute. Doses as high as 20microgram/kg/minute have been used in intensive care.

RENAL HYPERKALAEMIA

This indication is unlicensed.

All ages, *IV injection*, 4microgram/kg.

Nebulised, 2.5-5mg as a single dose, repeat as necessary.

Administration: Slow IV injection over 5 minutes or IV infusion, dilute if required with sodium chloride 0.9% or glucose 5%.

Notes:

a) Inhaled therapy is the preferred method of administration and should be used whenever possible. Oral salbutamol is much less effective and has more systemic side effects.

b) Children under 10 years are usually incapable of using inhalers and children under 4 years are usually incapable of using diskhalers. Nebuliser therapy may be ineffective in children under 18 months.

c) A Volumatic® spacer is available for use with the aerosol inhaler. If this is not available, for emergency use only, a hole just large enough for the inhaler mouthpiece can be cut in the bottom of a polystyrene cup. The inhaler is fitted into this and the cup can then be placed over the child's nose and mouth, however larger doses may be required.

d) The rotahaler requires a high inspiratory flow of approximately 60L/minute, therefore either the aerosol inhaler, preferably with a volumatic, or nebuliser should be used during acute exacerbations.

e) Salbutamol liquid (Ventolin®) is sucrose and dye free.

f) See management guidelines for acute and chronic asthma page 241 and 244.

SALMETEROL

Preparations: INHALER 25microgram/metered inhalation.

Dosage: **ASTHMA THERAPY**

ON CONSULTANT ADVICE ONLY

This indication is unlicensed for use in children under 4 years.

Inhaled,

Under 4 years   25 microgram   twice a day

Over 4 years   50 microgram   twice a day

Increase dose according to response up to 100microgram twice a day.

Notes:

a) **Note:** Salmeterol is not for immediate relief of acute attacks and existing corticosteroid therapy should not be withdrawn or reduced.

b) Children under 10 years are usually incapable of using inhalers. If a dry powder device is required eformoterol turbohaler (page 93) should be prescribed for children over 4 years.

c) A Volumatic® spacer (and mask) is available for use with the aerosol inhaler.

d) See chronic asthma management guidelines page 241.

SENNA

Preparations: TABLETS containing sennoside B 7.5mg.

LIQUID containing sennoside B 7.5mg in 5ml.

GRANULES containing sennoside B 15mg in 5ml.

Dosage: **CONSTIPATION**

Orally,

2 - 6 years   2.5-5ml at night

Over 6 years   5-10ml or 1-2 tablets at night

In severe constipation much higher doses may be necessary.

Notes:

Senna (Senokot®) liquid contains 3.3g of sucrose in 5ml and 7% v/v alcohol. Senna (Senokot®) granules are chocolate flavoured and contain 1.64g of sucrose in 5ml.

SERTRALINE

Preparations:	TABLETS 50mg and 100mg.
Dosage:	*OBSESSIVE COMPULSIVE DISORDER*

SEEK EXPERT ADVICE BEFORE PRESCRIBING

This indication is unlicensed for use in children.

Orally, initially, 0.5-1mg/kg/day rounded to the nearest half tablet (25mg). Increase dose according to response to 1-2mg/kg/day. Maximum 200mg/**day**.

Doses of **150mg/day** and above are not recommended to continue for more than 8 weeks.

OR

initially,

6 - 12 years	25mg once a day
12 years and over	50mg once a day

Notes:

a) Patients should be monitored weekly for side effects whilst dose is being established.
b) Sertraline tablets taste bitter but can be dispersed in water, orange juice or blackcurrant squash for ease of administration. They can also be crushed and mixed with soft food.
c) Avoid abrupt withdrawal. Sertraline should be withdrawn over approximately 4 weeks.

SIMPLE LINCTUS B.P (ADULT AND PAEDIATRIC)

Preparations:	The paediatric preparation is one quarter the strength of the adult preparation (**Extemporaneously prepared**).
Dosage:	*COUGH*

Under 5 years	5-10ml of the paediatric preparation.
Over 5 years	5-10ml of the adult preparation.

Give the above dose 3-4 times a day as necessary.

Notes:

Simple linctus (Adult) contains 3g of sugar in 5ml.

SODIUM BENZOATE

Preparation:	LIQUID (**Extemporaneously prepared**).
	INJECTION 1g in 5ml (**Manufactured special**).
Dosage:	*TREATMENT OF UREA CYCLE DEFECTS AND NON KETOTIC HYPERGLYCINAEMIA*

SEEK SPECIALIST ADVICE FROM METABOLIC TEAM BEFORE PRESCRIBING

Orally, all ages, initially, 250mg/kg/day in 2 to 4 divided doses.

IV injection, total daily dose as a continuous infusion over 24 hours.

ACUTE HYPERAMMONAEMIA

Doses may be increased up to maximum of 500mg/kg/day.

Administration:	Dilute to 20mg in 1ml with glucose 10% or 5%, maximum concentration is 50mg in 1ml.

Administer as a continuous infusion (see note b).

Notes:

a) **Caution:** in neonates, due to increased risk of kernicterus.
b) Sodium benzoate and sodium phenylbutyrate may be administered together as an intravenous infusion.
c) Aim to maintain plasma concentration of ammonia below 60micromol/L and glutamine below 800micromol/L.
d) 1mmol of nitrogen is theoretically cleared by 1mmol of sodium benzoate (500mg = 3.5mmol).
e) Give with food to reduce nausea and vomiting.
f) Injection can be given orally.
g) 1g contains 7mmol of sodium.

SODIUM BICARBONATE

Preparations: TABLETS 600mg (7.14mmol of sodium and bicarbonate). INJECTION 4.2% (0.5mmol of sodium and bicarbonate in 1ml), 10ml; 8.4% (1mmol of sodium and bicarbonate in 1ml), 10ml. PREFILLED SYRINGE 8.4%, 50ml. POLYFUSOR 8.4%, 200ml. INFUSION 1.26% (0.15mmol of sodium and bicarbonate in 1ml), 500ml; 8.4%, 500ml.

Dosage: **TO CORRECT ACIDOSIS**

SEEK EXPERT ADVICE BEFORE PRESCRIBING

Check blood gases, repeat every 15 minutes or as required.

> Total number of mmol of bicarbonate required can be calculated by:
> F x base deficit (mmol/L) x weight (kg).

F represents the extracellular fluid: weight ratio. This is 0.5-0.6 in premature neonates, 0.4 in neonates and 0.3 in infants and children.

Only **half** the base deficit should be corrected initially and blood glucose, pH and electrolytes analysed before full correction.

RENAL ACIDOSIS

Orally,

Infants 1-2mmol/kg/day (1-2ml/kg/day of 8.4%).

Older children 70mmol/m²/day (70ml/m²/day of 8.4%).

RENAL HYPERKALAEMIA

Slow IV injection, all ages, 1mmol/kg (1ml/kg of 8.4%) as a single dose.

RESUSCITATION

Slow IV injection, 1ml/kg of 8.4% initially, followed by 0.5ml/kg if necessary. See page 234 for resuscitation guidelines.

Administration: Dilute with glucose 5% or sodium chloride 0.9%. For peripheral administration dilute to 1 in 10 or use 1.26% infusion. Dilute 1 in 5 for central administration and only give neat (i.e. 4.2% for neonates and 8.4% for infants and children) in an arrest or other emergency situations.

Notes:

a) The use of sodium bicarbonate in respiratory acidosis and resuscitation has become controversial.
b) If serum sodium levels are high THAM may be considered.
c) The 1.26% infusion is isotonic.
d) Sodium bicarbonate preparations suitable for dialysis are available.
e) Injection can be given orally.

SODIUM CALCIUM EDETATE

Preparations:	INJECTION 1g in 5ml.
Dosage:	TREATMENT OF LEAD POISONING

> IF IN ANY DOUBT CONTACT THE MEDICAL TOXICOLOGY UNIT
> ☎ 0171-635-9191 ☎

	IV injection, all ages, 30-40mg/kg twice a day for 5 days, repeated if necessary after 2 days. Any further courses should not be repeated for at least 7 days.
Administration:	IV infusion over 1 hour diluted with sodium chloride 0.9% or glucose 5% to 2-4mg in 1ml. In fluid restricted patients, maximum concentration is 30mg in 1ml.
Notes:	
	Sodium calcium edetate is renally cleared and therefore adequate urinary output must be established and maintained during treatment.

SODIUM CHLORIDE

Preparations:	MODIFIED RELEASE TABLETS 600mg (10mmol of sodium and chloride).
	LIQUID 1mmol in 1ml and 2mmol in 1ml (**Both manufactured specials**).
	INJECTION 0.9% (0.15mmol of sodium and chloride in 1ml) 2ml, 5ml, 10ml and 100ml. INJECTION 30% (5mmol of sodium and chloride in 1ml) 10ml.
	INFUSION 0.45% (0.075mmol of sodium and chloride in 1ml) 500ml, 0.9% 100ml, 250ml and 500ml, 1.8% (0.3mmol of sodium and chloride in 1ml) 500ml.
	EYE/NOSE DROPS sodium chloride 0.9% .
Dosage:	SODIUM SUPPLEMENTATION
	Adjust the dose according to serum levels.
	CHRONIC RENAL LOSS
	Orally, 1-2mmol sodium/kg/day.
	NASAL CONGESTION
	Instill, 1-2 drops of 0.9% sodium chloride into each nostril before feeds.
Notes:	

a) Injection can be given orally.
b) 2mmol in 1ml liquid is preserved with chloroform and is NOT suitable for infants under 3 months of age. The 1mmol in 1ml liquid is unpreserved, expiry is 7 days after opening.

SODIUM CROMOGLYCATE

Preparations: INHALER 5mg/metered inhalation 112 dose unit (Intal®). SPINCAPS 20mg for use with a spinhaler (**Non-formulary**). NEBULES 20mg in 2ml (**Non-formulary**). NASAL SPRAY 4% (5.2mg/metered dose) (Rynacrom®). EYE DROPS 2% (Opticrom®).

Dosage: ***ASTHMA THERAPY***
Inhaled,
Intal® inhaler: initially 10mg (2 puffs) 4 times a day. In severe cases increase to 6-8 times a day. It may be possible to reduce to a maintenance dose of 5mg (1 puff) 4 times a day.
Spincaps: Over 4 years, one spincap (20mg) 4 times a day.
Nebulised,
Under 1 year, 10-20mg 4 times a day.
Over 1 year, 20mg up to 4 times a day, increasing in severe cases to 6 times a day. Dilute to 3-4ml with sodium chloride 0.9%.

ALLERGIC RHINITIS
Nasal spray 4%: Over 1 year, one spray into each nostril 2-4 times a day.

ALLERGIC CONJUNCTIVITIS
Eye drops 2%: 1-2 drops in each eye 4 times a day.

Notes:

a) The use of sodium cromoglycate in the treatment of asthma is controversial but may be effective in 'atopic' children sensitive to a wide variety of allergenic substances.

b) Regular administration is necessary for effective use.

c) Children under 4 years are usually incapable of using Spinhalers. Children under 10 years are usually incapable of using inhalers.

d) The inhaler will roughly fit a Nebuhaler® and so can be used in young children.

e) Occasionally spincaps cause bronchospasm, and in these circumstances the aerosol inhaler may be used or salbutamol can be inhaled 5-10 minutes beforehand.

f) A whistle may be attached to the Spinhaler to aid compliance in young children.

g) The Spinhaler should be dismantled and washed thoroughly twice weekly. Allow to dry thoroughly before use.

h) Spincaps should be kept in original container. Stable for only 24 hours in carrying case.

i) See management guidelines for chronic asthma page 241.

SODIUM FUSIDATE

Preparations:	TABLETS 250mg sodium fusidate. LIQUID 250mg fusidic acid in 5ml which is therapeutically equivalent to 175mg sodium fusidate in 5ml. INJECTION 500mg sodium fusidate. VISCOUS EYE DROPS 1% fusidic acid (Fucithalmic®).
Dosage:	***EYE PREPARATIONS***

Instil, into the affected eye/s TWICE a day. See note a).

TREATMENT OF STAPHYLOCOCCAL INFECTION

Use in combination with another staphylococcal agent because resistance develops rapidly if used alone. Seek expert advice from microbiology before prescribing.

Orally,
(See note f).

Under 1 year	0.3ml/kg	3 times a day
1 - 5 years	5ml	3 times a day
5 - 12 years	10ml	3 times a day
Over 12 year	15ml or 2 tablets	3 times a day

Intravenous Infusion,
Neonates and Children less than 50kg, 6-7mg/kg of sodium fusidate three times a day.
Children over 50kg, 500mg of sodium fusidate 3 times a day.
Doses may be doubled in SEVERE infections.

Administration: Reconstitute vial with the 10ml phosphate-citrate buffer provided. Displacement volume is negligible. Further dilute to 1mg in 1ml with sodium chloride 0.9%, and infuse slowly over at least 6 hours. Can administer over 2 hours if via central line.

Notes:

a) Fusidic acid 1% viscous eye drops are recommended for initial treatment. Chloramphenicol eye preparations are only indicated for neonates (in NICU/SCBU) and when sensitivities show that fusidic acid is not appropriate.

b) Sodium fusidate absorption is very good, use the oral route whenever practicable.

c) No modification of dosage is necessary in renal failure, however 10ml of phosphate-citrate buffer contains 1.1mmol of phosphate. Sodium content is 3.1mmol when reconstituted.

d) Jaundice may occur, particularly with high doses and/or when intravenous infusions are infused at too high a concentration or too rapidly. This usually resolves if sodium fusidate is stopped.

e) Doses in excess of the recommended IV dose may result in hypocalcaemia due to the large amount of phosphate/citrate buffer administered.

f) Sodium fusidate displaces bilirubin from its albumin binding sites in vitro, however the clinical significance of this is uncertain.

g) Fusidic acid liquid (Fucidin®) contains 1.25g of glucose in 5ml.

SODIUM NITROPRUSSIDE

Preparations:	INJECTION 50mg, plus 2ml glucose 5% for reconstitution.
Dosage:	**VASODILATION**
	This indication is unlicensed for use in children.
	Initially 500nanogram/kg/minute increasing in increments of 200nanogram/kg/minute as necessary to a maximum of 8microgram/kg/minute. If treatment for more than 24 hours, maximum of 4microgram/kg/minute. Wean dose on withdrawal to avoid any rebound effects.
Administration:	Reconstitute contents of each vial with the 2ml **glucose 5%** provided then further dilute to a concentration of 200microgram in 1ml with glucose 5% or sodium chloride 0.9%. If fluid restricted, maximum concentration is 1mg in 1ml. Protect infusion from light and use an amber giving set. **Discard after 24 hours**. Discard if the solution changes from pale orange to dark brown or blue.
Notes:	

a) If treatment continues for more than 72 hours, measure serum thiocyanate levels which should be less than 100mg/L (1.7mmol/L).
b) In hypertensive encephalopathy a rapid reduction in blood pressure to normotensive levels can result in water shed cerebral infarction, blindness or death.
c) Use with caution in severe liver or renal impairment, impaired cerebral circulation and hypothyroidism.
d) Sodium nitroprusside can **only** be reconstituted with glucose 5%.

SODIUM PHENYLBUTYRATE

Preparations:	TABLETS 500mg (**Manufactured special**).
	INJECTION 1g in 10ml (**Manufactured special**).
Dosage:	**TREATMENT OF UREA CYCLE DEFECTS**

> **SEEK EXPERT ADVICE FROM METABOLIC TEAM BEFORE PRESCRIBING**

Orally, all ages, initially, 250mg/kg/day usually in 3 to 4 divided doses.
IV injection, total daily dose as a continuous infusion over 24 hours.
ACUTE HYPERAMMONAEMIA
Doses may be increased up to maximum of 500mg/kg/day.

Administration:	Dilute to 20mg in 1ml with glucose 10% or 5%, maximum concentration is 50mg in 1ml.
	Administer as a continuous infusion (see note a).
Notes:	

a) Sodium benzoate and sodium phenylbutyrate may be administered together as an intravenous infusion.
b) Aim to maintain plasma concentration of ammonia below 60micromol/L and glutamine below 800micromol/L.
c) 2mmol of Nitrogen is theoretically cleared by 1mmol of sodium phenylbutyrate (500mg = 2.7mmol).
e) Injection can be given orally.
d) Give with food to reduce nausea and vomiting and increase palatability.
f) 1g contains 5.4mmol of sodium.

SODIUM PICOSULPHATE

Preparations: SACHETS 10mg. LIQUID 5mg in 5ml.

Dosage: **BOWEL EVACUATION BEFORE ABDOMINAL PROCEDURES, CONSTIPATION**

Orally,

Sachets:

1 - 2 years	0.25 sachet	twice a day
2 - 4 years	0.50 sachet	twice a day
4 - 9 years	1 sachet	am and
	0.50 sachet	evening
Over 9 years	1 sachet	twice a day

Give the above dose in the morning and then again in the early evening, on the day prior to procedure.

For treatment of constipation use above dose only **once** a day.

Liquid:

For constipation,

2 - 5 years	2.5ml at night
5 - 10 years	2.5-5ml at night
Over 10 years	5-15ml at night

Notes:

a)   Initially powder should be mixed with 30ml of water, followed by approximately 120ml after 5 minutes once the heat generated in the solution cools off.

b)   Each sachet contains 0.33mmol of sodium.

c)   Oral powder is sugar free.

d)   Sodium picosulphate liquid (Dulcolax®/Laxoberal®) is sugar and aspartame free but contains 6.2% alcohol.

SODIUM VALPROATE

Preparations: CRUSHABLE TABLETS 100mg. ENTERIC COATED TABLETS 200mg and 500mg. MODIFIED RELEASE TABLETS (Epilim Chrono®) 200mg, 300mg and 500mg. LIQUID 200mg in 5ml. INJECTION 400mg.

Dosage: **EPILEPSY**

Orally,

Under 20kg Initially 20mg/kg/day in divided doses, increasing if necessary by increments of 5mg/kg at weekly intervals.

Over 20kg Initially 400mg a day in divided doses, increasing if necessary until control is achieved. Maintenance dose is usually within the range of 20- 30mg/kg/day in divided doses.

Higher doses have been used, if above 40mg/kg/day, regularly monitor biochemistry and FBC.

Modified release tablets may be useful if peak level effects are a problem. Total daily dose may be administered as a **single** dose.

Slow IV injection,

All ages, 10mg/kg 2 times a day. For patients on satisfactory oral maintenance doses, give the same dose IV.

Administration: Reconstitute each vial with 4ml of diluent provided to give a solution of **95mg in 1ml.** Give slowly over 3-5 minutes.

Notes:

a) Therapeutic drug monitoring: Dosage is determined by seizure control rather than plasma levels, however they may be of value when there is poor compliance and/or side-effects are suspected. Therapeutic range 40-100mg/L.

b) Whilst raised liver enzymes are not uncommon with sodium valproate treatment, liver dysfunction (including fatal hepatic failure) has occurred. Liver function monitoring may be advisable in the first 6 months of treatment in those most at risk i.e. under 3 years, with metabolic/degenerative disorders and on multiple antiepileptic drugs. Patient/carer should be advised to report any signs of liver disorder e.g. persistent nausea, vomiting, malaise, fever or jaundice.

c) During concomitant administration of phenobarbitone and sodium valproate, blood levels of phenobarbitone may be increased and sedation may occur. During concomitant administration with phenytoin or carbamazepine blood levels of sodium valproate may be reduced. Dosage of sodium valproate may need to be increased by 5-10mg/kg/day. Concomitant administration with lamotrigine requires a reduction in dosage of lamotrigine.

d) Sodium valproate has been associated with thrombocytopenia and inhibition of platelet aggregation. A full blood count should be considered prior to surgery.

e) Ancedotally, the sodium valproate liquid has been used rectally. It should be retained for at least 15 minutes. Suppositories (100mg and 300mg) can be imported on a "named patient basis".

f) Although Convulex® claims to be bioequivalent caution is needed when changing brands of sodium valproate preparations.

g) Sodium valproate liquid (Epilim®) is sucrose free.

SOMATROPIN

Preparations:	MULTI DOSE AND PENFILL VIALS 16 unit and 32 unit (for use in Pen device). **(Purchased on request)**.
Dosage:	**CHRONIC RENAL INSUFFICIENCY**

Subcutaneously, 1 unit/kg/week in 7 divided doses; adjustment may be required after 6 months.

INSUFFICIENT SECRETION OF GROWTH HORMONE

Subcutaneously, 0.5 to 0.7 units/kg/week in 5 to 7 divided doses.

GONADAL DYSGENESIS (TURNER SYNDROME)

Subcutaneously, 0.6 to 1 unit/kg/week in 5 to 7 divided doses.

Administration: Reconstitute each vial as directed. Do not shake vigorously as this may denature the growth hormone. Once reconstituted, the vial can be stored in a fridge for up to 2 weeks. The vials are intended for multidose use.

Notes:

a) This preparation is only available on prescription by consultants in paediatrics or endocrinology. The indications are usually limited to children with height below the third centile, currently retarded growth velocity, proven deficiency of growth hormone and open epiphyses.

b) Somatropin preparations are changing to be expressed as mass units instead of international units: 1 unit of somatropin = 0.33mg

1mg of somatropin = 3 units

SOTALOL

Preparations:	TABLETS 40mg and 80mg.
	LIQUID **(Extemporaneously prepared)**.
Dosage:	**ANTIARRHYTMIC**

SEEK EXPERT ADVICE BEFORE PRESCRIBING

This indication is unlicensed for use in children.

All ages, *orally*, 1-2mg/kg three times a day; up to maximum 4mg/kg three times a day.

IN RENAL FAILURE

Creatinine clearance (ml/min/1.73m^2)	Dosage
30 - 60	½ dose
10 - 30	¼ dose
<10	Not recommended

Notes:

a) QT interval must be documented before and with any change in dosage. Caution should be used if the QT_c exceeds 500msec, dose should be reduced or therapy discontinued if QT_c exceeds 550msec.

b) Therapeutic drug monitoring:
   i) Approx. time to steady state: 2-3 days.
   ii) Therapeutic range: 0.04 - 2.0mg/l.
   iii) Take trough blood sample immediately prior next dose.

c) **Warning:** concomitant administration of cisapride, phenothiazines, terfenadine, astemizole and any drugs which lengthen the QT interval may precipitate arrhythmias.

d) As bioavailability may vary by 20% depending on whether sotalol is administered in a fasting or non-fasting state give with food/feed.

SPIRONOLACTONE

Preparations:	TABLETS 25mg and 100mg.
	LIQUID 25mg in 5ml **(Manufactured special)**.
Dosage:	*DIURESIS, ASCITES*
	Orally, all ages, initially, 3mg/kg/day in 1-2 divided doses (see note b).
Notes:	

a) Spironolactone has been shown to be carcinogenic **in rats** when high doses are given over prolonged periods of time. The clinical significance of this remains uncertain.

b) Cardiac children being treated with frusemide are usually prescribed concomitant spironolactone at the same dose, on a mg/kg basis as the frusemide to maintain potassium levels.

c) Spironolactone may increase digoxin levels.

d) Spironolactone liquid is sugar-free.

STREPTOKINASE

Preparations:	INJECTION containing 1,500,000 international units of streptokinase.
Dosage:	*FEMORAL ARTERY THROMBOSIS POST CARDIAC CATHETERISATION*
	All ages, **IF** fibrinogen >1.5g/L then, *IV injection* 1,000 international units/kg over 30 minutes then 1,000 international units/kg/hr for up to 72 hours (Maximum of 6 days). Check fibrinogen levels every 4 hours. **IF** level <1g/L, stop streptokinase and start heparin at 40units/kg/hr until fibrinogen levels reach 1g/L, streptokinase can then be restarted.
Administration:	Reconstitute vial with 5ml sodium chloride 0.9%. Further dilute with glucose 5% or sodium chloride 0.9%.
Notes:	

a) Haemorrhage is the most common complication. Allergic reactions including chills, bronchospasm and urticaria which may be unresponsive to steroids are not uncommon. Pyrexia which may be related to degradation products of the thrombus is commonly seen.

b) Streptokinase should be used with caution if a surgical or invasive procedure has been performed within the last 10 days.

c) Streptokinase should not be given to patients who have received streptokinase before or who have had a proven streptococcal infection within the last 12 months due to the formation of antibodies.

STREPTOMYCIN

Preparations:	INJECTION 1g (**Named patient**).
Dosage:	*TUBERCULOSIS THERAPY*

> **SEEK EXPERT ADVICE BEFORE PRESCRIBING**

IM injection, 15mg/kg once a day (maximum dose 1g). Change the injection site for each dose. Reduce the dose in renal failure, adjusting according to blood levels. Only include if ethambutol is contraindicated and there is a high risk of resistant infection.

Administration: On reconstitution 1g displaces 0.8ml. Add 4.2ml water for injection to 1g vial to give 1g in 5ml.

Notes:

a) Higher doses can be used initially but are ototoxic and nephrotoxic if continued.

b) Therapeutic drug monitoring:
   i) Approx. time to steady state: 24 hrs.
   ii) Therapeutic plasma levels: trough < 3mg/L
   peak 20-40mg/L
   iii) Take trough sample immediately prior to next dose and peak sample 1 hour after dose.

c) In renal failure give first dose as above, then give further doses when plasma levels are <3mg/L. If the trough level exceeds 3mg/L, the dosage should be reduced.

SUCCIMER (DMSA)

Preparations:	CAPSULES 100mg (**Named patient**). 300mg (**Extemporaneously prepared**).
Dosage:	*TREATMENT OF LEAD POISONING*

> **IF IN ANY DOUBT CONTACT THE MEDICAL TOXICOLOGY UNIT**
> ☎ 0171-635-9191 ☎

Orally, all ages, 10mg/kg 3 times a day for 5 days then 10mg/kg twice a day for 14 days. The course may be repeated after an interval of at least 2 weeks.

Notes:

a) Succimer can increase the absorption of lead from the gut and therefore should not be administered until after a clear abdominal x-ray.

b) Capsules can be opened and contents mixed with food or drink.

SUCRALFATE

Preparations:	TABLETS 1g. LIQUID 1g in 5ml.
Dosage:	**STRESS ULCER PROPHYLAXIS**

This indication is unlicensed for use in children.

0 - 2 years	250mg	4 times a day
3 - 12 years	500mg	4 times a day
Over 12 years	1g	4 times a day

Maximum 8g/**day**.

Notes:

a) Tablets may be dispersed in 10-15ml of water immediately prior to administration.

b) Sucralfate may reduce the bioavailability of tetracycline, phenytoin, ciprofloxacin, cimetidine, digoxin and warfarin. Concurrent administration with any of these drugs should be separated by 2 hours.

c) Sucralfate, although a complex of aluminium hydroxide and sulphated sucrose, has very little antacid properties. If an antacid is required it should be given half an hour before or after sucralfate.

d) Use with caution in renal failure as small amounts of aluminium may be absorbed.

e) Sucralfate liquid is sugar-free.

SULPHASALAZINE

Preparations:	TABLETS 500mg. ENTERIC COATED TABLETS 500mg. LIQUID 250mg in 5ml (**Non-formulary**). SUPPOSITORIES 500mg.
Dosage:	**ULCERATIVE COLITIS AND CROHN'S DISEASE**

Warn all patients/carers to report immediately any sore throats, fever, malaise or non-specific illness.

This indication is unlicensed for use in children under 2 years, due to increased incidence of side effects.

Orally, over 1 year, 10mg/kg 4-6 hourly for an acute attack. Decrease the dose by 50% when possible, for maintenance therapy.

Notes:

a) Sulphasalazine should be used with caution in glucose-6-phosphate dehydrogenase (G6PD) deficiency and is contra-indicated in salicylate or sulphonamide hypersensitivity or megaloblastic anaemia.

b) Use with caution in renal and liver failure.

c) Side effects are more common in slow acetylators and include hepatotoxicity, skin rashes, blood dyscrasias and polyarteritis nodosa.

d) Sulphasalazine reduces serum levels of digoxin.

e) Urine and tears may be stained an orange colour.

f) Sulphasalazine liquid contains approximately 1.2g of sucrose in 5ml.

SUXAMETHONIUM

Preparations: INJECTION 100mg in 2ml.
Dosage: ***MUSCLE RELAXANT FOR INTUBATION***
     IV injection,
     Neonates and infants, initially 2mg/kg.
     Children, initially 1-2mg/kg.
     Maximum dose 2.5mg/kg.
     (Maximum adult dose in an hour is 500mg).
Notes:

a)   Suxamethonium is not recommended in severe liver disease, burns patients or Duchenne muscular dystrophy.

b)   **Caution:** may cause bradycardia, especially in children and following a second dose.

c)   Profound hyperkalaemia may occur especially in burns, trauma and renal failure patients.

d)   Can lead to prolonged paralysis due to low levels of pseudocholinesterase e.g. liver disease, or genetically determined variants of pseudocholinesterase.

TACROLIMUS

Preparations:	CAPSULES 1mg, 5mg. LIQUID (**Extemporaneously prepared**). INJECTION 5mg in 1ml.
Dosage:	***REFRACTORY RENAL ALLOGRAFT REJECTION, STEROID RESISTANT NEPHROTIC SYNDROME***

The treatment of nephrotic syndrome is an unlicensed indication.

SEEK EXPERT ADVICE BEFORE PRESCRIBING

Orally, initially, 100-150microgram/kg twice a day.

IV injection, initially, **50-100microgram/kg/day** as a continuous infusion.

Administration: Dilute with dextrose 5% or sodium chloride 0.9%. Tacrolimus is incompatible with PVC, administration should be via a syringe pump (with Plastipak® or Gillette Sabre® syringe) or via a rigid burette set with non-PVC tubing (Lectrocath® or Gloucester® tubing).

Notes:

a) Give on an empty stomach (i.e. 1 hour before or 3 hours after food) to increase absorption.

b) Therapeutic drug monitoring:
   i) Approx. time to steady state: 1-2 days.
   ii) Therapeutic whole blood levels: 5-20mg/L.
   iii) Take trough sample, immediately prior to next dose.

c) Tacrolimus is metabolised by the cytochrome P450 enzyme system and may have an inducing or inhibiting effect on these enzymes. Care should be taken with the concomitant administration of other drugs metabolised by these enzymes.
   Tacrolimus is also extensively bound to plasma proteins. For information on possible drug interactions contact the paediatric pharmacist by bleep or drug information on:

☎ Guy's ext. 3594, Lewisham ext. 3202, St Thomas' ext. 3069 ☎

d) Monitor ciclosporin levels after converting to tacrolimus as clearance of ciclosporin may be affected.

e) **CSM warning:** hypertrophic cardiomyopathy has been reported. ECG/echocardiology monitoring should be performed to observe for changes.

f) After opening, the contents of the ampoule should be used immediately.

g) Tacrolimus injection contains polyethoxylated castor oil which has been reported to cause anaphylactic reactions.

TEICOPLANIN

Preparations: INJECTION 200mg and 400mg.
Dosage:

> **SEEK ADVICE FROM MICROBIOLOGY BEFORE PRESCRIBING**

MODERATE INFECTION WITH GRAM POSITIVE ORGANISMS
Over 2 months:
Slow IV injection   10mg/kg every 12 hours for **3 doses**
                        THEN
                        6mg/kg once a day.

SEVERE INFECTIONS, NEUTROPENIC PATIENTS
Premature and term neonates:
IV infusion   16mg/kg as a **single dose**
                        THEN 24 hours later
                        8mg/kg once a day.

Over 2 months:
Slow IV Injection   10mg/kg every 12 hours for **3 doses**
                        THEN
                        10mg/kg once a day.

IN RENAL FAILURE

Dosage reduction is not required until the **fourth** day of treatment then

Creatinine clearance (ml/minute/1.73m^2)	Dosage
40-60	Half normal dose
< 40 or haemodialysis	Third normal dose

Teicoplanin is **not** removed by haemodialysis.

Administration: Reconstitute vial with the diluent provided. Roll vial gently to dissolve. If foaming occurs, allow to stand for 15 minutes. Resultant concentration of 200mg and 400mg vial is 200mg in 3ml and 400mg in 3ml respectively.
Give as slow IV injection, over 5 minutes or as an IV infusion over 30 minutes. Dilute if required with sodium chloride 0.9% or glucose 5%.

Notes:

a) Use with caution in patients with known hypersensitivity to vancomycin.
b) Ototoxicity and nephrotoxicity may be potentiated by concomitant administration of other drugs with these side-effects; including aminoglycosides, frusemide, cisplatin, ciclosporin and amphotericin.
c) Therapeutic drug monitoring:
These are not routinely done as a relationship between toxicity and serum level has not been demonstrated, but may be of benefit in optimising therapy especially in renal failure.
   i)   Approx. time to steady state: after loading completed.
   ii) Therapeutic levels: trough   >10mg/L
                               peak   20-50mg/L
   iii) Take trough sample immediately prior to next dose and peak sample 1 hour after dose.

TEMAZEPAM - (CD)

Preparations: TABLETS 10mg. LIQUID 10mg in 5ml.
Dosage: **PREMEDICATION**
Orally, all ages, 0.5-1mg/kg, 1 hour prior to procedure. Maximum 30mg/**dose**.

Notes:
a) Temazepam liquid (Pharmacia/Rosemont) are sucrose free.
b) See premedication guidelines page 250.

TERBINAFINE

Preparations: TABLETS 250mg. CREAM 1%.
Dosage: **TREATMENT OF DERMATOPHYTES, MOULDS AND SOME FUNGAL INFECTIONS**

SEEK EXPERT ADVICE BEFORE PRESCRIBING

These indications are unlicensed for use in children.
Orally, over 1 year old, 3 - 6 mg/kg once a day.
OR

Less than 20kg	62.5mg once a day
20 - 40kg	125mg once a day
Greater than 40kg	250mg once a day

Recommended treatment duration is 4-8 weeks for tinea capitis, 6 weeks for fingernail onchomycosis and 12 weeks for toe-nail onchomycosis.
Topically, apply the cream twice a day for up to 2 weeks for tinea corporis or 1 week for tinea pedis.

IN RENAL OR HEPATIC FAILURE
If creatinine clearance is less than 50ml/minute/$1.73m^2$ or if in stable, chronic liver failure then reduce dose by 50%.

Notes:
a) Taste disturbances have been reported. This usually resolves slowly on discontinuation of drug.
b) Plasma levels are reduced by rifampicin and increased by cimetidine.

TERBUTALINE

Preparations: INHALER 250microgram/metered inhalation, 400 dose unit.
TURBOHALER 500microgram/metered inhalation, 100 dose unit.
RESPIRATOR SOLUTION 10mg in 1ml (**Non-formulary**).
RESPULES 5mg in 2ml.
INJECTION 500microgram in 1ml and 2.5mg in 5ml

Dosage: ***ASTHMA THERAPY***

Inhaled initially 250-500microgram up to 4 times a day. In some cases higher doses may be necessary - seek expert advice.
Turbohaler over 4 years, 1 dose up to 4 times a day.
Respirator solution 200-250microgram/kg 2-4 times a day, see note a).
OR

<3 years	0.2ml (2mg)	) up to
3 - 5 years	0.3ml (3mg)	) 4 times
6 - 8 years	0.4ml (4mg)	) a day
>8 years	0.5ml (5mg)	)
Respules		
<25kg	use solution	) use 2-4 times
>25kg	1 respule (5mg)	) a day (see note a)

Dilute with sodium chloride 0.9% to maximum of 4ml.
Injection SC, IM or slow IV injection (preferred routes SC or IM) 2 - 15 years, 10microgram/kg up to 4 times a day. Maximum total dose of 300microgram.

Notes:

a) Terbutaline may be nebulised more frequently in hospital under close supervision.
b) Terbutaline may not be effective in children under 1 year of age.
c) Children under 10 years are usually incapable of using inhalers, however children over 4 years may be able to use the turbohaler.
d) The turbohaler is a breath activated device which is effective at low respiratory flow rates, 30L/minute.
e) A Nebuhaler® spacer (with or without mask) is available for use with the aerosol inhaler. If a Nebuhaler® or mask is not available, in an emergency situation, a hole just large enough for the inhaler mouthpiece can be cut in the bottom of a polystyrene cup. The inhaler is fitted into this and the cup can then be placed over the child's nose and mouth, however larger doses may be required.
f) See management guidelines for acute asthma page 244 and chronic asthma page 241.

TESTOSTERONE

Preparations: CREAM 5% (**Manufactured special**). DEPOT INJECTION (Sustanon 100®) equivalent to 74mg of testosterone.

Dosage: **MICROPHALLUS**

Apply *topically* to the penis 3 times a day for 3 weeks.

TREATMENT OF DELAYED MALE PUBERTY

Deep IM injection, 1ml of Sustanon 100® every month for 3 doses.

Notes:

Depot injection contains arachis oil and is contraindicated in patients with peanut allergy.

TETANUS TOXOID

Preparations: INJECTION Adsorbed tetanus vaccine BP 0.5ml and 5ml, containing not less than 40i.u. of tetanus toxoid in 0.5ml.

Dosage: **PRIMARY IMMUNISATION**

Course of three *IM injections*, each of 0.5ml. Second dose after 4 weeks and third dose after a further 4 weeks. See immunisation guidelines page 261.

BOOSTER-DOSE

IM injection, 0.5ml 3 years after basic course (at school entry), then 10 years later (at school leaving). Two booster doses should give life long immunity.

IN THE EVENT OF TETANUS PRONE WOUND

IM injection, 0.5ml unless booster-dose has been given in the last 10 years.

Notes:

a) If the wound is thought to be 'tetanus-prone' and the child has not been previously immunised, then tetanus immunoglobulin is indicated.
b) **Caution:** Adsorbed vaccine is NOT for intradermal use.

TETRACOSACTRIN (TETRACOSACTIDE) (ACTH 1-24)

Preparations: INJECTION 250microgram in 1ml for IM or IV injection.
DEPOT INJECTION 1mg in 1ml for IM injection only.

Dosage: **STIMULATION TEST**

(Do **not** use depot injection).

Below 1 month, not suitable as indeterminate response seen due to immature liver function.

Over 1 month, note the plasma cortisol levels immediately before and 30 minutes after a single *IV injection* dose of 250microgram/1.73m^2 (145microgram/m^2).

ADRENOCORTICAL INSUFFICIENCY THERAPEUTIC DOSE
(Depot *IM injection*):

1 month-2 years,	Initially 250microgram once a day for up to 3 days.
	Maintenance 250microgram every 2-8 days.
2-5 years,	Initially 250-500microgram once a day for up to 3 days.
	Maintenance 250-500microgram every 2-8 days.
5-12 years,	Initially 250microgram-1mg once a day for up to 3 days.
	Maintenance 250microgram-1mg every 2-8 days.

INFANTILE SPASMS

This is an unlicensed indication.
(Depot IM injection)
IM injection, initially, 500microgram once a day.

Notes:

a) Plasma cortisol levels should be greater than 200nanomol/L (70microgram/L) 30 minutes after stimulation test.
b) In patients with a history of allergic disorders, tetracosactride should only be administered if no ACTH preparations have previously been given.
c) Tetracosactrin depot injection is best given into the buttock.
d) Depot injection is contraindicated in neonates.

THAM (TROMETAMOL)

Preparations: INJECTION 7.2% in 5ml (**Manufactured special**).
Dosage: ***TO CORRECT ACIDOSIS***

SEEK EXPERT ADVICE BEFORE PRESCRIBING

Check blood gases, repeat every 15 minutes or as required.

Total number of mmol of bicarbonate required can be calculated by: F x base deficit (mmol/L) x weight (kg).

F represents the extracellular fluid: weight ratio. This is 0.5-0.6 in premature neonates, 0.4 in neonates and 0.3 in infants and children.
Only **half** the base deficit should be corrected initially and blood glucose, pH and electrolytes analysed before correction of the remaining half.
As an approximate guide:
1ml of 7.2% THAM = 1mmol bicarbonate
Do not exceed a **total** dose of 15mmol/kg/24hours.

Administration: Dilute at least 1 in 2 with glucose 5% or water for injection. Can be given neat, in fluid restricted patients, via a central or long line. Do not exceed a rate of 5mmol/kg/hour.

Notes:

a) THAM should only be used where **sodium bicarbonate** is unsuitable e.g. when PCO_2 or sodium levels are raised.
b) Injection solution can be given orally.

THEOPHYLLINE

Preparations: MODIFIED RELEASE CAPSULES 60mg and 250mg (Slo-Phyllin®) and 125mg (**Non-formulary**).

MODIFIED RELEASE TABLETS 200mg (Uniphyllin Continus®) and 400mg (**Non-formulary**).

LIQUID theophylline sodium glycinate equivalent to theophylline hydrate 60mg in 5ml (Nuelin®).

Dosage: **ASTHMA THERAPY**

This indication is unlicensed for use in children under 2 years.

Oral liquid theophylline dosage:
Initially, all ages, 5mg/kg 3-4 times a day.

Oral slow release preparation dosage:

1 - 7 years	12mg/kg	twice a day
8 - 12 years	10mg/kg	twice a day
Over 12 years	8mg/kg	twice a day

Maximum of 500mg per dose.

OR

2 - 6 years	60-120mg	twice a day
6 - 12 years	125-250mg	twice a day
Over 12 years	250-500mg	twice a day

TAKE TROUGH BLOOD SAMPLE AT LEAST **8** HOURS AFTER SLOW RELEASE FORMULATIONS OR IMMEDIATELY PRIOR TO THE NEXT DOSE FOR THE LIQUID.

Serum concentration at steady state	Suggestion
Below 7.5mg/L	Increase dose by about 25%. ❶
7.5-10mg/L	Increase dose by about 25% if tolerated.
10-20mg/L	Maintain dose if tolerated; repeat serum assay 6-12 monthly.
20-25mg/L	Decrease dose by at least 10%. ❶
25-30mg/L	Omit next dose, decrease later ones by at least 25%. ❶
Over 30mg/L	Omit next 2 doses, halve later ones. ❶

❶ Repeat serum assay 3-7 days later.

Notes:

a) When prescribing oral theophylline start with the lowest recommended dose. This can be adjusted at 3-7 day intervals according to clinical response or the development of unwanted effects.

b) 80mg theophylline is equivalent to 100mg aminophylline.

c) As a guideline, for every 1mg/kg of theophylline administered as a loading dose, serum concentrations will rise by approximately 2mg/L.

d) Cimetidine, erythromycin and ciprofloxacin may increase blood levels of xanthine derivatives.

e) Barbiturates, carbamazepine, phenytoin and rifampicin may reduce blood levels of xanthine derivatives.

f) Slo-Phyllin® capsules contain individual slow-release granules and young children may find the loose granules (which can be sprinkled on a spoonful of soft food e.g. yoghurt) easier to swallow than capsules or tablets. However the loose granules must not be chewed.

g) Theophylline liquid (Nuelin®) contains 3.5g of sucrose in 5mls.

THIOPENTONE SODIUM

Preparations: INJECTION 500mg and 2.5g, plus water for injection for reconstitution.

Dosage: **INDUCTION OF ANAESTHESIA**

IV injection,

neonates 2mg/kg over 10-15 seconds

over 1 month 4-6mg/kg over 10-15 seconds

STATUS EPILEPTICUS

This indication is unlicensed for use in children.

ENLIST THE AID OF ANAESTHETIST

IV injection, initially, 4-8mg/kg followed by a maintenance *IV infusion* of 1-8mg/kg/hour, adjusted as necessary to control convulsions.

Administration: Reconstitute with water for injection provided to give 25mg in 1ml (20ml to 500mg vial and 100ml to 2.5g vial). Dilute if required with sodium chloride 0.9%.

Notes:

a) Use of doses exceeding 5mg/kg/hour may be associated with the possibility of hypothermia and cerebral shut down.

b) Use is not generally continued for more than 48 hours, as delayed recovery of consciousness has been encountered with prolonged use.

c) Ventilation must be available when used for status epilepticus.

d) Sulphonamides potentiate the effects of thiopentone.

e) Blood levels of thiopentone and pentobarbitone should be measured, and the ratio compared. The ideal ratio is 1:4 respectively.

f) Caution, injection is alkaline, therefore very irritant.

g) Acute intermittent porphyria is a contra-indication to use.

h) Thiopentone sodium injection contains 2.3mmol sodium per 500mg.

THYROXINE SODIUM

Preparations: TABLETS 25microgram, 50microgram and 100microgram.

CAPSULES 12.5microgram (**Manufactured special**).

LIQUID (**Extemporaneously prepared**).

Dosage: **CONGENITAL HYPOTHYROIDISM**

Initially 5microgram/kg a day, increasing by 5microgram/kg/day at intervals of 2-4 weeks, (see note a).

JUVENILE MYXOEDEMA

Under 1 year as above.

Over 1 year, initially 2.5-5microgram/kg/day, then increase as above.

Notes:

a) Dose may be adjusted by increasing until mild toxic symptoms occur then dose is reduced slightly. Dose is guided by clinical response, growth and plasma thyroxine and thyroid stimulating hormone levels.

b) Thyroxine may potentiate the effects of anticoagulants and side effects of salbutamol may be aggravated. Thyroxine may also increase requirements for hypoglycaemic drugs and insulin.

c) Administration of intravenous phenytoin to patients receiving thyroid hormones may induce supraventricular tachycardia.

d) 20microgram of liothyronine (intravenous) is equivalent to 100microgram of thyroxine.

TINZAPARIN

Preparations: PREFILLED SYRINGES 3500 units in 0.3ml, 10,000 units in 0.5ml, 14,000 units in 0.7ml, 18,000 units in 0.9ml.
INJECTION 5000units in 0.5ml.
(Guy's & St Thomas' only)

Dosage: *TREATMENT OF DEEP VEIN THROMBOSIS AND PULMONARY EMBOLISM*

These indications are unlicensed for use in children.

Subcutaneous injection, 175units/kg once a day for at least 6 days and until a therapeutic INR is reached.

Tinzaparin therapy does not require routine monitoring in patients with normal renal and hepatic function.

IN RENAL FAILURE

> **SEEK EXPERT ADVICE BEFORE PRESCRIBING**
> **CONTACT THE HAEMOPHILLIA REFERENCE CENTRE**
> ☎ ST THOMAS' EXT 3324 OR ONCALL HAEMATOLOGIST ☎

Patients with severe renal failure may require reduced doses. Monitor peak and trough anti-Xa activity on a daily basis. Take peak sample 3-4 hours after dose and trough sample immediately prior to next dose. Peak values should be between 0.8 to 1 units/ml and trough values around 0.2units/ml. Reduce dose if anti-Xa activity exceed 1unit/ml and extend dosage interval if trough exceeds 0.2units/ml.

Notes:

   a)   Anti Xa samples need to be taken from fast flowing venous blood and packed in ice immediately. Send samples to haemostatis laboratory.

   b)   Tinzaparin (Innohep®) injection contains sulphites which may lead to hypersensitivity (with bronchospasm and shock) especially in asthma patients.

TOBRAMYCIN

Preparations: INJECTIONS 40mg in 1ml and 80mg in 2ml **(Both Lewisham only)**.

Dosage: *TREATMENT OF INFECTION*

> Gentamicin is the preferred aminoglycoside. Tobramycin should be limited to treatment of cystic fibrosis and used on the basis of sensitivities.
> Seek microbiology advice before prescribing.

IV bolus,
Premature and full term neonates up to 7 days, 2mg/kg every 12 hours.
Neonates over 7 days and children, 2-2.5mg/kg every 8 hours.

CYSTIC FIBROSIS
Dose may need to be increased to 8-10mg/kg/**day**.
Use in combination with another antibiotic active against *Ps aeruginosa* or *S. aureus*.

Monitor blood levels and increase dose interval according to the table below:

Creatinine clearance (ml/minute/1.73m^2)	Dosage Interval (hours)
40-70	12
20-40	18
10-20	24
5-10	36
<5	48

Nebulised dose for cystic fibrosis
40-80mg 2-3 times a day after physiotherapy, depending on the patient's age and clinical condition.

Administration: IV injection given over 3-5 minutes or IM injection.
IV infusion in sodium chloride 0.9% or glucose 5%, given over 20 minutes.

Notes:

a) Blood levels:
   i) Approx. time to steady state: 24 hours
                                       (Unless renal impairment)
   ii) Therapeutic range: trough <2mg/L
                                       peak 6-10mg/L
   iii) Take a trough level, immediately prior to next dose **and** a peak level, 1 hour after IV or IM injection or 30 minutes after infusion.

b) Tobramycin has been added to peritoneal dialysis fluids in a concentration of 4mg/L.

c) Concurrent therapy with potent diuretics or other aminoglycosides increases the risk of ototoxicity and nephrotoxicity.

d) Neuromuscular blockade and respiratory paralysis have occurred when aminoglycosides have been administered to patients who have received non-depolarizing muscle relaxants.

e) Aminoglycosides interact with many drugs in infusion solutions so they should be administered as an IV injection or separate infusion.

TOCOPHERYL ACETATE (VITAMIN E)

Preparations: Tablets 50mg. Liquid 100mg in 1ml (**Non-formulary**).
Dosage: ***Vitamin E defiency***
Orally, all ages, 2-20mg/kg once a day.
Abetalipoprotinaemia
Orally, all ages, 50-100mg/kg once a day.
Vitamin E deficiency secondary to chronic cholestasis
Orally, all ages, 150-200mg/kg once a day.
Cystic fibrosis
Orally,

Under 1 year	50mg/day
1 - 12 years	100mg/day
Over 12 years	100-200mg/day

Notes:

a) Gastrointestinal disturbances (diarrhoea and abdominal pain) may occur with large doses.
b) An increased risk of thrombosis has been reported.
c) Liquid is alcohol free and contains 1g of sucrose in 5ml.

TOLAZOLINE

Preparations:	INJECTION 25mg in 1ml (**Manufactured Special**). (**Lewisham only**).
Dosage:	*PULMONARY HYPERTENSION*
	IV injection, 1-2 mg/kg given over 5 minutes, watch hypotension, then continuous IV infusion 1-6microgram/kg/minute.
Administration:	IV injection, over 5-10 minutes or IV infusion, diluted with sodium chloride 0.9% or glucose 5%, via a central line.
Notes:	

a)   Tolazoline should only be reserved for those cases where alternative therapy is contraindicated or unavailable.

b)   Tolazoline may cause profound hypotension, continuous blood pressure monitoring required.

TOPIRAMATE

Preparations:	TABLETS 25mg and 100mg. 50mg and 200mg (**Non-formulary**).
Dosage:	*ADJUNCTIVE THERAPY FOR EPILEPSY*

This indication is unlicensed for use in children under 2 years.

Orally, initially, 0.5mg/kg once a day for one week, then 0.5mg/kg twice a day for one week, then 1mg/kg twice a day for one week, then 1.5mg/kg twice a day for one week, then 3mg/kg twice a day for one week, then 4.5mg/kg twice a day. However doses over **7mg/kg/day** may cause unacceptable drowsiness.

Dosage escalation should be determined by toleration of CNS side effects.

IN RENAL FAILURE

If creatinine clearance is less than 20ml/minute/$1.73m^2$ time to steady state is increased therefore allow two weeks between dosage increases. Titrate dose by efficacy and side effects.

Notes:

a)   Topiramate may increase blood levels of phenytoin. Topiramate may decrease digoxin blood levels.

b)   Carbamazepine and phenytoin may decrease blood level of topiramate.

c)   Topiramate may be associated with an increased risk of nephrolithiasis. Avoid concomitant administration of drugs which may cause nephrolithiasis. Ensure adequate hydration to reduce the risk.

d)   A suspension is not available as the tablets are very bitter, however the tablets may be crushed and mixed with a strong tasting drink or food.

TRANEXAMIC ACID

Preparations:	TABLETS 500mg. LIQUID 500mg in 5ml (**Non-formulary**).
	INJECTION 500mg in 5ml.
Dosage:	**HAEMORRHAGE**

Orally, 25mg/kg 2-3 times a day.
Slow IV injection, 10mg/kg 2-3 times a day.

IN RENAL FAILURE
Reduce the dose in renal failure, according to serum creatinine levels.

Creatinine clearance (ml/minute/1.73m^2)	Dose	Dose frequency
25-50	As above	Twice a day
15-25	As above	Once a day
< 15	Half the above dose	Once a day

As tranexamic acid is removed by haemodialysis, give the dose (5-10mg/kg) post-dialysis.

Administration:	Slow IV injection over 10 minutes. Dilute if required with sodium chloride 0.9% or glucose 5%.
Notes:	

Tranexamic acid liquid (Cyklokapron®) is sucrose free.

TRICLOFOS

Preparations:	LIQUID 500mg in 5ml.
Dosage:	**SEDATION FOR PAINLESS PROCEDURES**

This is an unlicensed indication.
Orally, over 1 month, single dose of 30-100mg/kg, 30-60 minutes before procedure. Maximum dose is 2g however up to 4g has been given.
OR

Sedation level	Age	Dose
2	3 months - 1year	30mg/kg
	1 - 6 years	50mg/kg
3	<3 months	50-75mg/kg
	3 months - 6 years	75-80mg/kg
4	<3 months	80mg/kg
	3 months - 6 years	100mg/kg

Notes:

a) Infants less than 3 months of age usually sleep in response to a feed immediately prior to the procedure.
b) **Caution:** children with obstructive sleep apnoea could be at risk from life threatening respiratory obstruction during sedation.
c) If sedation is not successful re-administer triclofos up to dosage at the next level. Do not exceed 100mg/kg or 4g total dose.
d) Liquid contains 3.3g of sucrose in 5ml.
e) See also sedation guidelines page 247.

TRIMEPRAZINE (ALIMEMAZINE)

Preparations:	TABLETS 10mg. LIQUID 7.5mg in 5ml and 30mg in 5ml.
Dosage:	***ANTIHISTAMINE***

This indication is unlicensed for use in children under 2 years.
Orally, over 6 months, 1mg/kg/day in 3-4 divided doses,
OR

6 months - 1 year	250microgram/kg	3-4 times a day
1 - 4 years	2.5mg	3-4 times a day
5 - 12 years	5mg	3-4 times a day
Over 12 years	10mg	2-3 times a day

Up to maximum 100mg/**day**.

SEDATION, PREMEDICATION

This indication is unlicensed for children under 2 years and over 7 years.
Orally, over 1 month, 2mg/kg/dose 30-60 minutes before procedure (e.g. MRI scan) in conjunction with triclofos (page 217). Maximum dose is 60mg.

Notes:

a) **Caution:** in infants under 6 months because of the possible association with 'cot deaths'.
b) In chronic eczema doses are often just given at night and higher doses may also be needed.
c) Trimeprazine liquid (Vallergan®) contains 2.6g of sucrose in 5ml and 4.8% w/v of alcohol.
d) See sedation guidelines page 247, premedication guidelines page 250.

TRIMETHOPRIM

Preparations:	TABLETS 100mg and 200mg. LIQUID 50mg in 5ml.
Dosage:	***URINARY TRACT INFECTION TREATMENT***

Orally, all ages, 4mg/kg twice a day,
OR

4 weeks - 1 year	4mg/kg	twice a day
1 - 5 years	50mg	twice a day
6 - 12 years	100mg	twice a day
Over 12 years	200mg	twice a day

LONG TERM PROPHYLAXIS

Orally, all ages, 1-2mg/kg at night. Dose may be given twice a day if patient is incontinent or has an urostomy tube.
OR

1 - 5 years	25mg	at night
5 - 12 years	50mg-75mg	at night
Over 12 years	100mg	at night

IN RENAL FAILURE

Creatinine clearance (ml/minute/1.73m^2)	Dosage
15-30	Normal dose for 3 days then reduce by half.
below 15	Reduce dose by half.

Notes:

a) There is a theoretical risk of folate deficiency with long term use. Calcium folinate supplements may be needed.
b) Trimethoprim appears to inhibit the hepatic metabolism of phenytoin, may decrease plasma levels of ciclosporin and has also shown synergistic nephrotoxicity with ciclosporin.
c) Trimethoprim liquids (Monotrim®, Trimopan®) are sucrose free.

TUBERCULIN TESTS

Preparations: INJECTION   10 units in 1ml (1 in 10,000)
100 units in 1ml (1 in 1,000)
1000 units in 1ml (1 in 100)
100,000 units in 1ml

Dosage: **MANTOUX (TUBERCULIN SKIN) TEST**

The following doses are given in succession. The second and subsequent injection is only given if a negative reaction is obtained from the previous injection.

Infants and Children

1.   0.1ml (1unit) of 10 units in 1ml *intradermally*❶
2.   0.1ml (10units) of 100 units in 1ml *intradermally*
3.   0.1ml (100units) of 1000 units in 1ml *intradermally*

Neonates, see BCG vaccine page 34.

❶This is the initial dose for patients in whom tuberculosis is suspected or are known to be hypersensitive to tuberculin, otherwise give step 2.

There should be at least 72 hours between the injections. Measure the diameter of the reaction (palpable induration) at 48-72 hours - a valid reading can be done up to 96 hours after injection:

4mm or less   negative test
5mm or more   positive test

HEAF TEST

Multiple puncture using the 100,000 units in 1ml strength.

Notes:

a) Mantoux test is the preferred test in hospital environment.
b) Heaf test should only be performed using the gun. It is ideal for multiple testing in the community.

TYROSINE - see Metabolic dietitian

UROKINASE

Preparations:	INJECTION 5,000units.
Dosage:	OCCLUDED ARTERIOVENOUS SHUNTS, PERITONEAL DIALYSIS CATHETERS AND INDWELLING CENTRAL LINES
	Instill the appropriate volume of 5,000units in 2ml solution into the catheter. The volume is dependent on the length and lumen size of the catheter. Refer to catheter manufacturer if lumen volume is unknown.
Administration:	Reconstitute vial with 2ml of sodium chloride 0.9%.
	Instill into the affected catheter, clamp off and retain for at least 4 hours. The lysate is then **aspirated**. DO NOT FLUSH until urokinase has been aspirated from the catheter.

URSODEOXYCHOLIC ACID

Preparations:	TABLETS 150mg.
Dosage:	BILIARY CIRRHOSIS, CHOLESTASIS*
	*This indication is unlicensed.
	Orally, all ages, 5-7.5mg/kg 2-3 times a day.
	Maximum 40mg/kg/**day**.

VALINE - see Metabolic dietitian

VANCOMYCIN

Preparations:	INJECTION 500mg and 1g. CAPSULES 125mg.
Dosage:	PSEUDOMEMBRANOUS COLITIS

Metronidazole is the preferred treatment in order to discourage emergence of vancomycin resistant organisms.
Seek microbiology advice before prescribing.

Orally, 40mg/kg/day in divided doses 6-8 hourly.
Total daily dose should not exceed 2g.

SYSTEMIC INFECTIONS

IV infusion, infants and children, loading dose of 15mg/kg followed by 10mg/kg every 6 hours.
Neonates (see note e).

Corrected gestational age (weeks)	Postnatal age (days)	Dose	Frequency
<26	up to 7	20mg/kg	36 hourly
	above 7	15mg/kg	24 hourly
26-30	up to 7	15mg/kg	24 hourly
	above 7	10mg/kg	12 hourly
30-36	up to 14	10mg/kg	12 hourly
	above 14	10mg/kg	8 hourly
>36	up to 7	10mg/kg	12 hourly
	above 7	10mg/kg	8 hourly

VENTRICULITIS OR MENINGITIS
Intrathecal injection 5-20mg once a day. Adjust dose according to CSF levels after 3-4 days. Patients with enlarged ventricles require the higher doses.

PROPHYLAXIS OF BACTERIAL ENDOCARDITIS
For special risk patients who are allergic to penicillins, (see endocarditis guidelines page 265).

IN RENAL FAILURE
Dose should be reduced in renal failure according to blood levels (see below). A loading dose is given as above, followed by maintenance dose when blood levels fall between 5-10mg/L. Peritoneal Dialysis, add to dialysis fluid: 25mg/L in every bag for 5 days **OR** 100mg/L in **one** bag only per day for 5 days. Not significantly removed by haemodialysis.

Administration: Reconstitute 500mg vial (Dumex) with 10ml water for injection to give 500mg in 10ml. For IV infusion further dilute with sodium chloride 0.9% or glucose 5% to 5mg in 1ml and infuse over **at least 1 hour**. In fluid restricted patients, maximum concentration is 10mg in 1ml, infused centrally if possible over **at least 1 hour.**

Notes:

a) Too rapid infusion may be associated with the 'red man' syndrome, a histamine mediated reaction.
b) Vancomycin must not be given by IM injection.
c) Therapeutic drug monitoring:
   i) Approx. time to steady state: 1-2 days
   ii) Therapeutic levels: Trough   5-10mg/L
                                        Peak   15-30mg/L
   iii) Take trough blood sample, immediately prior to next dose and peak blood sample, 1 hour after completion of infusion.
d) CSF levels: Take trough sample, immediately prior to next dose. Level should be less than 10mg/L.
e) Corrected gestational age = gestational age + postnatal age.
f) Injection can be given orally for a non-systemic effect.

VARICELLA VACCINE

Preparations: LIVE, ATTENUATED OKA STRAIN VACCINE containing not less than 2,000
                  PFU (Paster-Merieux MSD) or 10,000 PFU (Smith Kline Beecham)
                  (Both named Patient).

Dosage: *VACCINATION*

                  Test that patient is seronegative for VZV prior to vaccination.
                  Subcutaneous injection, 0.5ml.
                  Repeat dose at least 1 month after first dose. Test for antibodies
                  1 month after completion of course and then at 6 month intervals.

Notes:

a)   Patients under immunosuppressive treatment (including corticosteroid
     therapy) for malignant solid tumour or for serious chronic diseases (e.g.
     chronic renal failure, autoimmune diseases, severe bronchial asthma) are
     generally immunised when they are in complete haematological remission
     from the disease. The total lymphocyte count should be above 1,200 per
     mm^3 and there should be no other evidence of lack of cellular immune
     competence.

b)   When immunising patients in the acute phase of leukaemia maintenance
     chemotherapy should be stopped for 1 week before and 1 week after
     vaccination.

c)   If organ transplantation (e.g. kidney transplant) is being considered
     patient should be immunised and seroconversion demonstrated prior to
     transplantation.

d)   Varicella vaccine should not be administered within 3 months of varicella
     zoster immunoglobulin.

e)   Course must be completed using the same brand of vaccine.

VARICELLA-ZOSTER IMMUNOGLOBULIN (VZIG)

Preparations: INJECTION 250mg (**Named Patient**).
Dosage: ***PROPHYLAXIS OF CHICKENPOX OR SHINGLES INFECTION***

> **SEEK VIROLOGY ADVICE BEFORE PRESCRIBING**
> **SUPPLIES ARE EXTREMELY LIMITED**

See notes below before contacting virology
Intramuscular injection,

0 - 5 years	250mg
6 - 10 years	500mg
11 - 14 years	750mg
15 years and over	1000mg

Notes:

a) VZIG prophylaxis is only recommended for individuals who fulfil **all** of the following criteria:
   - Significant exposure to chickenpox or shingles within the past 10 days.
   - A clinical condition which increases the risk of severe varicella; this includes neonates, immunosuppressed patients (see notes below) and pregnancy.
   - No antibodies to varicella zoster virus on testing of recent blood sample.

b) VZIG is recommended for **neonates** whose mothers develop chickenpox (but not shingles) in the period 7 days before to 28 days after delivery. Also for VZ antibody negative infants exposed to either chickenpox or shingles in the first 28 days of life.
   Neonates who develop varicella, are especially at risk of severe disease and intravenous aciclovir is recommended see page 14.
   The following infants do not require VZIG since maternal antibody will be present:
   - Infants whose mothers have a positive history of chicken pox and/or a positive VZ antibody result;
   - Infants whose mothers develop shingles before or after delivery.

c) VZIG is recommended for **immunosuppressed** children, see the DoH "Green book" guidelines for full criteria. This includes children who within the previous 3 months have received prednisolone at a daily dose (or its equivalent) of 2mg/kg/day (or more than 40mg/day) for at least one week or 1mg/kg/day for one month. Patients on lower doses of steroids, given in combination with other immunosuppressant drugs are also included.

d) Varicella immunisation with the vaccine page 222 may be considered for susceptible immunosuppressed patients at long-term risk.

e) There may be a role for aciclovir prophylaxis where VZIG is warranted but not administered. Seek expert advice from the virologist on call.

f) **Caution:** Currently, all immunoglobulins prepared in the UK infer a theoretical risk of transmitting new variant CJD. Patient/carer should be informed of the theoretical risk.

VECURONIUM

Preparations:	INJECTION 10mg.
Dosage:	**NEUROMUSCULAR BLOCKADE FOR VENTILATION* AND SURGERY**

*This is an unlicensed indication.

> NEUROMUSCULAR CONDUCTION, USING A NERVE STIMULATOR, SHOULD BE MONITORED IN ALL PATIENTS IN WHOM REPEATED DOSES OR INFUSIONS ARE ADMINISTERED.

Initially *IV injection* 80-100microgram/kg, then 20-30microgram/kg according to patient's response. Test dose for infants under 4 months, 10-20microgram/kg.

IV infusion, 50-200microgram/kg/hour.

Administration: Reconstitute vial with 5ml water for injection to give a 2mg in 1ml solution.

For IV infusion, dilute if required with sodium chloride 0.9% or glucose 5%.

If fluid restricted, reconstitute vial with 2.5ml water for injection. Maximum concentration 4mg in 1ml.

Notes:

a) Doses must be reduced in neonates as they have an increased sensitivity to non-depolarising muscle relaxants.

b) The usual duration of action is 15-20 minutes in children, this is increased to 30-40 minutes in infants, so fewer supplementary doses are needed. The onset of action is quicker in infants and children compared to adults.

c) Prolonged recovery time has been observed in patients on continuous high dose infusions with moderate renal failure. This is not a problem when neuromuscular conduction is monitored with a nerve stimulator.

d) Aminoglycoside antibiotics, metronidazole, suxamethonium and calcium antagonists may prolong the effect of vecuronium.

VERAPAMIL

Preparations: TABLETS 40mg and 80mg. INJECTION 5mg in 2ml.
LIQUID 40mg in 5ml (**Manufactured special**).

Dosage: **SUPRAVENTRICULAR TACHYCARDIA TREATMENT**

Verapamil has been associated with fatal collapse during treatment of supraventricular tachycardia, especially under 1 year of age. Adenosine should be used first line for this condition.

CONSULT A CARDIOLOGIST BEFORE TREATMENT OF UNDER 1 YEAR OLDS.

IV injection, given very slowly over at least 15 minutes,

0-5 years	15microgram/kg
5-10 years	50microgram/kg
10-15 years	100microgram/kg

Blood pressure should be monitored. Treatment should be stopped if sinus rhythm occurs. If tachycardia worsens during administration stop immediately. If the blood pressure is low use DC shock rather than verapamil.

SUPRAVENTRICULAR TACHYCARDIA PROPHYLAXIS

Orally,

Neonates & infants	1-2mg/kg	3 times a day
Up to 2 years	20mg	2-3 times a day
Over 2 years	40-120mg	2-3 times a day

Adjust dose according to blood levels.

HYPERTENSION

Orally, up to 5mg/kg twice a day, according to severity of disease.

Notes:

a) **Note**: Verapamil is no longer treatment of choice in supraventricular tachycardia. ADENOSINE should be used first line, see page 16.

b) Verapamil should not be given concomitantly with quinidine. If given concomitantly with digoxin the dose of digoxin may need to be reduced. The concomitant use of IV verapamil with IV/PO beta-blockers is contra-indicated as it may cause hypotension and asystole. The concomitant use of oral verapamil and beta blockers may also be hazardous and should only be prescribed by experts and when myocardial function is well preserved. Verapamil interacts with many drugs, contact your clinical pharmacist.

c) Injection can be given orally.

d) A modified release preparation is available for use in adults (120mg and 240mg tablets). These preparations are not effective for prophylaxis or treatment of arrhythmias because of pre-systemic metabolism of the isomer that is active on the heart. It can be used in hypertension.

VIGABATRIN

Preparations: TABLETS 500mg. SACHET 500mg.
Dosage: **EPILEPSY**

ON NEUROLOGIST ADVICE ONLY

Orally, initially, 20-40mg/kg once or twice a day increasing to 80-100mg/kg/day **OR**,

10-15kg	1-2 tablets/day
15-30kg	2-3 tablets/day
30-50kg	3-6 tablets/day
>50kg	4-8 tablets/day

INFANTILE SPASMS (WEST SYNDROME)

Orally, 60-100mg/kg/day. Doses up to 150mg/kg/day have been used with good tolerability.

IN RENAL FAILURE

Dose should be reduced if creatinine clearance is less than 60ml/minute/1.73m^2, and patients should be monitored for adverse effects such as sedation and confusion.

Notes:

a) Warning: Vigabatrin has been associated with persistent visual field defects. Base line perimetry should be performed before or as soon as possible after starting vigabatrin and every 6 months thereafter, in children able to co-operate (usually 9 years old and over). Patient/carer should be warned to report any new visual problems.

b) Other adverse effects are mainly CNS related. Any drowsiness decreases with continuing treatment. However excitation and agitation may also be seen in children.

c) Vigabatrin should only be prescribed first-line in infantile spasms associated with Tuberous Sclerosis.

d) There is no direct correlation between blood levels and efficacy.

e) Vigabatrin may cause a gradual reduction of about 20% in plasma phenytoin levels, however this is unlikely to be clinically significant.

f) Sachet contents, dissolved in water, may be kept for 24 hours. If sachets are not available tablets can be crushed and then dispersed in water or squash **OR** they can be crushed and mixed with soft food.

VINCRISTINE

Preparations:	INJECTION 1mg in 1ml and 2mg in 2ml.
Dosage:	**NEPHROTIC SYNDROME**

This is an unlicensed indication.

> **SEEK EXPERT ADVICE BEFORE PRESCRIBING**

IV injection, 1.5mg/m^2 (maximum 2mg dose), once a week for 6-8 weeks. In overweight or grossly oedematous patients, ideal body weight must be used for calculating dose.

Child must have satisfactory white cell count before administering.

Administration:

> **VINCRISTINE MUST ONLY BE GIVEN INTRAVENOUSLY.**
> **INTRATHECAL INJECTION IS USUALLY FATAL.**

Vincristine is a cytotoxic drug therefore it will be prepared in the oncology pharmacy department.

> ☎Guy's ext. 5418, Lewisham ext. 3201, St Thomas' ext. 3851☎

Administer as a injection, over approximately 2 minutes, through the side port of a fast running (approximately 150-200ml/hour) infusion of sodium chloride 0.9% or glucose 5%.

Do not administer with any other fluid or drug as precipitation of vincristine may occur.

Notes:

a) **CAUTION: VINCRISTINE IS A VESICANT.** Avoid extravasation during administration of injection.
b) If extravasation occurs stop infusion immediately, aspirate as much fluid as possible and leave needle in situ. Apply moderate warmth, DO NOT APPLY ICE, to the site and contact a member of the Plastics team immediately.
c) If accidental contamination of skin or eyes occurs wash thoroughly and immediately with water or sodium chloride 0.9% (use polyfusor). Seek urgent medical advice.
d) Dose may need to be reduced in hepatic dysfunction.
e) Use with caution in patients concurrently taking drugs known to inhibit the hepatic cytochrome P450 isoenzymes in the CYP 3A subfamily (i.e. itraconazole). For further advice contact paediatric pharmacist by bleep or drug information on:

> ☎Guy's ext. 3594, Lewisham ext. 3202, St Thomas' ext. 3069☎

WARFARIN

Preparations:	TABLETS 1mg (brown), 3mg (blue) and 5mg (pink).
	LIQUID (**Extemporaneously prepared**).
Dosage:	***ANTICOAGULATION***

This indication is unlicensed for use in children.

SEEK EXPERT ADVICE BEFORE PRESCRIBING

Orally, loading doses:

Day 1   200microgram/kg once a day (see notes a and b). Maximum dose 10mg.

Day 2-4   Once a day according to INR. (See table below).

INR	Dose (mg)
1.1 - 1.3	Repeat Day 1 dose
1.4 - 1.9	50% of Day 1 dose
2.0 - 3.0	50% of Day 1 dose
3.1 - 3.5	25% of Day 1 dose
>3.5	Stop until INR <3.5; restart at 50% of previous dose

Maintenance doses:

Once a day (see note a) according to INR (see table below); approximately 100microgram/kg/**day**.

INR	Dose (mg)
1.1 - 1.4	Increase dose by 20%
1.5 - 1.9	Increase dose by 10%
2.0 - 3.0	No change
3.1 - 3.5	Decrease dose by 10%
>3.5	Stop until INR <3.5; restart at 80% of previous dose

Notes:

a) Warfarin should be given at the same time each day and this is usually **6pm**. INR should be checked the following morning.

b) Loading doses may need to be altered according to condition, concomitant interacting drugs and if baseline INR is greater than 1.3.

c) The anticoagulant effect of warfarin takes up to 36-48 hours to develop, whilst the antithrombotic effect may take at least 3 days. Heparin infusion, if prescribed, should be continued until INR in therapeutic range for 2 consecutive days.

d) The current INR therapeutic ranges are:
Prophylaxis of DVT: 2 - 2.5
Treatment of DVT and pulmonary embolism: 2 - 3
Recurrent DVT, pulmonary embolism; arterial grafts and mechanical cardiac prosthetic valves: 3 - 4.5

e) Warfarin interacts with many drugs. The INR should be monitored whenever a drug is added to, or withdrawn from, the patient's therapeutic regimen. Check for interactions carefully, the following is not an exhaustive list.
Warfarin effect is **potentiated** by erythromycin, imidazoles, ciprofloxacin, metronidazole, co-trimoxazole, cimetidine, dipyridamole, amiodarone, thyroxine, aspirin and other non-steroidal anti-inflammatory analgesics.
Warfarin effect is **reduced** by barbiturates, rifampicin, griseofulvin, carbamazepine and phytomenadione.
Warfarin effect may be **reduced** or **potentiated** by phenytoin, corticosteroids or cholestyramine.

ZIDOVUDINE

Preparations:	CAPSULES 100mg and 250mg. LIQUID 10mg in 1ml. INJECTION 200mg in 10ml.
Dosage:	**PROPHYLAXIS FOR NEONATES** Neonates, see note a), start within 12 hours of birth, *Orally,* 2mg/kg every 6 hours for 4 weeks. *IV injection,* only if oral route not available, 1.5mg/kg, over 30minutes, every 6 hours. **MANAGEMENT OF HIV DISEASE** *Orally,* over 3 months old, 120-180mg/m^2 every 6 hours. Maximum dose 200mg every 6 hours. *IV injection,* 80-160mg/m^2, over 60minutes, every 6 hours. **IN RENAL FAILURE** In advanced renal failure use doses at the lower end of the dosage range. Zidovudine is not significantly removed by haemodialysis or peritoneal dialysis.
Administration:	IV injection over 30-60minutes, dilute with glucose 5% to 2mg in 1ml or 4mg in 1ml.
Notes:	

a) As part of a regimen to reduce the risk of vertical transmission of HIV, the mother (see Adult Formulary page section 5.3b or ward protocol) and neonate (doses above) should receive zidovudine.
b) A baseline full blood count should be performed and then repeated every 2 weeks for the first 3 months and then once a month. Reduce doses (short term) or interrupt treatment if haemoglobin level falls to between 7.5-9g/dL or neutrophil count falls to between 0.75-1.0 x 10^9/L.
c) Vitamin B$_{12}$ deficiency increases the risk of neutropenia.
d) In neonates with hyperbilirubinaemia requiring treatment other than phototherapy or with transaminases of over 5 times the upper limit of normal, seek expert advice before prescribing.
e) 120mg/m^2 intravenously is approximately equivalent to 180mg/m^2 orally. To convert oral dose to intravenous doses multiply the oral dose by a factor of 0.67.
f) Zidovudine liquid (Retrovir®) is sugar free.

TREATMENT GUIDELINES

These guidelines should be tailored where necessary to individual patient needs and do not replace the need for consultation with senior staff and/or referral for expert advice.

GASTRO-OESOPHAGEAL REFLUX DISEASE

Gastro-oesophageal reflux disease is most common in infancy with symptoms resolving around 12-18 months of age but can occur in children.
Gastro-oesophageal reflux disease is basically a clinical diagnosis. In older infants and children diagnosis may be confirmed by pH monitoring and/or a barium swallow. Endoscopy may be performed if severe gastro-oesophageal reflux disease is suspected.

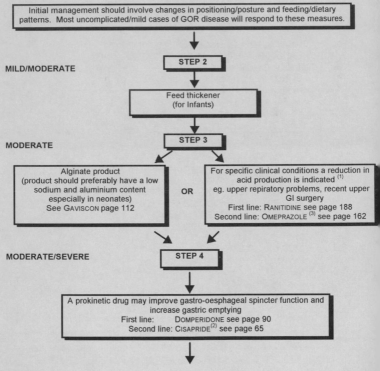

MILD

STEP 1

Initial management should involve changes in positioning/posture and feeding/dietary patterns. Most uncomplicated/mild cases of GOR disease will respond to these measures.

MILD/MODERATE

STEP 2

Feed thickener
(for Infants)

MODERATE

STEP 3

Alginate product
(product should preferably have a low sodium and aluminium content especially in neonates)
See GAVISCON page 112

OR

For specific clinical conditions a reduction in acid production is indicated [1]
eg. upper repiratory problems, recent upper GI surgery
First line: RANITIDINE see page 188
Second line: OMEPRAZOLE [3] see page 162

MODERATE/SEVERE

STEP 4

A prokinetic drug may improve gastro-oesophageal spincter function and increase gastric emptying
First line: DOMPERIDONE see page 90
Second line: CISAPRIDE [2] see page 65

SEVERE

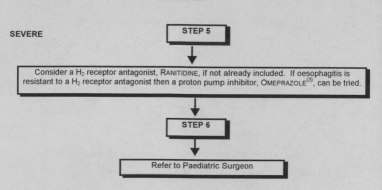

STEP 5

Consider a H_2 receptor antagonist, RANITIDINE, if not already included. If oesophagitis is resistant to a H_2 receptor antagonist then a proton pump inhibitor, OMEPRAZOLE[3], can be tried.

STEP 6

Refer to Paediatric Surgeon

NOTE: (1) Alginates may be less effective in the presence of decreased acid production.
(2) Check **cautions** and **warnings** carefully before prescribing.
(3) It is not advisable to use Ranitidine and Omeprazole concomitantly.

CARDIOPULMONARY RESUSCITATION (CPR)

A successful outcome is dependent on restoring a stable circulation rapidly. Unless action is taken within 3-4 minutes, damage to vital organs, especially the brain, will occur. All doctors and nurses should be familiar with the basic life support techniques of mouth-to-mouth resuscitation and external cardiac massage.

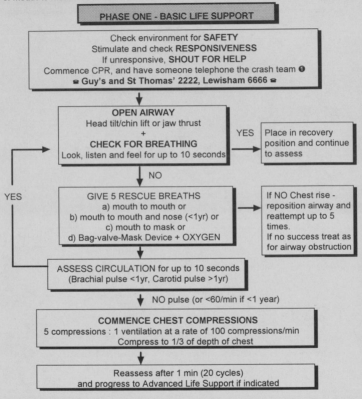

PHASE ONE - BASIC LIFE SUPPORT

Check environment for **SAFETY**
Stimulate and check **RESPONSIVENESS**
If unresponsive, **SHOUT FOR HELP**
Commence CPR, and have someone telephone the crash team ❶
☎ Guy's and St Thomas' 2222, Lewisham 6666 ☎

OPEN AIRWAY
Head tilt/chin lift or jaw thrust
+
CHECK FOR BREATHING
Look, listen and feel for up to 10 seconds

YES → Place in recovery position and continue to assess

NO

YES

GIVE 5 RESCUE BREATHS
a) mouth to mouth or
b) mouth to mouth and nose (<1yr) or
c) mouth to mask or
d) Bag-valve-Mask Device + OXYGEN

→ If NO Chest rise - reposition airway and reattempt up to 5 times.
If no success treat as for airway obstruction

ASSESS CIRCULATION for up to 10 seconds
(Brachial pulse <1yr, Carotid pulse >1yr)

↓ NO pulse (or <60/min if <1 year)

COMMENCE CHEST COMPRESSIONS
5 compressions : 1 ventilation at a rate of 100 compressions/min
Compress to 1/3 of depth of chest

Reassess after 1 min (20 cycles)
and progress to Advanced Life Support if indicated

❶ If you are alone, not near a telephone and no-one responds to your call for help, perform resuscitation for 1 minute then go to the nearest telephone and call the crash team. Return immediately to child and reassess ABC, continuing BLS as necessary. If telephone unavailable, continue resuscitation until you are exhausted or child improves.

PHASE TWO - ADVANCED LIFE SUPPORT

CONTINUE CARDIAC COMPRESSION AND BAG-VALVE MASK VENTILATION WITH **100%** OXYGEN WITHOUT INTERRUPTION AND INTUBATE WHEN POSSIBLE.

Doses of the most common drugs used in CPR are given in a table at the end of this section.

The following steps should ideally take place **SIMULTANEOUSLY**:

1) **Note time of arrest.**
2) **Attach an ECG monitor as soon as possible.**
3) **Diagnose rhythm on the monitor as being:**

Non VF/Non VT Non ventricular fibrillation or non pulseless ventricular tachycardia i.e. **Asystole** or **Pulseless Electrical Activity**. Note: PEA ≡ EMD Follow algorithm on page 236.	**OR**	**VF/VT** **Ventricular fibrillation or ventricular tachycardia** Follow algorithm on page 237.

Continue to monitor rhythm during any interventions. **Other rhythms should not be treated until the patient is stable and on PICU.** Tachycardia guidelines are on page 239.

4) **Establish vascular access for drugs and fluids** - insert a large venous line rapidly. If not successful within 90 seconds, insert an intraosseous line.

   If IV/IO access is unattainable, the endotracheal route can be used to administer epinephrine (adrenaline).

5) **Give appropriate drugs** according to rhythm. Suggested treatment for these rhythms is outlined below.

DO NOT STOP CPR UNTIL A SATISFACTORY CARDIAC OUTPUT IS ACHIEVED OR DISCONTINUATION OF RESUSCITATION ATTEMPT HAS BEEN AGREED.

235

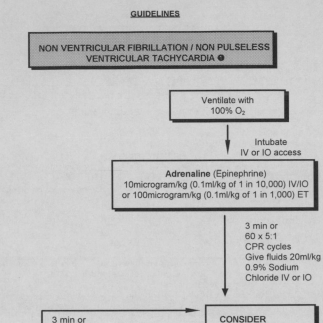

NON VENTRICULAR FIBRILLATION / NON PULSELESS VENTRICULAR TACHYCARDIA ❶

Ventilate with
100% O₂

Intubate
IV or IO access

Adrenaline (Epinephrine)
10microgram/kg (0.1ml/kg of 1 in 10,000) IV/IO
or 100microgram/kg (0.1ml/kg of 1 in 1,000) ET

3 min or
60 x 5:1
CPR cycles
Give fluids 20ml/kg
0.9% Sodium
Chloride IV or IO

3 min or
60 x 5:1 CPR cycles

CONSIDER
Hypovolaemia
Hypoxia
Tension pneumothorax
Cardiac tamponade
Drug overdose
Electrolyte imbalance
Hypothermia
and treat appropriately

Adrenaline (Epinephrine)
100microgram/kg (0.1ml/kg of 1 in 1,000) IV/IO/ET

If no output

❶ Non VF/VT includes :   Asystole and Bradycardia
                             (<60 beats per minute if <1yr).
                     :   Pulseless Electrical Activity
                             (Electro Mechanical Dissociation)

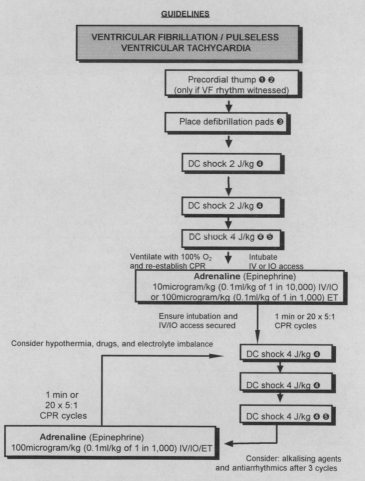

VENTRICULAR FIBRILLATION / PULSELESS VENTRICULAR TACHYCARDIA

Precordial thump ❶ ❷
(only if VF rhythm witnessed)

↓

Place defibrillation pads ❸

↓

DC shock 2 J/kg ❹

↓

DC shock 2 J/kg ❹

↓

DC shock 4 J/kg ❹ ❺

Ventilate with 100% O₂ and re-establish CPR   Intubate IV or IO access

Adrenaline (Epinephrine)
10microgram/kg (0.1ml/kg of 1 in 10,000) IV/IO
or 100microgram/kg (0.1ml/kg of 1 in 1,000) ET

Ensure intubation and IV/IO access secured   1 min or 20 x 5:1 CPR cycles

Consider hypothermia, drugs, and electrolyte imbalance

DC shock 4 J/kg ❹

↓

DC shock 4 J/kg ❹

↓

DC shock 4 J/kg ❹ ❺

1 min or 20 x 5:1 CPR cycles

Adrenaline (Epinephrine)
100microgram/kg (0.1ml/kg of 1 in 1,000) IV/IO/ET

Consider: alkalising agents and antiarrhythmics after 3 cycles

❶ Precordial thump: a thump to sternum with clenched fist; two fingers if newborn.
❷ Recheck pulse if change in rhythm seen on monitor.
❸ Defibrillation pads need to be changed when becoming dry.
❹ Announce "CHARGING DEFIBRILLATOR" and then "STAND CLEAR; OXYGEN AWAY" before each shock (High flow oxygen is a combustion risk). **Check rhythm after each shock.**
❺ Return paddles to defibrillator after every 3rd shock.

237

POST-RESUSCITATION MANAGEMENT

Once spontaneous cardiac output has been established, frequent clinical reassessment must be carried out to detect deterioration or improvement with therapy. All patients should be monitored for the following:

- Pulse rate and rhythm.
- Oxygen saturation.
- Core temperature.
- Skin temperature.
- Blood pressure.
- Urine output.
- Arterial pH and gases.

    Additionally some patients will require:

- CO_2 monitoring.
- Invasive BP monitoring.

RESUSCITATION SCHEDULE

This dosage schedule is designed as a guide only. It is grouped by age and weight.

AGE	NEWBORN	6 MONTHS	1 YEAR	4 YEARS	8 YEARS
WEIGHT	**3kg**	**6kg**	**10kg**	**15kg**	**25kg**
Mask	0 or 1	1	1 or 2	1 or 2	3
ET tube	2.5 or 3	3.5 or 4	4 or 4.5	5	6 or 6.5
Maintenance Fluid/hour	12ml	25ml	40ml	50ml	65ml
Adrenaline (Epinephrine) 10microgram/kg IV/IO 1 in 10,000	0.3ml	0.6ml	1ml	1.5ml	2.5ml
Adrenaline (Epinephrine) 100microgram/kg IV/IO 1 in 1,000	0.3ml	0.6ml	1ml	1.5ml	2.5ml
Atropine	100 microgram	120 microgram	200 microgram	300 microgram	500 microgram
Calcium Chloride 10%	0.3ml	0.6ml	1ml	1.5ml	2.5ml
Calcium Gluconate 10%	0.6ml	1.2ml	2ml	3ml	5ml
Isoprenaline 200micrograms in 10ml	0.75ml	1.5ml	2.5ml	3.75ml	6.25ml
Lidocaine (Lignocaine) 1%	0.3ml slowly	0.6ml slowly	1.0ml slowly	1.5ml slowly	2.5ml slowly
Sodium Bicarbonate 8.4%	-	6ml slowly	10ml slowly	15ml slowly	25ml slowly
Sodium Bicarbonate 4.2%	6ml slowly	-	-	-	-

TACHYCARDIA

MANAGEMENT

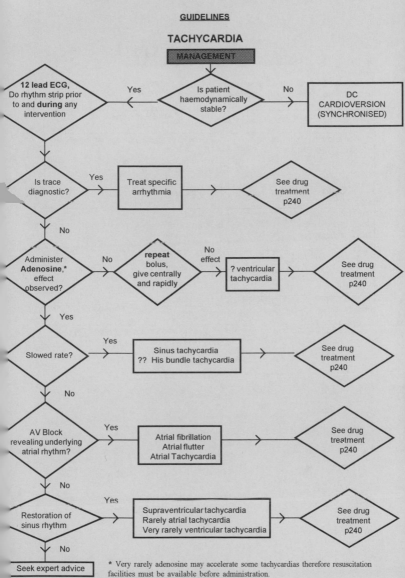

12 lead ECG, Do rhythm strip prior to and **during** any intervention ← Yes — Is patient haemodynamically stable? — No → DC CARDIOVERSION (SYNCHRONISED)

Is trace diagnostic? — Yes → Treat specific arrhythmia → See drug treatment p240

No ↓

Administer **Adenosine,*** effect observed? — No → **repeat** bolus, give centrally and rapidly — No effect → ? ventricular tachycardia → See drug treatment p240

Yes ↓

Slowed rate? — Yes → Sinus tachycardia ?? His bundle tachycardia → See drug treatment p240

No ↓

AV Block revealing underlying atrial rhythm? — Yes → Atrial fibrillation Atrial flutter Atrial Tachycardia → See drug treatment p240

No ↓

Restoration of sinus rhythm — Yes → Supraventricular tachycardia Rarely atrial tachycardia Very rarely ventricular tachycardia → See drug treatment p240

No ↓

Seek expert advice

* Very rarely adenosine may accelerate some tachycardias therefore resuscitation facilities must be available before administration.

DRUG TREATMENT

The following are only guidelines as to the initial treatment of a specific arrhythmia, expert advice should be sought before prescribing or if there is a lack of response.

Arrhythmia	Initial treatment
Supraventricular tachycardia	1. Adenosine, repeat bolus when necessary 2. Digoxin 3. Esmolol * 4. Verapamil *
Sinus tachycardia	Find underlying cause
Atrial fibrillation Atrial flutter Atrial tachycardia	1. Digoxin 2. Propranolol 3. Amiodarone
Ventricular tachycardia	1. Lignocaine 2. Amiodarone 3. Magnesium
Wolf-Parkinson-White Syndrome with Atrial fibrillation	1. Amiodarone DO **NOT** GIVE digoxin or verapamil

* See contraindications in esmolol (page 100) and verapamil (page 225) monographs.

CHRONIC ASTHMA

Start at the step most appropriate to initial severity; consider 'rescue' course of prednisolone at any time and at any step.

Once control is achieved consideration should be given to stepping down therapy.

STEP 1   **Occasional use of Short Acting Beta₂ - agonist bronchodilators** e.g. Salbutamol/Terbutaline. Inhaled whenever possible.
(<1year Ipratropium Bromide may be more effective).

↕

STEP 2   **Regular Inhaled Low Dose Corticosteroid**
e.g. Budesonide/Beclomethasone   <5years up to 200microgram B.D.
                                           >5years up to 400microgram B.D.
plus P.R.N short acting Beta₂ agonist
See notes ❶

↕

STEP 3   **Regular Inhaled Low Dose Corticosteroid & Inhaled Long Acting Beta₂ agonist**
e.g.Budesonide/Beclomethasone   <5years up to 200microgram B.D.
                                           >5years up to 400microgram B.D.
plus Salmeterol/Eformoterol plus P.R.N short acting Beta₂ agonist

OR

Regular Inhaled High Dose Corticosteroid
e.g. Budesonide   <5years up to 400microgram B.D.
                                           >5years up to 1mg B.D.
plus P.R.N short acting Beta₂ agonist
See notes ❷, ❸ & ❹

↕

STEP 4   **Regular High Dose Inhaled Corticosteroid & Regular Bronchodilators**
Budesonide/fluticasone plus P.R.N short acting Beta₂ agonist
plus sequential trial of one or more of the following:
     i)   inhaled salmeterol/eformoterol
     ii)   oral S.R. theophylline/aminophylline
     iii)   montulekast (see note (4).
     iv)   nebulised Beta₂ - agonist
     v)   regular inhaled ipratropium bromide

NOTES

❶ Sodium Cromoglycate may be used at step 2 before low dose inhaled corticosteroids. If no response, replace with low dose inhaled corticosteroids.

❷ Salmeterol is available as a metered dose inhaler. Eformoterol is included as an inhaled powder device. (Turbohaler®). (N.B. Eformoterol is not licensed <12years and salmeterol is not licensed <4years).

❸ Budesonide is the inhaled corticosteroid of choice for high dose therapy. Fluticasone propionate (Flixotide®) may be used in place of budesonide, on the advice of a consultant, if high dose corticosteroid therapy is not effective or side-effects are a problem. N.B. Fluticasone propionate is approximately twice as potent as budesonide.

❹ At present the place of the leukotriene antagonists in paediatric asthma therapy is uncertain. Montulekast is licensed as add-on therapy in children (>6years) with mild/moderate asthma inadequately controlled on inhaled corticosteroids, but it may be tried at Step 3 or Step 4.

CHOICE OF INHALER DEVICES FOR CHILDREN

Age (years)

	1 - 2	3 - 5	>5
MDI + Large volume spacer + mask	1st Choice	2nd Choice	---
MDI + Large volume spacer	2nd Choice	1st Choice	2nd Choice
Dry Powder Inhaler i.e. Turbohaler	INAPPROPRIATE	OCCASIONALLY USEFUL	1st Choice

USE & CARE OF LARGE VOLUME SPACER DEVICES

1) All children using a metered dose inhaler (MDI) for bronchodilator therapy, should try and use a large volume spacer, unless inhaler technique has been assessed as competent.

2) All children receiving inhaled corticosteroids via an MDI should use a large volume spacer as lung deposition is improved and oropharyngeal deposition is reduced.

3) The appropriate spacer device for the inhaler should always be used:

   Volumatic +/- mask: Beclomethasone,   Fluticasone,   Salbutamol, Salmeterol, Ipratropium
   Nebuhaler +/- mask: Budesonide, Terbutaline
   If more than one inhaler is prescribed, inhalers which fit a common spacer should be chosen, whenever possible e.g. Budesonide & Terbutaline

4) The aerosol half life after actuation is often less than 10 seconds. Patients should inhale as soon as possible after aerosol actuation. If more than one aerosol puff is required for a dose, inhalation from the spacer should be performed after each puff.

5) The spacer should be washed and rinsed each week and allowed to dry naturally. Wiping dry can create static and reduce drug delivery.

6) The spacer should be replaced every 6-12 months or sooner if necessary.

Adapted from British Thoracic Society Guidelines on Asthma Management (1997).

ACUTE SEVERE ASTHMA

RECOGNITION OF ACUTE SEVERE ASTHMA

Remember:
- in pre-school children there are other important causes of cough, breathlessness and wheeze
- if you think a child has severe asthma, give Beta$_2$ agonist at once
- Too breathless to talk/feed
- Respirations
  <5 years >50 breaths/min
  >5 years >40 breaths/min
- Pulse
  <5 years >140 beats/min
  >5 years >120 beats/min

No other investigations are needed for immediate management. Blood gas estimations are rarely helpful in deciding initial management in children.

- Use of accessory muscles of breathing
- PEF <50% best or predicted after inhaled bronchodilator

LIFE THREATENING FEATURES

CAUTION: **Children with severe attacks may not appear distressed; assessment in the very young may be difficult. The presence of any of the features below should alert the doctor.**
- Cyanosis, silent chest or poor respiratory effort
- Fatigue or exhaustion
- Agitation or reduced level of consciousness
- PEF <33% best or predicted after inhaled bronchodilator

MANAGEMENT OF A SEVERE ASTHMA ATTACK

Immediate treatment

- High flow oxygen via non rebreathe mask
- Salbutamol 5mg (2.5mg <5 years) via an oxygen driven nebuliser
- Prednisolone 1-2mg/kg orally (maximum 40mg)
- Pulse oximetry is helpful. SaO$_2$ <92% in air may indicate the need for admission.

IF LIFE THREATENING FEATURES ARE PRESENT:
- Give intravenous salbutamol **OR** aminophylline (consider high dependency or intensive care unit)
  Salbutamol 4-6microgram/kg over 5 minutes then a continuous infusion at 0.6-1microgram/kg/minute
  Aminophylline 5mg/kg over 20 minutes then a continuous infusion at 900microgram/kg/hour. **Omit loading dose if child receiving oral aminophylline or theophylline.**
- Give intravenous hydrocortisone 4-8mg/kg (maximum 200mg), followed by 6 hourly doses of 2-4mg/kg (maximum 100mg).
- Add nebulised ipratropium 0.25-0.5mg (0.125-0.25mg <5 years)
- Use pulse oximetry to assess response to treatment. If SaO$_2$ <92% consider chest radiography if first attack or clinical condition indicates.

Subsequent management

IF THE CHILD IS IMPROVING, CONTINUE:
- High flow oxygen to maintain SaO_2 >92%
- Nebulised salbutamol 1-4 hourly
- Corticosteroids (Prednisolone orally or hydrocortisone intravenously)
- Other treatment already commenced e.g. intravenous salbutamol, nebulised ipratropium

IF THE CHILD IS NOT IMPROVING AFTER 15-30 MINUTES:
- Continue oxygen and corticosteroids
- Give nebulised salbutamol more frequently (up to every 30 minutes or even continuously (back to back) if indicated)
- Add nebulised ipratropium (if not started already). Repeat 6 hourly until improvement starts
- Consider need for chest radiography

IF THE CHILD STILL NOT IMPROVING START:
- Intravenous salbutamol **OR** aminophylline (if not already started)
  Salbutamol: 4-6microgram/kg over 5 minutes then a continuous infusion at 0.6-1microgram/kg/min
  Aminophylline: 5mg/kg over 20 minutes then a continuous infusion at 900microgram/kg/hour

Monitoring treatment

- Pulse oximetry: maintain SaO_2 >92%
- Note clinical features at regular intervals
- Repeat PEF measurement 15-30 minutes after starting treatment (if appropriate)
- Chart PEF (if appropriate) before and after inhaled $Beta_2$ agonists and at least 4 times daily throughout hospital stay

When to transfer to Paediatric Intensive Care Unit

Transfer child to Paediatric Intensive Care Unit accompanied by a doctor prepared to intubate if there is:

- Worsening or persisting hypoxia or hypercapnia or a deteriorating PEF
- Exhaustion, feeble respirations, confusion or drowsiness
- Coma or respiratory arrest

Discharge

When discharged from hospital children should have:

- been stable on discharge medication for 12-24 hours
- had inhaler technique checked and recorded
- if recorded, PEF >75% best or predicted, and PEF diurnal variability of <25%
- if appropriate, own PEF meter (available from pharmacy)
- completed a minimum of 3-5 days of corticosteroids or have sufficient prescribed for the course to be completed after discharge
- if appropriate, inhaled corticosteroids prescribed at twice the preadmission dose for at least 4 weeks
- instructions to use inhaled short acting Beta$_2$ agonist regularly for up to 7 days
- written instructions for parents and a self-management plan if appropriate
- GP or hospital follow up arranged with direct readmission for any deterioration within 24 hours

Adapted From British Thoracic Society Guidelines On Asthma Management (1997)

SEDATION FOR PAINLESS PROCEDURES

These sedation guidelines are for painless procedures that require conscious sedation.

Conscious sedation is a medically controlled state of depressed consciousness that:

1. Allows protective reflexes to be maintained.
2. Retains the patients ability to maintain a patent airway independently and continuously.
3. Permits appropriate responses by the patient to physical or verbal commands.

(American Academy of Paediatrics, 1992).

The ideal sedative is one that provides adequate and safe sedation for the minimum duration required. Chloral hydrate and triclofos are good sedatives with minimal cardiac and respiratory depressant effects. However, they have an active half-life of about 8 hours and can cause gastric irritation (lower incidence with triclofos). Midazolam has a very short half life of approximately 2 hours, but may cause respiratory depression especially if given intravenously. Opiates are inappropriate as analgesia is not required. Barbiturates and other benzodiazepines often oversedate, have long half lives and may cause respiratory and cardiac depressant effects.

It should always be remembered that sedation should not be considered the 'norm' and that it should not take the place of adequate preparation of the infant or child.
Infants under 3 months of age will usually be adequately sedated if they are fed prior to the procedure. **Children over 6 years of age** should be fully prepared before the procedure and only sedated if after preparation they are still anxious or unable to stay motionless.
Children between 3 months and 6 years of age may need to be sedated as adequate preparation of the child is often not possible due to their level of understanding.

- Child must be fit to sedate.   (Monitor T.P.R; also oxygen saturation if level 4 sedation required).
- Child must not have a compromised airway or a decreased level of consciousness. **Seek expert advice before prescribing in these conditions**.
- Child must be accompanied by a parent or carer and where appropriate medical or nursing staff.

SEDATION SCALE

The following sedation scale can be used to determine the level of sedation required to provide optimum and safe sedation. Triclofos is initially the sedative of choice and dosage is determined by the level of sedation required (see page 217). It must, however, be remembered that this is only a guideline and that every child is an individual and the dose should be tailored to their individual needs.

LEVEL	SEDATION	TYPE OF PROCEDURE
1	Awake	All procedures with co-operative child
2	Drowsy	This level is often inappropriate as it can produce an unexpected response
3	Asleep, moves spontaneously	ECG, Echocardiogram, CT Scan, BSER
4	Asleep, responds to stimulation	MRI
5	Hard to rouse	This is deep sedation. Contact doctor immediately.

Adapted from Lloyd-Thomas A. R. et al. *BMJ* 1992;**304**:1175.

NOTE
- Triclofos is usually the first choice sedative as it is more palatable and causes less gastric irritation, than chloral hydrate.
- For some procedures e.g. insertion of catheters for urodynamics, oral midazolam is used first line as its short half-life is an advantage.
- Children on anti-epileptic drugs may require a lower dose of sedative due to the sedative effects of their drugs.
- Children with behavioural problems and special needs may require an increased dose of sedative to provide the same level of sedation.
- **Level 5** sedation should only be performed by an anaesthetist. If sedation score is assessed as level 5 after sedative administered contact doctor immediately.

TREATMENT FAILURES

- Ensure adequate time has elapsed from administration to allow triclofos to work. The peak effect is usually seen 30-60 minutes after an oral dose.
- Maximum dose of triclofos (see page 217) should be administered before addition of another drug.
- If triclofos sedation has failed, midazolam (see page 151) is the preferred sedative to add in. It has a short duration of action and may be given orally, intranasally or parenterally. **Caution:** midazolam may cause respiratory depression. Intravenous midazolam results in level 5 sedation and must only be used with concurrent pulse oximetry and with flumazenil and resuscitation facilities at hand.
- "A failure rate of 10-20% should be accepted as this prevents the use of excessive doses of sedatives".

Ferguson and Ball, *Br J Hosp Med* 1996.

POST SEDATION ASSESSMENT

- Monitor respiration rate until child fully awake. If level 4 sedation given, also monitor oxygen saturation until child awake.
- Give a drink, and something to eat if appropriate.
- Give 'who to contact' and safety advice to parent or carer.
- Discharge when bright and alert.

PREMEDICATION

Premedication is usually given to alleviate anxiety. In addition it may facilitate the induction of anaesthesia or the process of an unpleasant procedure (e.g. central I.V. line insertion) or give a pre-emptive dose of analgesic. The premedication, itself should not induce anxiety or distress.

ELECTIVE CASES

Oral premedication is preferable because of the distress caused by I.M. injections. However, for ENT procedures, I.M. atropine (20microgram/kg) is preferred as absorption is more predictable than after oral administration.

AGE	RECOMMENDED PREMEDICATION
< 1 year	EMLA
	+ Atropine p.o. 30microgram/kg
> 1 year	EMLA alone or add
	Temazepam p.o. 0.5mg/kg
	+/- Atropine p.o. 30microgram/kg

Alternative sedatives include midazolam, triclofos and trimeprazine (see monographs for details).

URGENT SURGERY

Premedication may be difficult to administer at an appropriate time before urgent surgery. If the wait for surgery is 4 hours or longer, an I.V. cannula should be inserted and I.V. fluids prescribed.

If premedication is necessary, oral drugs are less useful because absorption is unpredictable. I.M. atropine (20microgram/kg) with or without I.M. morphine (100-200microgram/kg) may be appropriate.

FASTING GUIDELINES

The fasting guidelines for elective surgery for all ages, are:

milk and solids   up to 4 hours before surgery
clear liquid°   up to 2 hours before surgery

° Clear liquid does not include orange juice and fizzy drinks.

NOTES

1. The insertion of a peripheral IV line is usually part of the procedure. This should be covered by **EMLA CREAM,** applied a minimum of 1 hour prior to the needle puncture, on at least visible veins. Every child above 1 month should have EMLA applied if time permits.
2. No sedation should be given in children with compromised airway or consciousness, or head injury.
3. For ENT/dental surgical cases the administration of pre-operative opiates is not recommended.

PAIN

The purpose of these guidelines is to advise prescribers with regard to providing optimum and safe analgesia for children. However, it should be remembered that analgesia represents only one component of effective pain management. Every child is an individual and therefore analgesia must be tailored and titrated to their individual requirements.

It is also important to remember that all children, including babies, are capable of feeling pain and should never be left without appropriate analgesia. The fear of opioid induced respiratory depression in neonates and infants can mostly be overcome by using appropriate dosage schedules. Anticipating and preventing pain is far more effective than trying to relieve established pain. Breakthrough pain can adversely affect a child's future pain coping strategies.

POST OPERATIVE PAIN MANAGEMENT

Post operative pain and anxiety may be reduced by the pre-operative preparation of the child. This should include a full explanation of the procedure or operation to be undertaken, including what the child can expect to come back with from theatre e.g. drips, drains, catheters. All children and parents should therefore be seen pre-operatively by the surgeon, the anaesthetist and a member of recovery nursing staff. The need for and type of pre-medication and post-operative analgesia can be discussed at this time.

Decisions regarding **post operative** analgesia must take note of any analgesics (particularly opioids) that have been given intra-operatively and in the recovery room, and the type of operation that has been performed, especially if the patient's airway is compromised e.g. ENT procedures. This information must be clearly documented on the anaesthetic sheet, drug chart or operation notes BEFORE transfer to the ward.

PRESCRIBING IN PAIN MANAGEMENT

Prescriptions with variable doses or routes of administration should be avoided, as they are confusing and do not give adequate information as to the analgesia being provided. Where pain is expected to last 12-24 hours the analgesia of choice should be written up in the regular section with an appropriate valid period. "PRN" analgesics are inappropriate as they are only given if the patient is "complaining" of pain, and often lead to suboptimal analgesia.

The route of administration should in itself not be frightening or painful. It is well documented that children find IM injections frightening and will avoid them at all costs, leading to suboptimal analgesia. If an infusion is deemed inappropriate then the use of the subcutaneous, oral or rectal routes is preferable to using IM injections.

For **subcutaneous** administration either a butterfly needle or intravenous cannula should be inserted and strapped down, if appropriate, whilst the child is still anaesthetised. Subcutaneous access should not be positioned on the distal part of a limb as these areas may be inadequately perfused resulting in poor analgesic absorption and ineffective analgesia. The site of administration should be changed every 2-3 days. The use of intravenous bolus doses of opioids, without a back up opiate infusion or that are not part of a PCA programme, are not as effective in producing sustained, adequate analgesia as a subcutaneous injection and carry an increased risk of inducing respiratory depression. The oral route should be used where possible or as soon as it can be tolerated.

The efficacy of the analgesic regimen should be regularly assessed, although this may often be difficult in the young. The degree of pain is usually underestimated by observers. Pain and sedation scores should be used.

GUIDELINES FOR MONITORING CHILDREN RECEIVING AN OPIOID INFUSION

- Patient must be nursed on the open ward, not in a cubicle.
- Pain and sedation score must be done with T.P.R and B.P monitoring; the frequency depending on the clinical status. The pain score is assessed using table 1 below:

Table 1   Pain Score

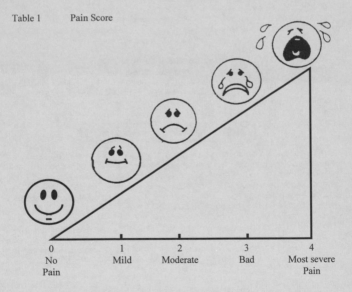

0	1	2	3	4
No Pain	Mild	Moderate	Bad	Most severe Pain

Table 2 below, adapted from Lloyd-Thomas A. R. et al *BMJ* 1992;304:1175 should be used to assess the pain and sedation score and to take the appropriate action. Ideally patients should have a low sedation score **and** a low pain score.

LEVEL	SEDATION	PAIN
0	Awake	Pain free
1	Drowsy	Comfortable except on moving
2	Asleep but moves spontaneously	Uncomfortable
3	Asleep responds to stimulation	Mild distress but can be comforted
4	Hard to rouse	Distressed
LEVEL	ACTION	ACTION
1	**Level 1:** No action	**Level 1:** NCA - give bolus PCA - encourage bolus (10 minutes before activity) Epidural - increase rate
2	**Level 2:** No action	**Level 2:** NCA - give bolus PCA - encourage bolus
3	**Level 3:** Stop infusion until return to level 3, restart infusion at lower dose	**Level 3:** NCA - give bolus and increase background infusion. Epidural - give bolus and increase rate
4	**Level 4:** Stop infusion. Call doctor.	**Level 4:** Contact doctor
	NCA = Nurse controlled analgesia	PCA = Patient controlled analgesia

- Naloxone (Narcan®) and Oxygen **must** be readily available.
- All patients receiving an opioid infusion must be prescribed naloxone on the 'when necessary' section of their drug chart.
- Caution: do not administer any other bolus drugs through the same line as the opioid infusion. If this is essential then an extension set with a non return valve must be used.

WITHDRAWAL OF OPIOIDS

Where opioids have been used continuously for more than a week, the withdrawal of these drugs should be gradual. This is particularly important if the opioid has a short elimination half life e.g. fentanyl, as tolerance and dependence are seen earlier than in opioids with a longer half life e.g. morphine.

A stepping down method could involve giving oral morphine initially at an equivalent dose as the intravenous one for 24 hours and then reducing.

GUIDELINES FOR THE MANAGEMENT OF SKELETAL MUSCLE SPASM POST ORTHOPEDIC SURGERY

Skeletal muscle spasm in cerebral palsy children following orthopaedic surgery can be difficult to manage and can delay recovery.

In the immediate post operative period the child should be maintained on their pre-operative antispasmodic (e.g. baclofen) and prescribed appropriate regular analgesics for the surgical procedure performed (see recommended analgesics). Diazepam (see page 84) should also be prescribed on an as required basis for any breakthrough spasm.

If the child was not previously on antispasmodics, regular baclofen (see page 34) should be prescribed along with appropriate regular analgesics and diazepam on an as required basis for any breakthrough spasm.

The management of the spasm should then be determined using the spasm scores detailed in the table below. The amount and frequency of diazepam administered per day should also be assessed as regular administration may warrant the patient being assessed as having a higher spasm score.

Patients on opiate infusions should be assessed using the guidelines on page 253 rather than those below.

LEVEL	SPASM	SEDATION/MUSCLE TONE
0	Spasm free	Awake with good tone
1	Spasm on moving	Asleep/Drowsy - rousable and manageable tone
2	Intermittent spontaneous spasm	Asleep/Drowsy - rousable but floppy
3	Continuous spasm	Hard to rouse
LEVEL	ACTION	ACTION
0	**Level 0:** No action	**Level 0:** No action
1	**Level 1:** Administer diazepam - if requiring regular doses increase baclofen	**Level 1:** Stop diazepam PRN - consider decreasing baclofen dose
2	**Level 2:** Increase baclofen - if patient on alternative/additional antispasmodics, start or increase baclofen	**Level 2:** Decrease baclofen - do not administer further doses of diazepam until adequate tone returns
3	**Level 3:** Seek expert advice	**Level 3:** Contact doctor immediately

RECOMMENDED ANALGESICS

The following guidelines provide recommendations as to the level of analgesia required for the management of pain. The severity of pain is individual and should be determined using a pain assessment tool rather than the procedure performed. The latter may however be useful for initiating analgesic therapy. It must always be remembered that every child is an individual and that the following represents guidance which can be used to tailor therapy. The individual drug monographs should be referred to for full prescribing advice.

CAUSE OF PAIN	SEVERITY ❶	RECOMMENDED TREATMENT ❷	ALTERNATIVE or ADDITIONAL TREATMENT ❸	COMMENTS
Post operative (general'). Trauma. If patient has unstable neuro-observations, consult neurologist before prescribing opioids.	Mild	Paracetamol		
	Mild/Moderate	Ibuprofen	Paracetamol with codeine phosphate tablets or dihydrocodeine elixir	Use rectal route until oral tolerated. Prescribe concomitant laxative with regular administration of opioid.
	Moderate/Severe	Diclofenac (suppository/tablets) or Naproxen (liquid/tablets)	Morphine. Buprenorphine	Prescribe analgesic regularly. DO NOT USE 'PRN'
	Severe	Morphine	Add diclofenac (suppository/tablets) or naproxen (liquid/tablets). Seek expert advice	**Caution:** Check operation notes for intraoperative opioids before administering a loading dose. Consider concomitant anti emetic and laxative therapy.

❶ Determine using a pain assessment tool.
❷ Non steroidal anti-inflammatory drugs should not be prescribed in children with renal failure, severe liver failure, abnormal clotting or asthmatics with known sensitivity to NSAIDs.
❸ There is no benefit in using more than one agent from the same class of analgesic e.g. opioid, NSAID.

255

CAUSE OF PAIN	SEVERITY ❶	RECOMMENDED TREATMENT ❷	ALTERNATIVE or ADDITIONAL TREATMENT ❸	COMMENTS
Post operative (specific) - caudal/epidural ❹ - wound infiltration		Bupivicaine	Lignocaine	As the local anaesthetic wears off start alternative analgesia May require combination with opioid to provide some sedation. If epidura opioid used, systemic infusion is contra-indicated. Seek advice from paediatric anaesthetist.
Post operative skeletal muscle spasm - orthopedic related	Mild	Diazepam PRN	Baclofen	Add in regular baclofen if diazepam required regularly.
	Moderate	Baclofen + Diazepam PRN	Morphine	Increase baclofen dose if diazepam required regularly
	Severe	Baclofen + Morphine	Seek expert advice	

❶ Determine using a pain assessment tool.
❷ Non steroidal anti-inflammatory drugs should not be prescribed in children with renal failure, severe liver failure, abnormal clotting or asthmatics with known sensitivity to NSAIDs.
❸ There is no benefit in using more than one agent from the same class of analgesic e.g. opioid, NSAID.
❹ Epidural infusions must only be used in designated areas with suitably trained staff.

CAUSE OF PAIN	SEVERITY ❶	RECOMMENDED TREATMENT ❷	ALTERNATIVE or ADDITIONAL TREATMENT ❸	COMMENTS
Fracture or bone related	Mild/Moderate	Ibuprofen ± Paracetamol	Paracetamol with codeine phosphate tablets or dihydrocodeine elixir.	Prescribed analgesic regularly for 24-48 hours and then PRN.
	Moderate/Severe	Diclofenac (suppository/tablets) or Naproxen (liquid/tablets)	Morphine Buprenorphine	Prescribe analgesic regularly. DO NOT USE 'PRN'
	Severe	Morphine	Add diclofenac (suppository/tablets) or naproxen (liquid/tablets). Seek expert advice	Give loading dose before commencing infusion. Caution: Check operation notes for intraoperative opioids.
Sickle cell crisis	Mild/Moderate	Ibuprofen	Paracetamol	
	Moderate/Severe	Diclofenac (suppository/tablets) or Naproxen (liquid/tablets)	Morphine	Prescribe regularly.
	Severe	Morphine	Add diclofenac (suppository/tablets) or naproxen (liquid/tablets). Seek expert advice	
Renal Colic	Mild/Moderate	Hyoscine N butyl bromide		
	Moderate	Diclofenac (suppository/tablets) or Naproxen (liquid/tablets)	Pethidine	
	Severe	Pethidine	Pethidine	

❶ Determine using a pain assessment tool.
❷ Non steroidal anti-inflammatory drugs should not be prescribed in children with renal failure, severe liver failure, abnormal clotting or asthmatics with known sensitivity to NSAIDs.
❸ There is no benefit n using more than one agent from the same class of analgesic e.g. opioid, NSAID.
❹ Do not use NSAIDs for pain during peritoneal dialysis if renal function is recoverable.

257

CAUSE OF PAIN	SEVERITY ❶	RECOMMENDED TREATMENT ❷	ALTERNATIVE or ADDITIONAL TREATMENT ❸	COMMENTS
Pain during peritoneal dialysis	Mild/Moderate	Paracetamol Ibuprofen ❹	Lignocaine in dialysis	
	Moderate/Severe	Diclofenac (suppository/tablets) or Naproxen (liquid/tablets) ❹	Buprenorphine Morphine	Prescribe regularly during dialysis sessions.
	Severe	Morphine	Add diclofenac (suppository/tablets) or naproxen (liquid/tablets). Seek expert adviceSeek expert advice	? peritonitis, position of catheter
Bladder muscle spasm	Mild/Moderate	Oxybutinin	Propantheline	Ibuprofen may also reduce residual pain
	Moderate/Severe	Oxybutinin ± Diclofenac	Oxybutinin ± Morphine	
Renal biopsy or other ward procedure	Moderate/Severe for short period	Ketamine + midazolam	Fentanyl or Morphine + midazolam	This procedure must only be performed with resuscitation facilities and antagonists e.g. Flumazenil/Naloxone at hand.

❶ Determine using a pain assessment tool.

❷ Non steroidal anti-inflammatory drugs should not be prescribed in children with renal failure, severe liver failure, abnormal clotting or asthmatics with known sensitivity to NSAIDs.

❸ There is no benefit in using more than one agent from the same class of analgesic e.g. opioid, NSAID.

ANTIBIOTIC TREATMENT

GENERAL PRINCIPLES

This guide gives recommendations for common infections, it is not intended to be comprehensive. Antibiotics are usually started **before** microbiology results are available. This guide is designed to give information on the initial treatment of common conditions. Treatment may have to be modified depending upon the child's progress and bacterial sensitivities.

Isolation of bacteria from a specimen does not automatically mean antibiotic treatment is required.

Before prescribing any antibiotic ASK child and/or carer about ALLERGIES. Do not assume records in the notes are accurate.

If possible, specimens for microbiological examination should be taken before starting antimicrobial therapy.

RECOMMENDATIONS WHEN INITIATING ANTIBIOTIC THERAPY

1. Consider the severity of the condition to be treated.
2. Consider the possible infecting pathogen(s).
3. Choose the route of administration, remembering that oral therapy is often appropriate.
4. Monitor the child's response and consider changing from IV therapy (if used initially) to oral therapy when possible.
5. For most bacterial infections other than those involving bone, joint or heart valve **5 days** treatment is enough.

RESTRICTED ANTI-INFECTIVE AGENTS

A number of antibiotics included in the formulary are restricted for a variety of reasons including efficacy, toxicity and cost. The use of these agents should be discussed with a microbiologist before prescribing.

ORAL ANTIBIOTIC THERAPY

Oral antibiotics can often be substituted for IV therapy without loss of efficacy. Many, but not all, oral antibiotics are rapidly and well absorbed, for example, ciprofloxacin, metronidazole and co-amoxiclav are well absorbed after oral administration.

CONTACT NUMBERS FOR MICROBIOLOGY ADVICE:		
St Thomas' Hospital:	Prof S. Eykyn ext 2578	or *microbiologist Bleep* 0132
Guy's Hospital:	Dr W. Gransden ext 4513	or *microbiologist Bleep* 1300
Lewisham Hospital:	Dr G. Rao ext 3264	or *microbiologist Bleep 219*

If in doubt ASK - advice is always available from microbiology doctors.

SUGGESTED INITIAL TREATMENTS

CONDITION	AGE	LIKELY ORGANISMS	INITIAL ANTIBIOTICS	NOTES
Bacterial meningitis	Neonate	Group B Streptococcus Escherichia coli Listeria monocytogenes	Cefotaxime + Amoxycillin	
	1-3 months	as for > 3months + neonatal pathogens	Cefotaxime + Amoxycillin	For prophylaxis of meningitis contacts see page 264
	> 3 months	Neisseria meningitidis Streptococcus pneumoniae ❷ Haemophilus influenzae ❶	Cefotaxime	
"Sepsis" (Fever without obvious source)	Neonates < 48 hours old "Early Onset"	Group B Streptococcus Escherichia coli	Benzylpenicillin + Gentamicin	Coagulase negative staphylicoccal infections are common however vancomycin should only be prescribed after positive culture.
	Neonates > 48 hours old	As above and various hospital acquired organisms	Varies according to isolates and sensitivities. Seek Microbiology advice.	
	Infants and children (non-immuno compromised)	Neisseria meningitidis Streptococcus pneumoniae ❷ Haemophilus influenzae ❶	Cefotaxime	
Pneumonia Community Acquired	< 5 years	Usually viral Streptococcus pneumoniae ❷ Haemophilus influenzae ❶	Cefuroxime (IV) or Co-Amoxiclav (PO)	
	> 5 years	Streptococcus pneumoniae ❷ Mycoplasma pneumoniae Respiratory viruses	Cefuroxime (IV) or Amoxycillin or Erythromycin (if Mycoplasma suspected)	
Pneumonia Hospital Acquired		Many possible pathogens	Seek Microbiology advice	

If in doubt ASK - advice is always available from microbiology doctors.

❶ Haemophilus influenzae infection is rare in fully immunised children.
❷ Strep. pneumoniae exhibiting intermediate penicillin resistance is being seen with increasing frequency (5.7% in 1997).

260

SUGGESTED INITIAL TREATMENTS

CONDITION	AGE	LIKELY ORGANISMS	INITIAL ANTIBIOTICS	NOTES
Urinary tract infections	< 3 months and/or acutely ill	*Escherichia coli* *Proteus* species *Klebsiella* species	Gentamicin or Cefotaxime	Prophylaxis until imaging complete Hospital acquired gram negative bacilli infections maybe trimethoprim resistant. Seek Microbiology advice.
	> 3 months and mildly unwell	*Escherichia coli* *Proteus* species *Klebsiella* species	Trimethoprim (PO)	
Necrotizing Enterocolitis	Neonates	*Escherichia coli* *Klebsiella spp* *Enterobacter spp.* *Clostridium perfringens*	Benzylpenicillin + Gentamicin + Metronicazole	
Febrile Neutropenia	All	Aerobic Gram negative bacilli e.g. *Pseudomonas aeruginosa* *Staphylococcus aureus* Fungi	Azlocillin + Gentamicin	Adjust therapy to response, isolates and sensitivities. Seek Microbiology advice.
Sickle Cell Crisis (if infection suspected)	All	*Streptococcus penumoniae* [2] *Haemophilus influenzae* [1]	Cefuroxime (IV) or Co-Amoxiclav (PO)	

If in doubt ASK - advice is always available from microbiology doctors.

[1] *Haemophilus influenzae* infection is rare in fully immunised children.
[2] *Strep. pneumoniae* exhibiting intermediate penicillin resistance and being seen with increasing frequency (5.7% in 1997).

SUGGESTED INITIAL TREATMENTS

CONDITION	AGE	LIKELY ORGANISMS	INITIAL ANTIBIOTICS	NOTES
Pseudomembranous colitis (antibiotic associated)	All	Toxin producing strain of *Clostridium difficile*	Stop other antibiotics. Metronidazole (PO)	
Helicobacter pylori positive gastritis or duodenal ulcer	All	*Helicobacter pylori*	Amoxycillin + Metronidazole + Omeprazole	
Human bites	All	Upper respiratory tract aerobes and anaerobes	Co-Amoxiclav	Consider tetanus toxoid
Animal bites	All	*Pasteurella multocida* *Capnocytophaga canimorsus (DF2)* Anaerobes	Co-Amoxiclav	Consider tetanus toxoid
Cellulitis/Impetigo	All	*Streptococcus pyogenes* *Staphylococcus aureus*	Amoxycillin (IV) + Flucloxacillin (IV) or Erythromycin (PO)	
Periorbital Cellulitis	All	*Streptococcus pyogenes* *Staphylococcus aureus* Anaerobes *Haemophilus influenzae* ❶	Co-Amoxiclav	Seek ENT advice.

If in doubt ASK - advice is always available from microbiology doctors.

❶ *Haemophilus influenzae* infection is rare in fully immunised children.

❷ *Strep. pneumoniae* exhibiting intermediate penicillin resistance and being seen with increasing frequency (5.7% in 1997).

SUGGESTED INITIAL TREATMENTS

CONDITION	AGE	LIKELY ORGANISMS	INITIAL ANTIBIOTICS	NOTES
Acute septic arthritis/Osteomyelitis	< 5 years	Staphylococcus aureus Streptococcus pneumoniae ❷ Streptococcus pyogenes Haemophilus influenzae ❶	Co-Amoxiclav	Seek advice from Microbiology and Orthopaedics
	> 5 years	Staphylococcus aureus Streptococcus pneumoniae ❷ Streptococcus pyogenes	Flucloxacillin	Seek advice from Microbiology and Orthopaedics
Tonsillitis	All	Group A Streptococcus Viruses	Phenoxymethylpenicillin (PO) or Benzylpenicillin (IV)	
Pharyngitis	All	Usually viral Group A Streptococcus	If bacterial infection suspected Phenoxymethylpenicillin (PO) or Benzylpenicillin (IV)	
Acute Epiglottitis	Infants and children	Streptococcus pneumoniae ❷ Haemophilus influenzae ❶	Cefotaxime	
Acute otitis media Sinusitis	Infants and children	Streptococcus pneumoniae ❷ Haemophilus influenzae ❶	Amoxycillin (Co-Amoxiclav if recurrent)	

If in doubt ASK - advice is always available from microbiology doctors.

❶ Haemophilus influenzae infection is rare in fully immunised children.
❷ Strep. pneumoniae exhibiting intermediate penicillin resistance and being seen with increasing frequency (5.7% in 1997).

263

ANTIBIOTIC PROPHYLAXIS

GENERAL PRINCIPLES

1. Prophylaxis should be used where the procedure, condition or contact commonly leads to infection, or if infection would result in a serious illness.
2. The antimicrobial agent should be bactericidal and directed against specific organisms with predictable sensitivities.
3. Surgical prophylaxis is usually given to prevent wound infection.
   Doses and further information can be found in the individual drug monographs.

MEDICAL PROPHYLAXIS

INDICATION	COMMON PATHOGENS	RECOMMENDATION
Meningitis: patient and close domestic or very close medical contacts	*Neisseria meningitidis*	Ciprofloxacin Rifampicin Pregnant contacts: Ceftriaxone
	Haemophilus. influenzae	Rifampicin
Whooping cough: unvaccinated contact < 1 year	*Bordetella pertussis*	Erythromycin for 7-10 days
Tuberculosis Child <2 years and not BCG vaccinated in contact with sputum-positive tuberculosis	*Mycobacterium tuberculosis*	Isoniazid for 3-6 months. A BCG vaccination is then needed **after** a negative tuberculin test.
Prophylaxis of UTI	*Escherichia coli* *Proteus* species *Klebsiella* species	Trimethoprim
Tetanus prone wound	Tetanus and secondary infection	Tetanus toxoid or anti-tetanus immunoglobulin may be required (see page 210) + Phenoxymethylpenicillin or Amoxycillin
Sickle cell or splenectomy patients	*Streptococcus pneumoniae* *Haemophilus influenzae* *Neisseria meningitidis*	Phenoxymethylpenicillin and vaccination with pneumovax, meningococcal vaccine and Hib vaccine

SURGICAL PROPHYLAXIS

INDICATION	COMMON PATHOGENS	RECOMMENDATION
Acute appendicitis and other abdominal surgery	Anaerobes Coliforms	Cefuroxime + Metronidazole up to 48 hours post op.
Cardiac surgery	*Staphylococcus epidermidis* *Staphylococcus aureus* Coliforms	Cefuroxime stat & for up to 48 hours post op.
Urological procedures	*Escherichia coli* Coliforms	Gentamicin stat and for up to two doses post op depending upon renal function.

ANTIBIOTIC PROPHYLAXIS OF INFECTIVE ENDOCARDITIS

These guidelines are based on the Working Party Report of the British Society for Antimicrobial Chemotherapy (*Lancet* 1990; i 88-89 and revised in *Lancet* 1992; 339: 1292-1293 and again in *J. Antimicrob. Chem.* 1993; 31: 437-453).

Warning cards for susceptible children are available free of charge, from the British Heart Foundation or pharmacy.

CHILDREN AT RISK

- Children with congenital or acquired cardiac defects or prosthetic heart valves and those with a past history of infective endocarditis.
- **Special risk children are those who:**
- Need a general anaesthetic **and** have received a penicillin more than once in the previous month **or** have a prosthetic valve **or** are allergic to penicillin.
- All patients who have previously had endocarditis.
- When clindamycin is used, periodontal or other multistage procedures should only be repeated after an interval of at least 2 weeks.

PROCEDURES TO BE COVERED

- **Dental treatment** with gingival bleeding: dental extractions, deep scaling and periodontal surgery. Plan the dental treatment to reduce the need for antibiotic cover. Try to do as much as possible under the same antibiotic cover. For appropriate antibiotic regimen see page 267.
- **Other procedures**.

PROCEDURE	VALVE	REGIMEN (as in diagram for dental treatment see page 267)	
Genito-urinary instrumentation	Damaged native valve or prosthetic valve.	No penicillin allergy:	Regimen D
		Penicillin allergy:	Regimen E
GI endoscopy, barium enema	Prosthetic valves.	No penicillin allergy:	Regimen D
		Penicillin allergy:	Regimen E
Tonsillectomy/ adenoidectomy	a) Damaged native valve.	No penicillin allergy:	Regimen C
		Penicillin allergy:	Regimen E
	b) Prosthetic valves.	No penicillin allergy:	Regimen D
		Penicillin allergy:	Regimen E

ADMINISTRATION AND TIMING OF ANTIBIOTICS

The administration and timing of antibiotic theapy varies according to the regimen required:

- **Oral amoxicillin** should be given under supervision at the times stated.
- I.M. and I.V. antibiotics should be given immediately before the procedure. I.V. **vancomycin** should be infused over 120 minutes and followed by **gentamicin**. I.V. **teicoplanin** or **clindamycin** should be given at the time of induction of anaesthesia or 15 minutes before the surgical procedure.
- **Oral clindamycin** should be given under supervision as a single dose 1 hour before procedure.
- **IV clindamycin** must be diluted to at least 6mg in 1ml with sodium chloride 0.9% or 5% glucose and adminstered over at least 10 minutes.

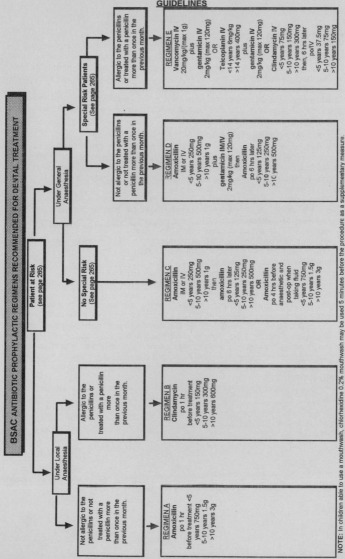

BSAC ANTIBIOTIC PROPHYLACTIC REGIMENS RECOMMENDED FOR DENTAL TREATMENT

GUIDELINES

Patient at Risk (see page 265)

Under Local Anaesthesia

Not allergic to the penicillins or not treated with a penicillin more than once in the previous month.

REGIMEN A
Amoxicillin
po 1 hr
before treatment <5
years 750mg
5-10 years 1.5g
>10 years 3g

Allergic to the penicillins or treated with a penicillin more than once in the previous month.

REGIMEN B
Clindamycin
po 1 hr
before treatment
<5 years 150mg
5-10 years 300mg
>10 years 600mg

Under General Anaesthesia

No Special Risk (See page 265)

REGIMEN C
Amoxicillin
IM or IV
<5 years 250mg
5-10 years 500mg
>10 years 1g
then
amoxicillin
po 6 hrs later
<5 years 125mg
5-10 years 250mg
>10 years 500mg
OR
Amoxicillin
po 4 hrs before
anaesthetic and
post-op when
taking fluid
<5 years 750mg
5-10 years 1.5g
>10 years 3g

Special Risk Patients (See page 265)

Not allergic to the penicillins or not treated with a penicillin more than once in the previous month.

REGIMEN D
Amoxicillin
IM or IV
<5 years 250mg
5-10 years 500mg
>10 years 1g
plus
gentamicin IM/IV
2mg/kg (max 120mg)
then
Amoxicillin
po 6 hrs later
<5 years 125mg
5-10 years 250mg
>10 years 500mg

Allergic to the penicillins or treated with a penicillin more than once in the previous month.

REGIMEN E
Vancomycin IV
20mg/kg/(max 1g)
plus
gentamicin IV
2mg/kg (max 120mg)
OR
Teicoplanin IV
<14 years 6mg/kg
>14 years 400mg
plus
gentamicin IV
2mg/kg (max 120mg)
OR
Clindamycin IV
<5 years 75mg
5-10 years 150mg
>10 years 300mg
then, 6 hrs later
po/IV
<5 years 37.5mg
5-10 years 75mg
>10 years 150mg

NOTE: In children able to use a mouthwash, chlorhexidine 0.2% mouthwash may be used 5 minutes before the procedure as a supplementary measure.

267

INSULIN

Insulin preparations are principally classified by their absorption characteristics after subcutaneous injection. The majority of insulin used in the UK is human sequence and is a standard strength of 100units/ml (U100).

Children rarely require porcine or bovine insulin and human insulin is the treatment of choice. Occasionally, children from abroad may be using unusual strengths of insulin e.g. 40 or 80 units/ml.

ABSORPTION CHARACTERISTICS

The duration of action of different insulin preparations varies considerably and needs to be assessed for every Individual patient. The figures below are average values and significant variations occur between and within individual children. The effects of insulin may vary further in children with hepatic or renal failure or hypothyroidism.

a) **Short Acting Insulins:** Soluble Human Insulin (Human Actrapid, Humulin S)

Soluble Insulin is the only insulin suitable for intravenous administration. Following IV injection the effects are seen very rapidly, the active half-life is 5 minutes and the effects last less than 30 minutes.

After subcutaneous injection the onset of action is 15-60 minutes, the peak effect is seen after 2-4 hours and the duration of actiont is 6-8 hours.

b) **Intermediate Acting Insulins:**
- Isophane Human Insulin (Human Insulatard ge, Humulin I)
- Insulin Zinc Suspension (Mixed) (Human Monotard)

c) **Premixed Insulin Mixtures:**

The mixing of short with intermediate - acting insulins at the time of injection offers the greatest flexibility of dosage, but such mixtures have to be injected immediately and may be less convenient than fixed proportion premixed insulins. These are available in a variety of combinations of soluble insulin and isophane insulin often in cartridges suitable for use with pen injectors. If a child uses a premixed insulin solution they should keep a vial of soluble insulin in the home to be used in case of febrile illness etc. (See Insulin monograph page 129).

IMMUNOGENICITY

Since the advent of highly purified insulins, these immunological phenomena are a rarity.

ADMINISTRATION

RECOMMENDED INSULIN REGIMES

- Short-acting insulin mixed with Intermediate-acting insulin: twice daily (before breakfast and evening meal).
- Intermediate-acting insulin with or without Short-acting insulin: twice daily (before breakfast and evening meal).
- Short-acting insulin: three times daily (before meals).
  Intermediate-acting insulin: at bedtime.

The regime chosen depends upon the particular needs, motivation and understanding of the child and parents or carers.

INJECTION TECHNIQUE AND SITE

Good injection technique is important to minimise avoidable variations in absorption after subcutaneous injection.

The upper, outer aspects of arms and thighs, the buttocks and the central abdomen are all suitable sites for subcutaneous injection of insulin. At rest, absorption is faster from the abdomen than the limbs. However, absorption from the limbs is faster if an injected-limb is exercised. Vigorous or sustained exercise can lower blood glucose for up to 18 hours.

The site of injection should be rotated on a daily basis as repeated injection into the same site can lead to accumulation of fat and fibrous tissue, which disrupts insulin absorption and worsens glycaemic control.

The depth of injection also influences insulin absorption. If too shallow, absorption is slowed, and if given I.M. (often painful), absorption is more rapid. To ensure the correct depth of injection:

- a 6 or 8mm pen needle or a U30, U50 or U100 microfine insulin syringe should be used;
- the skin at the injection site should be pinched between the thumb and fore finger before injection and
- the needle should be inserted at right angles to the injection site

INSULIN PENS & SYRINGES

NovoPens and the BD pen are portable devices that can be used in place of syringes and offer children with diabetes a considerable degree of freedom and convenience.

Most insulin preparations are available as pen cartridges and the majority of children now use a pen device. The pens are free of charge but needles must be purchased by patients.

MONITORING WHEN WELL

Blood glucose monitoring is essential to ensure good control of diabetes. The frequency required varies but when well, blood glucose should be monitored a minimum of twice daily before meals. In well motivated or poorly controlled patients this may be increased to four times daily. A blood test in the middle of the night should be performed occasionally especially if morning blood glucose levels are elevated. Urinary ketones should be measured if blood sugars are elevated or child is unwell.

SUBCUTANEOUS INSULIN DOSE

A child's total daily insulin requirement can only be assessed when the child is at home. However, when commencing subcutaneous insulin an initial dose must be estimated and then adjusted according to response. The method of calculating this initial dose depends upon the child's previous exposure to insulin. If a child has received an IV insulin infusion, some degree of control can be achieved by calculating their 24 hour soluble insulin dose and using this as a basis for initial subcutaneous therapy. If no intravenous insulin has been administered, a reasonable starting dose of subcutaneous insulin is 0.5units/kg/day.

If the child is commenced on a twice daily regime of mixed intermediate and short-acting insulin before breakfast and dinner, two thirds of the estimated daily dose should be given in the morning and one third in the evening. The proportion of these doses given as intermediate and short-acting insulins is variable. However giving 30% of the dose as short-acting and 70% as intermediate-acting is reasonable e.g. Human Mixtard 30ge, Humulin M3.

Close monitoring of blood glucose is essential to tailor the predicted initial dose to a child's actual insulin requirement. The distribution of insulin doses and overall requirement varies according to the child's diet and degree of activity on a daily basis. Well-informed and confident children and/or parents/carers should be able to learn to adjust insulin doses and/or diet to match the child's activities and/or diet and in response to blood glucose measurements.

IN ILLNESS

Even when a child is not eating, their insulin requirements will be the same or greater than normal and injections must not be omitted. Under these conditions blood glucose comes mainly from the liver. The child must continue to have an adequate fluid and calorie intake, given intravenously if necessary, with appropriate adjustments to insulin dose (based on blood glucose readings).

- **Child reasonably well and eating**
  Monitor blood glucose regularly during mild or moderate intercurrent illness. Increase dose of insulin in 10% increments should hyperglycaemia develop.
- **Child reasonably well, but off food**
  Give regular carbohydrate-rich drinks (e.g. fruit juice, milk, milkshakes, Lucozade, non-diet fizzy drinks, non-diet squash) in small amounts each hour to ensure an adequate glucose intake throughout the day. Balance insulin requirement against carbohydrate intake.
- **Child severely ill and insulin-treated or less ill but unable to maintain an adequate carbohydrate intake**
  Treat with insulin infusion and intravenous glucose. (See Major Surgery Protocol page 272).

ACUTE HYPOGLYCAEMIA

If the child is conscious, give fast acting carbohydrate orally e.g. orange juice or lucozade, followed by slower acting carbohydrate e.g. biscuits or bread. Review after 30 minutes.

If the child's level of consciousness is depressed, give **25% glucose** intravenously (<2 years 25mls, >2 years 50mls). If intravenous access is not available and cannot be sited quickly give glucagon I.M. (see page 115). Glucagon may be less effective in poor nutritional states and/or hepatic impairment due to reduced liver glycogen storage. If no response is seen 10-15 minutes after glucagon injection, I.V. glucose should be given.

DIABETES MELLITUS (PERI-OPERATIVE MANAGEMENT)

These guidelines can also be used for sick children and those who are nil by mouth. The following recommendations are for guidance only. Each child must be assessed and their management based on normal insulin requirements, diabetic control and the operative procedure.

For major surgery and/or prolonged periods of 'nil by mouth' (NBM) it may be necessary to run glucose and insulin infusions separately for safe control of blood glucose.

Ideally, diabetic control should be optimised before admission, IV insulin and glucose replacement needs to start when the child first omits insulin injection and a meal.

MAJOR SURGERY

MORNING LIST

Nil by mouth from midnight.
Give usual subcutaneous insulin on evening before operation.
At 06.00 to 08.00 start intravenous infusion of 5% glucose (or glucose/saline) with added potassium (20mmol/l). See table1 for maintanance rates.
Table 1:

Body weight	Fluid volume
1st 10kg	4ml/kg/hr
10-20kg	add 2ml/kg/hr
>20kg	add 1ml/kg/hr

SLIDING SCALE (IV INFUSION)
At the same time start an IV infusion of soluble INSULIN (Human Actrapid) 50units made up to 50ml with sodium chloride 0.9% in a syringe pump. (1ml = 1unit insulin) Flush giving set with insulin solution **before** connecting to the child.
Table 2:

Blood Glucose (mmol/l)	Insulin Infusion (unit/kg/hr) (ml/kg/hr)
0-5	0
6-10	0.05
11-15	0.1
16-20	0.15
>20	0.2

Measure blood glucose at bedside as soon as insulin pump is started and adjust infusion rate to keep blood glucose between 4 and 11 mmol/l. Measure blood glucose each hour before surgery and every 30 minutes during the operation.
Be prepared to adjust scale if insulin infusion is not controlling blood glucose levels adequately.

Post operatively, measure blood glucose 2 hourly until stable, then 6 hourly.
Check urine for ketones if laboratory values for glucose are below 4 or above 17mmol/l.

272

AFTERNOON LIST

Give patients **half** usual pre-breakfast dose of **soluble insulin only** (omit all intermediate or long-acting insulins) with a light breakfast.
Mid morning start IV dextrose and insulin as in above regimen.
Once food and drink can be taken normally, resume patients previous treatment.

DO NOT STOP INFUSION OF INTRAVENOUS INSULIN UNTIL AFTER A SUBCUTANEOUS DOSE HAS BEEN ADMINISTERED.

MINOR SURGERY

If possible, admit the child 24 hours pre-op for assessment of diabetic control. Check BM's pre-meals and then 2-4 hourly.

MORNING LIST

- Ensure child is 1st on the list
- **"Nil by mouth"** from midnight.
- Omit morning insulin.
- At 0600 start I.V. infusion of 4% glucose/0.18% saline (dextrose/saline)

On return from theatre
Check BM's at bedside 2 hourly until midday. If the child is well enough to eat and drink, then do the following:
If BM <12 pre-meal: give meal, check BM's 2 hourly and consider stopping dextrose/saline infusion.

If BM >12 pre-meal: give 2 units Human Soluble Insulin S.C., give meal and consider stopping dextrose/saline infusion.

Later in the afternoon
If BM's 6-12 and child is well, give usual subcutaneous insulin dose prior to evening meal and if still well after meal, discharge.
If BM's less than 6   } discuss with
or BM's greater than 12   } a senior doctor

If child unable to eat or drink at any time, refer to major surgery protocol and discuss with a more senior doctor.

AFTERNOON LIST

- Ensure child first on the list

In the morning
- Administer short acting insulin S.C. at the child's usual dose, before a light breakfast.
- Omit any medium/long acting insulin.
- Place the child 'Nil by Mouth'.
- Start I.V. infusion of 4% glucose/0.18% saline (dextrose/saline).
- Check BMs hourly before theatre.

On return from theatre
Check blood glucose at bedside 2 hourly. If the child is well enough to eat and drink, do the following:

BM <12 pre-meal: give meal, check BM's 2 hourly and consider stopping dextrose/saline infusion.

If BM >12 pre-meal: give child their usual subcutaneous dose of short acting insulin and give meal. Check BM's 2 hourly and consider stopping the dextrose/saline infusion.

Keep child in overnight and discuss with a more senior doctor how much extra insulin to give overnight and what type (i.e. short or long acting).

If the child is unable to eat or drink at any time, then refer to major surgery protocol, but discuss with a more senior doctor first anyway.

DIABETIC KETOACIDOSIS (EMERGENCY TREATMENT)

The following recommendations are guidelines. Individual children's requirements may vary and frequent reassessments are always necessary.

Children who are more than 5% dehydrated and/or drowsy and/or acidotic will usually require intravenous fluid and electrolyte correction. Those not in this group may tolerate oral rehydration and subcutaneous insulin.

The leading causes of mortality associated with diabetic ketoacidosis are: cerebral oedema, hypokalaemia and inhalation of vomit.

MANAGEMENT RECOMMENDATIONS

1. **Notify registrar and consultant on call.**

2. **Assess vital signs**
   Conscious level, perfusion, TPR, blood pressure, oxygen saturation.

3. **Establish/maintain airway**
   Ensure patency. Insert airway if comatose or recurrent vomiting. Give oxygen if necessary.

4. **Insert NG tube,** aspirate and leave on open drainage.

5. **Establish IV access**

6. **Confirm diagnosis**
   a)   blood glucose (bedside - BM stix).
   b)   acidosis (urinary, ketones and blood gases).
   c)   urea & electrolytes (request urgent potassium).
   d)   other blood tests (FBC and differential, PCV, CRP, LFT, blood cultures, serum osmolality).

7. **ECG monitor**
   Look for large T waves on ECG.

8. **Assess degree of dehydration**

   a)   weigh the child and compare with last clinic weight.

1kg of weight loss = 1 litre of fluid loss

   b)   clinical assessment: mild dehydration (5%)
                                    moderate/severe (10%) with poor perfusion, the early pulse etc.

9. **Monitor urinary ketones and glucose**
   Record all urine output.

SPECIFIC TREATMENT RECOMMENDATIONS

Shocked children need immediate treatment. If tachycardic, poor capillary refill time and hypotensive give 10ml/kg sodium chloride 0.9%. Repeat as necessary.
Rehydrate, by calculating child's fluid requirement.

fluid requirement = maintenance + deficit + continuing losses

Maintenance	=	1500ml/m^2/24 hours
		OR
0 - 2 years	=	100ml/kg/24 hours
3 - 5 years	=	90ml/kg/24 hours
6 - 9 years	=	75ml/kg/24 hours
> 10 years	=	50ml/kg/24 hours
Deficit (ml)	=	calculated weight loss in milligrams
		OR
	=	dehydration (%) x body weight (kg) x 1,000

(NOTE: Maximum dehydration used is 10%)

Hourly rate of fluid replacement = $\dfrac{\text{Maintenance + deficit}}{24 \text{ hours}}$

Continue to replace losses ml for ml

Infuse sodium chloride 0.9% at calculated hourly rate. Unless child is anuric add 20ml of potassium chloride to each 500ml intravenous fluid. Check potassium levels every 2-4 hours for the first 24 hours and use ECG monitor. Alter potassium supplements to keep potassium levels between 4-5mmol/l.

Continue under observation until blood glucose <12mmol/l. Then convert to 4% dextrose/0.18% saline with or without potassium.

Check serum sodium every 2-4 hours and maintain between 145-155mmol/l. Serum sodium levels must be brought down slowly, avoiding rapid shifts which may be associated with cerebral oedema.

Insulin: start IV infusion of soluble insulin (Human Actrapid 1unit/ml).

Initial rate of infusion: 0.1unit (0.1ml)/kg/hour reduce to
0.05unit (0.05ml)/kg/hour if rate of blood glucose fall is greater than or equal to 5mmol/hour.

If rate of fall is greater than 5mmol/hour this can lead to cerebral oedema due to changes in osmolality.

Reduce the insulin infusion rate when blood glucose is below 12mmol/l and 4% dextrose/0.18% saline has been started. Vary the rate of administration to maintain a blood glucose between 10-11mmol/l.

If blood glucose falls <7mmol/l, do **not** stop insulin. Give additional IV dextrose.

Continued acidosis is usually a sign of incomplete resuscitation. Consider bicarbonate if child is profoundly acidotic (pH ≤6.9) and shocked with circulatory failure or has distressing hyperventilation (Kussmaul respiration). Avoid rapid changes in pH.

Discuss with registrar or consultant before administering bicarbonate.

Introduce oral feeds as soon as child is able to tolerate them. Reduce IV infusion as appropriate. When child is free of ketonuria and maintaining an adequate oral intake discontinue IV insulin infusion after first dose of subcutaneous insulin has been given. Seek advice from paediatric dietitian.

CYTOTOXIC-INDUCED EMESIS

Nausea and vomiting can cause considerable distress. It should be anticipated and therefore, if possible, prevented by antiemetic treatment tailored to the regimen and the patient's response.

This guide should be used to prescribe the appropriate first line treatment. Dosages for the drugs recommended can be found in the appropriate monographs.

EMETOGENIC GRADING OF CHEMOTHERAPY AGENTS

The following are guidelines as to the emetogenic potential of the more commonly prescribed cytotoxic agents at Guy's and St Thomas'.

LOW EMETOGENIC POTENTIAL

Cyclophosphamide(po) - page 75
Methotrexate - page 147
Vinca alkaloids - page 227

MODERATE EMETOGENIC POTENTIAL

Cyclophosphamide (IV) - page 75
Etoposide

SEVERE EMETOGENIC POTENTIAL

Carboplatin   Doxorubicin
Cisplatin   Mustine - page 154
Daunorubicin

ANTIEMETIC GUIDELINES

The antiemetic prescribed first line should be based on the emetogenic potential of the chemotherapy prescribed. If more than one cytotoxic agent is to be prescribed then the antiemetic prescribed should be based on the cytotoxic with the greatest emetogenic potential. If two or more cytotoxic agents of the same emetogenic potential are to be administered together then it may be prudent to prescribe an antiemetic regimen from a higher emetogenic potential.

LOW EMETOGENIC POTENTIAL

a)   No antiemetics required
          OR
b)   prochlorperazine/domperidone (po/pr) ❶ ❷

MODERATE EMETOGENIC POTENTIAL

a) granisetron (po) for 24 hours❶
    OR
b) granisetron (IV) pre chemotherapy❷
    then (po) for 24 hours

SEVERE EMETOGENIC POTENTIAL

a) granisetron (po) for 48 hours❶
    OR
b) granisetron (IV) pre chemotherapy❷
    then (po) for 48 hours
❶ PO/PR administration should be at least 30-60 minutes before chemotherapy commences.
❷ Metoclopramide or granisetron (IV) may be administered immediately prior to chemotherapy.

ANTIEMETIC FAILURE GUIDELINES

EARLY ANTIEMETIC FAILURE

Severe nausea, retching or vomiting limited to the first 24-48 hours.
If treated with option a) in the guidelines above, give option b) in the same emetogenic potential band. If the option b) has failed, treat:

low   emetogenic chemotherapy treat as if **moderate,**
moderate   emetogenic chemotherapy treat as if **high** and for
high   emetogenic chemotherapy give granisetron IV and consider adding dexamethasone (IV), immediately before chemotherapy and orally, for 48 hours afterwards.

LATE ANTIEMETIC FAILURE

Severe nausea, retching or vomiting for 72 hours or more should be treated as for early antiemetic failure **plus** dexamethasone (for 6 days post chemotherapy) **and** domperidone or prochlorperazine (for 2-6 days post chemotherapy) should be added.
$5HT_3$ antagonists e.g. granisetron, whilst excellent at treating symptoms of early onset have no proven benefit over the older antiemetics (e.g. prochlorperazine) for treatment of symptoms of late onset.
In patients where antiemetic therapy has failed, the antiemetics for subsequent courses of chemotherapy should be one stage higher than the emetogenic potential suggests.

ANTICIPATORY EMESIS

This should initially be treated with diazepam or lorazepam given the night before chemotherapy is due. If emesis continues consider starting antiemetic regimen 24 hours earlier.

It should always be remembered that these are guidelines for antiemetic therapy and that the patient's response must always determine the actual therapy required.

PARENTERAL NUTRITION
AT GUY'S AND ST THOMAS'

The purpose of these guidelines is to give background information and practical advice on prescribing Total Parenteral Nutrition (TPN) for neonates and children. Guidance differs from adult practice as a result of two important patient characteristics: **age and the need to support growth.**

Age has a profound effect on protein and nutrient requirements, particularly in early infancy. For this reason standard feeds are not usually suitable and TPN is individualised. The TPN composition must be calculated to allow for normal requirements plus previous deficiencies, clinical condition, concurrent therapy and/or abnormal losses.

Advice may be sought from the Paediatric Parenteral Nutrition Team: at Guy's contact Dr Fox (bleep 1134), a paediatric pharmacist (bleep 1348/1376) or a manufacturing pharmacist (bleep 1114); at St Thomas' contact the pharmacy aseptic unit (extension 3051).

GENERAL PRESCRIBING INFORMATION

PRESCRIBING AT GUY'S & ST THOMAS'

Paediatric TPN prescriptions (see pages 285-286) are available on all the paediatric and neonatal units in the trust. They should be completed and sent to pharmacy with the ward pharmacist, **before 11am.** The TPN will be delivered to the ward that evening.

TPN FLUID VOLUME

First calculate the child's total fluid requirement taking into account the patient's age and gestation (in neonates), clinical condition and any abnormal fluid losses. Calculate the proportion of this available for TPN by subtracting from the total requirement all other fluids being administered. **Multiple infusions should be carefully accounted for during this process.**

TPN COMPOSITION

The paediatric TPN prescriptions contain suggested basic requirements for:
a) neonates, and infants up to 10kg (see page 285).
b) infants and children over 10kg (see page 286).

Protein, carbohydrate and lipid are prescribed on a g/kg/day basis. The quantities are gradually built up to full requirements in premature neonates but can be increased more rapidly in term infants and children. If a child has been maintained on IV fluids before starting TPN, the constituents of these fluids e.g. glucose, electrolytes should be considered when prescribing TPN.

It is rarely appropriate to increase the fat content above 3.5g/kg/day or protein above 2.5g/kg/day. Increments should not be greater than 0.5g/kg/day for fat and protein and not greater than 2g/kg/day for carbohydrate. Such increases are not usually made more frequently than every 2-3 days.

The regimens stated on the TPN prescription sheets automatically limit the amounts of Peditrace, Additrace, Solivito N and Vitlipid N Infant to their maximum total daily dose. The other constituents are not automatically limited and care needs to be exercised particularly when prescribing for children >25-30kg.

Children receiving TPN for greater than 2 weeks may require the addition of extra trace elements, depending upon blood levels. All premature neonates <32 weeks gestation or <1500g routinely receive double the standard selenium dose.

INGREDIENTS

AMINO ACIDS

In addition to the 9 essential amino acids in adults (leucine, isoleucine, valine, lysine, methionine, phenylalanine, threonine, tryptophan and histadine), it is likely that taurine, tyrosine and cysteine are essential during infancy. Alanine and proline may also be 'semi-essential'. The neonate also has a limited ability to metabolise an excessive intake of phenylalanine and tyrosine (important in possible excessive neurotransmitter formation). Solutions used are:

1) **Under 6 months**

Vaminolact where the amino acid profile is based on breast milk protein which includes cysteine, taurine and tyrosine essential for premature neonates (Electrolyte free).

2) **Over 6 months**

Vamin 9 glucose where the amino acid profile is based on egg protein but with added cysteine; it also contains Na 50mmol/l, K 20mmol/l, Ca 2.5mmol/l and Mg 1.5mmol/l.

CARBOHYDRATE

Carbohydrate is supplied in the form of **glucose** which provides 4kCal/g. Adequate carbohydrate must be supplied, otherwise the amino acids will be used as energy and not converted to protein. If hyperglycaemia develops a soluble insulin infusion should be considered to maintain normoglycaemia. A reasonable starting dose is 0.05 units/kg/hour with early and frequent review.

LIPID

Lipid is provided as a soya bean oil emulsion, **Intralipid 20%**, supplying 10kcal/g. It is important to include lipid as it:
- is a concentrated source of calories (contributing 30-50% of energy).
- is a vehicle for fat soluble vitamins.
- prevents the development of essential fatty acid deficiency.
- is isotonic with blood and may be infused peripherally.

Intralipid 20% with added vitamins is given as a separate infusion to the vamin. The infusion rates quoted for both are based on delivery over 24 hours. No attempt should be made to 'catch up' the Intralipid infusion if it is running behind, as lipid may be inadequately cleared from the blood at higher infusion rates (particularly in neonates).

NOTE when lipid is contra-indicated - water soluble vitamins are put in Vamin Bag but fat soluble vitamins are omitted.

CIRCUMSTANCES WHERE THE REGIMEN MAY NEED TO BE ALTERED

Poor weight gain
May require increased protein and calories.
Phototherapy
Consider increasing daily fluid allowance by 30ml/kg/day.
Overhead Radiant Heating
Consider increasing daily fluid allowance by 30ml/kg/day.
Heart failure
If the patient is in heart failure, fluid allowance may need to be reduced.
Renal failure
Seek expert advice.
Jaundice
Lipid intake should be decreased to 0.5g/kg/day in newborn infants with levels of unconjugated bilirubin exceeding 75% of the exchange transfusion level.
Hepatic failure
Seek expert advice.
Infection\Sepsis
Consider reducing lipid to 0.5g/kg/day, check triglyceride levels more frequently and increase lipid accordingly.
Fluid restriction
In severely fluid restricted patients the volume prescribed may be insufficient to prepare the prescribed TPN regimen. Pharmacy will inform the clinician when this situation arises.
Hypocalcaemia/Hypophosphataemia
Any alteration to be made to either calcium or phosphate content of the regimen should be discussed with pharmacy.
Inborn errors of metabolism
Seek expert advice.
Catabolic states
Any infant or child who is catabolic (e.g. burns) will need more calories than the basic regimen provides. This should be discussed with the Paediatric Parenteral Nutrition Team.

TECHNIQUES FOR ADMINISTRATION OF PARENTERAL NUTRITION

ACCESS FOR TPN

TPN should be administered via a dedicated central line. If central access cannot be secured and TPN is imperative, solutions containing less than 12.5% glucose may be infused peripherally. Central access must be gained as soon as possible since thrombophlebititis is likely and extravasation causes tissue burns.

The central line should be reserved for TPN unless a multi-lumen line has been inserted, when the same lumen should be used for TPN at all times.
NOTE
- **Nothing** else should be given down the TPN line unless there is no alternative i.e. treatment is essential and alternative access is unobtainable.
- Blood must **not** be taken through the TPN line at any time.
- The **giving set** should be changed with full aseptic precautions.

INFUSION

The TPN infusions supplied by pharmacy contain an overage (an additional volume of fluid) to allow the priming of the attached giving sets without reducing the volume available for infusion into the patient. The Requisition for Parenteral Nutrition (the manufacturing sheet) is sent to the ward with the TPN. It specifies the rates of Vamin and Lipid (ml/hr) to run over 24 hours. The clear plastic outer bag in which the TPN is dispensed is simply protective and is not a sterility barrier.
In-line filters are currently recommended for all neonatal TPN. A 0.2micrometre filter (white) is used for the Vamin and a 1.2micrometre filter (blue) is used for the lipid. These are changed every 48 hours and accordingly neonatal TPN is dispensed with filters attached every other day. On the days in between, no filters are dispensed and the TPN should be infused through the existing filters. Care must be taken to connect the lipid to the lipid filter and the Vamin to the Vamin filter.

STORAGE

Whenever possible all TPN solutions should be protected from light to prevent the formation of free radicals. Once made all TPN solutions should be stored in the fridge.

MONITORING

The Biochemical investigations required and their recommended frequencies are set out below. If patients are stabilised on TPN these investigations may be performed less often:

BLOOD TESTS	
DAILY	U&E
	Creatinine
	LFT
	Calcium & Phosphate
	Glucose (usually more frequent)
TWICE WEEKLY	Triglycerides
	Magnesium
FORTNIGHTLY	Trace Elements

NOTE: Bloods should be taken early morning and sent as an urgent request.

Bloods for trace elements should be sent directly to Medical Toxicology at New Cross and results obtained by phoning 0171-771-5372. Pharmacy can advise on trace element supplementation.

WEEKENDS and BANK HOLIDAYS

TPN is not manufactured in pharmacy at weekends. On Fridays, it is therefore necessary to decide on the parenteral nutrition requirements for the weekend ahead. For existing patients 3 days TPN must be prescribed on Friday. If you plan to start TPN over the weekend this should be arranged on the Friday before 11am. If TPN is needed outside normal working hours contingency arrangements are laid out below.

Bank holiday arrangements will be negotiated with the TPN team and clinicians advised appropriately.

EMERGENCY TPN REGIME

In many instances TPN may be delayed until the next working day without adversely affecting the patient. However, if TPN is needed, it is recommended that a regime of glucose, electrolytes and protein is used (see notes 1). The required maintenance glucose and electrolyte infusion should be prepared on the ward and administered in addition to a protein infusion (Vaminolact) run at the rates outlined in the tables below. **Vaminolact is an electrolyte free solution which provides protein only.**

NEONATES AND INFANTS (less than 10Kg)

	Day 1	Day 2	Day 3
Vaminolact ml/kg/hr	0.3	0.5	0.7
Protein content (g/kg/24hrs)	0.4	0.7	1

CHILDREN (over 10kg)

	Day 1	Day 2	Day 3
Vaminolact ml/kg/hr	0.7	1	1
Protein content (g/kg/24hrs)	1	1.4	1.4

NOTE 1:   The above prescription for emergency TPN may not be appropriate for renal, hepatic or metabolic patients.   Seek expert advice before prescribing.

STOPPING TPN

For patients who are prescribed TPN long term, i.e. 2 weeks or over, the TPN must be reduced gradually over at least two or three days when stopping.   Full TPN should still be prescribed but the solutions run at a reduced rate.   When weaning, the vamin and lipid should be reduced in proportion i.e. run at a similar percentage of the full rate.   Under these circumstances a TPN bag may be infused over up to 48 hours. It is advisable to discuss the patient with the paediatric dietitian in order to determine the best route and type of enteral nutrition.

PAEDIATRIC TOTAL PARENTERAL NUTRITION (TPN) PRESCRIPTION
(For infants and children, <10kg)

Name: Hospital No: Date of Birth:	GUY'S & ST THOMAS' HOSPITAL TRUST Pharmacy Manufacturing Department GUY'S HOSPITAL Extension: 3712 Bleep: 1114 ST THOMAS' HOSPITAL Extension: 3051 Bleep 0428 TO BE COMPLETED BY 11:00AM

Ward: Consultant: Pact Code:

Feeding weight: Gestation: Reason for TPN:

Regime: Regimen 1 to 5 are used for the first 5 days, regimen 6 from day 6. The Paediatric Parenteral Nutrition Team will review prescription regimes every Wednesday. Please contact Pharmacy Manufacturing if there are any problems.

ALL FIGURES ARE PER Kg PER 24 HOURS

Date						
Regimen	1	2	3	4	5	6
❶ Total daily fluid (ml)						
❷ Total other fluids (ml)						
❶-❷ Fluid for TPN (ml)						
Protein (g) ❸	0.5	0.8	1.0	1.5	2.0	2.5
Carbohydrate (g)	8	10	10	12	12	14
Peditrace (ml) ❹[max 10ml]	1	1	1	1	1	1
Sodium (mmol) ❺	5	5	5	5	5	5
Potassium (mmol)	2.5	2.5	2.5	2.5	2.5	2.5
Phosphate (mmol) ❻	0.4	0.4	0.4	0.4	0.4	0.4
Calcium (mmol) ❻	0.6	0.6	0.6	0.6	0.6	0.6
Magnesium (mmol)	0.3	0.3	0.3	0.3	0.3	0.3
Solivito N (ml) [max 1 vial]	1	1	1	1	1	1
Vitlipid N Inf (ml)[max10ml]	4	4	4	4	4	4
Fat (g)	1	1	2	2	3	3.5
Additive (mmol)						
Doctors signature:						
Bleep no:						
Pharmacist:						

❸   Vaminolact in infants < 6 months, Vamin 9 Glucose in infants > 6 months.
❹   Selenium is doubled in preterm neonates (<1500g or <32/40).
❺   Sodium requirements in preterm neonates (<32/40) will vary greatly.
❻   Phosphate in preterm neonates (<32/40) is 1.5mmol/kg/24 hours and calcium is 1.5mmol/kg/24 hours.

Revised Dec 1998

PAEDIATRIC TOTAL PARENTERAL NUTRITION (TPN) PRESCRIPTION
(For infants and children, >10kg)

Name:		GUY'S & ST THOMAS' HOSPITAL TRUST
Hospital No:		Pharmacy Manufacturing Department GUY'S HOSPITAL Extension: 3712 Bleep: 1114
Date of Birth:		ST THOMAS' HOSPITAL Extension: 3051 Bleep: 0428 TO BE COMPLETED BY 11:00AM

Ward: Consultant: Pact Code:

Feeding weight: Gestation: Reason for TPN:

Regime: Regimen 7 and 8 are for day 1 and 2 respectively, regimen 9 from day 3 onwards.

The Paediatric Parenteral Nutrition Team will review prescription regimes every Wednesday. Please contact Pharmacy Manufacturing if there are any problems.

ALL FIGURES ARE PER Kg PER 24 HOURS

Date						
Regimen	7	8	9	9	9	9
❶ Total daily fluid (ml)						
❷ Total other prescribed fluids (ml)						
❶-❷ Fluid for TPN (ml)						
Protein (g)	1	1.5	1.5	1.5	1.5	1.5
Carbohydrate (g)	3	4	6	6	6	6
Additrace (ml) [max 10ml]	0.2	0.2	0.2	0.2	0.2	0.2
Sodium (mmol)	3	3	3	3	3	3
Potassium (mmol)	2.5	2.5	2.5	2.5	2.5	2.5
Phosphate (mmol) ❸	0	0	0	0	0	0
Calcium (mmol)	0.1	0.2	0.2	0.2	0.2	0.2
Magnesium (mmol)	0.1	0.2	0.2	0.2	0.2	0.2
Solivito N (ml) [max 1 vial]	1	1	1	1	1	1
Vitlipid N Inf (ml) [max 10ml]	1	1	1	1	1	1
Fat (g)	1	1.5	2	2	2	2
Additive (mmol)						
Doctors signature:						
Bleep no:						
Pharmacist:						

❸   Phosphate in Intralipid is assumed to be bioavailable.   Monitor patients plasma phosphate level.

Revised Dec 1998

METABOLIC DISORDERS

INTERCURRENT ILLNESS IN INBORN ERRORS OF INTERMEDIARY METABOLIC

Diet is the mainstay of treatment for many inborn errors of intermediary metabolism. However an emergency regimen may need to be started, and feeds stopped, at times of metabolic stress such as an intercurrent infection.

The basic emergency regimen is essentially the same for all disorders. A solution of glucose polymer e.g. Maxijul®, is used as the major energy source because it is simple, palatable and usually well tolerated. Fat emulsions can provide additional energy but are less well tolerated. Fat delays gastric emptying, may cause vomiting and is not routinely used. It is also contra-indicated in some disorders.

EMERGENCY REGIMEN

Age	% Glucose polymer	Energy kcal/100ml	Fluid allowance ml/kg
0 - 5 months	10	40	150 - 200
6 -11 months	10	40	120 - 150
1 - 2 years	15	60	95
3 - 6 years	20	80	85 -95
7 - 10 years	20	80	75
> 10 years	25	100	50 - 55

Give the drink as oral or nasogastric boluses every 2 to 3 hours or as a slow continuous feed if child is vomiting. There is some flexibility in the frequency of the drinks particularly in older children and during recovery. However, it is important not to allow a gap of longer than 4 hours between feeds, particularly during the night.

This regimen should not be continued for long periods of time as it does not supply adequate nutrition.

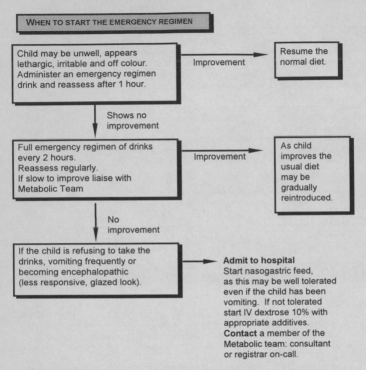

WHEN TO START THE EMERGENCY REGIMEN

Child may be unwell, appears lethargic, irritable and off colour. Administer an emergency regimen drink and reassess after 1 hour. — Improvement → Resume the normal diet.

Shows no improvement ↓

Full emergency regimen of drinks every 2 hours.
Reassess regularly.
If slow to improve liaise with Metabolic Team — Improvement → As child improves the usual diet may be gradually reintroduced.

No improvement ↓

If the child is refusing to take the drinks, vomiting frequently or becoming encephalopathic (less responsive, glazed look). →

Admit to hospital
Start nasogastric feed, as this may be well tolerated even if the child has been vomiting. If not tolerated start IV dextrose 10% with appropriate additives.
Contact a member of the Metabolic team: consultant or registrar on-call.

NOTE 1: The emergency regimen should not be continued for longer than 24-48 hours without discussion with the metabolic team.

NOTE 2: In addition to the emergency regimen the usual medication should continue to be administered, including arginine/citrulline if these are being given with the diet. The medications may need to be given by another route e.g. intravenously, if not tolerated orally. If uncertain about dosage conversion, seek advice. For some disorders it may be appropriate to increase the usual medication however this will need to be done in conjunction with the metabolic team.

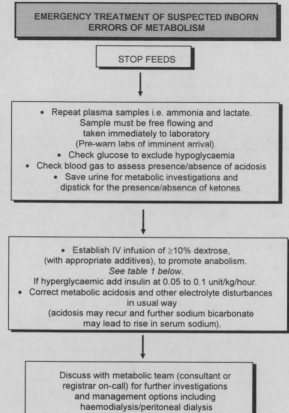

EMERGENCY TREATMENT OF SUSPECTED INBORN
ERRORS OF METABOLISM

STOP FEEDS

- Repeat plasma samples i.e. ammonia and lactate.
  Sample must be free flowing and
  taken immediately to laboratory
  (Pre-warn labs of imminent arrival).
- Check glucose to exclude hypoglycaemia
- Check blood gas to assess presence/absence of acidosis
- Save urine for metabolic investigations and
  dipstick for the presence/absence of ketones.

- Establish IV infusion of ≥10% dextrose,
  (with appropriate additives), to promote anabolism.
  See table 1 below.
  If hyperglycaemic add insulin at 0.05 to 0.1 unit/kg/hour.
- Correct metabolic acidosis and other electrolyte disturbances
  in usual way
  (acidosis may recur and further sodium bicarbonate
  may lead to rise in serum sodium).

Discuss with metabolic team (consultant or
registrar on-call) for further investigations
and management options including
haemodialysis/peritoneal dialysis
and other medication.

TABLE 1.

AGE (years)	INFUSION RATE
<1	150ml/kg/day
1 - 2	100ml/kg/day
3 - 6	1200 - 1500ml/day
>6	1500 - 2000ml/day

SKIN DISORDERS

THE MANAGEMENT OF ATOPIC ECZEMA AND DRY SKIN

Around 50% of children with atopic eczema also have xerosis (dry skin). In the vast majority of cases treatment is straightforward.

GENERAL MEASURES

These include avoidance of soap, wearing cotton clothing next to the skin, avoidance of potential allergens where possible, (e.g. pets should be kept out of the bedroom) and keeping the child cool (e.g. avoid excessive central heating).

EMOLLIENTS

Prescribe a bath oil (e.g. Alpha Keri®, Balneum®) 2-3 capfuls in the bath water of an adult size bath and a soap substitute (e.g. aqueous cream or emulsifying ointment) to use instead of soap. Some bath oils (e.g. Oilatum Plus®) include an antiseptic which can be useful in children prone to episodes of infected eczema. Balneum Plus® may be useful in eczema with pruritus. Emollients need to be applied **at least** twice a day and more frequently in severe cases. They vary in the degree of greasiness from very greasy such as 50% white soft paraffin in 50% liquid paraffin to those that are hardly greasy at all such as E45® cream or aqueous cream. The aim is to prescribe an emollient that the patient/parent will use and that moisturises the skin adequately. Emollients are best applied after a bath. Topical corticosteroids should be applied after the emollient. Ideally this should be 10-15minutes after the emollient although this may be difficult to achieve in practice. An infant may require up to 250g and a child 500g of emollient every week.

TOPICAL CORTICOSTEROIDS

Topical corticosteroids are the mainstay of treatment for atopic eczema even in infancy. Failure to manage eczema adequately often results from inadequate use of topical steroid. Hydrocortisone 1% is safe to use and will not give rise to significant local or systemic side effects. Start with hydrocortisone 1% ointment applied twice a day to all the affected areas. Only use anything stronger than this on the face at the recommendation of a dermatologist. If hydrocortisone 1% ointment is not adequately controlling the eczema on the body, increase the strength to 2.5% or use one of the moderately potent steroids (e.g. Eumovate®) for a short period (usually 3-5 days) until the disease is under control and then return to maintenance therapy. Ointments are preferable to creams for the treatment of eczema however creams may be easier to apply on very hairy areas. Always use the weakest possible steroid to control the disease.

ANTIHISTAMINES

Sedative antihistamines (e.g. Trimeprazine see page 218) can be useful at night, particularly if the child has difficulty sleeping. Administer one hour before bedtime. Topical antihistamines should be avoided as the risk of skin sensitisation is unacceptably high.

ANTI-INFECTIVE AGENTS

Secondary infection is very common in eczema and the majority of children with eczema have skin colonised by *Staphylococcus aureus* and occasionally *Group A streptococcus*. In cases where there is clinical evidence of infection treat with combined topical steroid and antibiotic (e.g. Fucidin H®) and if necessary systemic antibiotics. Erythromycin is a good choice, for community acquired infections, since it covers both streptococcal and staphylococcal infections.

WET WRAPS

Occasionally, in cases of severe eczema, emollient and topical steroid can be applied under occlusion with 'wet wraps'. This involves the use of a layer of wet, followed by a layer of dry Tubifast® to the affected areas i.e. limbs and trunk. The benefits are probably due to cooling by evaporation, relieving pruritus, enhanced absorption of the topical steroid and physical protection of the skin from excoriation. As the risk of local and systemic toxicity from topical steroids is increased the choice of topical steroid must be appropriate. A 1:10 dilution of Propaderm® ointment in white sort paraffin is recommended.

TOPICAL THERAPY IN CHILDREN

Parent/carers are often unsure of how much topical therapy, particularly corticosteroids, are needed to treat a particular area of a child's body. This can be quantified for parents/carers using the 'Adult Fingertip Unit' (FTU) as a guide. **Emollients may be applied in quantities greater than those suggested.**
One FTU is the amount of cream or ointment expressed from a tube applied from the distal skin crease to the tip of the palmar aspect of an adult's index finger. The table below shows how many FTUs are required to cover each area of a child's body.

Age	Face & Neck	Arm & Hand	Leg & Foot	Trunk (Front)	Trunk (Back) inc. Buttocks
	Number of FTUs/area				
3-6 months	1	1	1½	1	1½
1-2 years	1½	1½	2	2	3
3-5 years	1½	2	3	3	3½
6-10 years	2	2½	4½	3½	5

(Adapted from C. C. Long et al. British Journal of Dermatology 1998;138:293-296).

MANAGEMENT OF IMPETIGO

There are 2 forms of impetigo, a bullous form caused by infection with *Staphylococcus aureus* and a non-bullous form which may be caused by infection with *Staph. aureus* or group A *streptococci*. The causative organism should be identified by taking skin swabs from affected sites.

Localised infection may be adequately treated with topical mupirocin ointment which is active against infection due to either organism. More severe or generalised cases should be treated with systemic antibiotics according to the sensitivities of the causal organism but erythromycin or flucloxacillin are generally suitable.

MANAGEMENT OF TINEA CAPITIS (SCALP RINGWORM)

All suspected cases of tinea capitis should be confirmed by appropriate mycological examination prior to commencing treatment.

Systemic treatment is necessary to treat scalp ringworm. At present griseofulvin (see page 118) is the treatment of choice. Treatment should be for 8 weeks in the first instance at which point the child should be re-assessed.

Topical treatment with ketoconazole shampoo may be useful in reducing cross infection to other children by reducing the spread of fungal spores in some types of fungal infection.

Treatment failures should be discussed with a dermatologist.

MANAGEMENT OF VIRAL WARTS

The majority of viral warts do not require treatment however when treatment is indicated it depends upon site:

SITE	TREATMENT
Feet	Salicyclic acid (Occlusal®) applied accurately to warts each day after rubbing off thick surface.
Hands	Salicylic acid (Occlusal®) applied accurately to warts each day after rubbing off thick surface.
Face	Cryotherapy or surgical removal. Seek expert advice.
Anogenital❶	Seek expert advice.

❶ The mode of acquisition must be queried in all cases of anogenital warts in children.

HEAD LICE

Head lice are small insects, roughly the size of a match head when fully grown. They spread by clambering from head to head. Anyone with hair can catch them. It is estimated that one in ten primary school children are affected by head lice every year.

Head lice feed by sucking blood through the scalp of the child. The female lays eggs in sacs (nits) glued to hair where the warmth of the scalp will hatch them. The eggs take 7-10 days to hatch and are small and dull in colour. Empty egg sacs (nits) are white and shiny and may be found further along the hair shaft as the hair grows out. Lice take 7-14 days to become fully grown and able to reproduce.

GUIDELINES FOR PREVENTION AND DETECTION OF HEAD LICE

1. Comb hair each day with a fine tooth comb. Good grooming enables early detection of head lice.
2. Wet comb hair weekly to detect live head lice if present. Wash hair with normal shampoo, rinse and follow up with conditioner. Rinse and then wet comb hair, section by section, with a detection comb (fine toothed comb),over a white surface. If live lice are present, follow 'Guidelines for treatment of head lice'.

GUIDELINES FOR TREATMENT OF HEAD LICE

Lambeth, Southwark and Lewisham Health Authority Guidelines do not recommend a rotational policy for insecticide treatment of head lice. Mosaic prescribing/supply is recommended (i.e. an alternative preparation is used if after repeat administration of the initial preparation there are still live lice) and no one chemical treatment is recommended.

1. Alcoholic lotions are the preparations of choice. However, they are unsuitable for children <6 months of age, asthmatics and those with skin problems. For these children, malathion aqueous liquid (Suleo-M®) and Malathion aqueous lotion (Derbac-M®) and routinely stocked by the pharmacy departments. Shampoos are ineffective as they are too dilute and have an insufficiently short contact time.
2. Ensure hair is dry before commencing treatment.
3. Rub lotion gently into scalp until all the hair and scalp is thoroughly moistened (50mls is usually required).
4. Comb hair and allow to dry naturally.
5. After a minimum of 12 hours, remove chemical by washing hair.
6. 3-7 days after treatment, a detection comb should be used to check hair for traces of lice and eggs. Action required is outlined below:

On Inspection after 3-7 days	Action
No adult lice, nymphs only	Survival of eggs - repeat same treatment
Range of lice found: adult, nymphs and new eggs	Treatment incorrectly used or resistance. Check correct use. Repeat application, try alternative or try wet combing (see below).
Adult lice only, no nymphs	Re-infection. Check contacts and repeat treatment.

7. If live lice continue to be detected seek expert advice.
8. Household contacts should not be treated routinely. Treat only if infestation has occurred.
9. Treat all patients with live lice at the same time to prevent re-infection within the household.
10. Prophylactic use of an insecticide is not recommended.

PHYSICAL REMOVAL

Wet Combing is a method of physical removal of lice and requires full understanding and motivation to be effective. It is suitable for all hair types. 'Bug Busting' is the wet combing method developed by the charity Community Hygiene Concern (CHC). 'Bug Busting' kits can be obtained from CHC (Tel: 0181-341 7167) or community pharmacies. The kit includes all the required equipment.

Method
1. Wash hair with ordinary shampoo.
2. Apply lots of conditioner and comb hair while still wet with an ordinary wide/tooth comb.
3. Section hair and comb from roots with a fine tooth comb. The teeth of the comb must be no more than 0.25mm apart.
4. Clear comb of lice between each stroke. The lice are viable and should be disposed of appropriately.
5. Comb entire head.
6. If lice found, repeat routine every 3-4 days for 2 weeks to remove lice hatching from eggs.
7. Finding large lice after/during treatment indicates re-infection.

SCABIES

Scabies is an infection caused by the scabies mite Sarcoptes Scabei, a parasitic mite, which burrows into the skin. The mites are usually found in the epidermis of the hands and wrists, and may also occur on the face and scalp of small children. A secondary eczematous response is common and may not always appear to correspond to the sites of infestation.

GUIDELINES FOR THE TREATMENT OF SCABIES

1. Wash, dry and allow skin to cool.
2. Apply malathion aqueous lotion to whole body, including head. Avoid contact with the eyes and mouth. Take particular care to apply under the finger nails and to the soles of the feet.
3. If hands or any other parts of the body must be washed during the treatment period reapply lotion immediately.
4. Wash off lotion thoroughly after 24 hours.
5. Repeat application after 1-2 days to ensure areas that may have been missed are covered.
6. After treatment, itching may take between some weeks to subside - further applications of insecticide should not be used. Consider the use of 1% hydrocortisone ointment to treat associated eczema. Treatment for secondary infection may also be necessary.
7. Members of the same household, and other close contacts, should be treated at the same time, whether or not they are infected.
8. Change and launder sheets, towels and any clothing including gloves worn next to the skin during the past week. It is not necessary to clean outwear or furniture as the mites survive only briefly away from the human host.

IMMUNISATION

"It is every child's right to be protected against infectious diseases. No child should be denied immunisation without serious thought as to the consequences, both for the individual child and the community. Where there is any doubt, advice should be sought from a Consultant Paediatrician or Consultant in Communicable Disease Control".

From: Immunisation against Infectious Disease, Department of Health (1996) ('Green Book').

If further information is required concerning immunisation, please refer to the 'Green Book' or seek advice from the virology or pharmacy department.

Immunity can be induced, either **actively** (long term) or **passively** (short term), against a variety of bacterial and viral agents.

ACTIVE IMMUNISATION

Vaccines are used to induce active immunity and are of three types:
1. **a live attenuated** form of a virus (e.g. MMR vaccine or varicella vaccine) or mycobacteria (e.g. BCG vaccine).
2. **inactivated** preparations of the virus (e.g. influenza vaccine) or bacteria, or
3. **extracts of,** (e.g. Haemophilus influenzae B vaccine), or **detoxified exotoxins** (e.g. tetanus toxoid), produced by, a micro-organism.

SPECIAL RISK GROUPS
Children with certain conditions which increase the risk of complications from infectious diseases should be immunised as a matter of priority. These conditions include: asthma, congenital heart disease, Down's Syndrome, Human immunodeficiency Virus (HIV) Infection (seek further advice), premature and growth retarded neonates. Neonates of all gestational ages should be immunised according to the standard protocol from two months of age.

Children with no spleen or functional hyposplenism are at increased risk of bacterial infections especially those caused by encapsulated bacteria. In addition to antibiotic prophylaxis and standard vaccination schedule, such children should receive pneumococcal vaccine (over two years of age), Hib vaccine (irrespective of age), meningococcal A and C vaccine and influenza vaccine.

GENERAL CONTRAINDICATIONS
Children suffering from an acute illness should have immunisation postponed unless the child has a minor infection without fever or systemic upset.

Immunisation should not be carried out in individuals who have a definite history of a **severe** local or general reaction to a preceding dose. Appropriate further advice should be sought if there is any doubt.

Hypersensitivity to egg contraindicates influenza vaccine; previous anaphylactic reaction to egg contradindicates influenza and yellow fever vaccines. There is increasing evidence that MMR vaccine can be safely given even to children with a history of anaphylaxis after egg ingestion.

LIVE VACCINES - SPECIAL RISK GROUPS

Some children may be at risk if given live vaccines. Inactivated vaccines are not dangerous to these patients but may be ineffective. These children include:

- all those receiving cytotoxic chemotherapy or generalised radiotherapy, or within 6 months of terminating such treatment.
- all those receiving immunosuppressive therapy e.g. after organ transplantation.
- all those receiving high-dose corticosteroids i.e. the equivalent of prednisolone at an oral dose of 2mg/kg/day or 40mg/day for at least 1 week or 1mg/kg/day for 1 month. Postpone live vaccines for at least 3 months after stopping treatment or after non-immunosuppressive doses have been reached.
- children with immunodeficiency states (seek further advice). For HIV infection, see below.

HIV Infection

HIV-positive children (with or without symptoms) should receive all vaccines apart from BCG and yellow fever. Vaccine efficacy may however be reduced. In HIV-positive, symptomatic children, inactivated polio vaccine may be substituted for oral polio vaccine. For information regarding the use of varicella vaccine in HIV infection see monograph page 222.

THE FOLLOWING ARE NOT CONTRAINDICATIONS FOR IMMUNISATION:

a) Family history of any adverse reactions following immunisation.
b) Previous history of pertussis, measles, rubella or mumps infection.
c) Prematurity: immunisation should not be postponed.
d) Stable neurological conditions such as cerebral palsy and Down's syndrome.
e) Contact with an infectious disease.
f) Asthma, eczema, hay fever or 'snuffles'.
g) Treatment with antibiotics or locally-acting (e.g. topical or inhaled) steroids.
h) Child's mother is pregnant.
I) Child being breast fed.
j) History of jaundice after birth.
k) Under a certain weight.
l) Over the age recommended in immunisation schedule.
m) Child taking 'replacement' corticosteroids.

MMR Vaccine

The Department of Health can find no established causal link between MMR vaccine and inflammatory bowel disease or autism and recommend the continued use of MMR vaccine.

There is no evidence to support the use of separate doses of monovalent vaccines of measles, mumps and rubella over MMR in this situation. Indeed monovalent measles and mumps vaccines are no longer available.

There is increasing evidence that MMR vaccines can be given safely to children who have had an anaphylactic reaction to food containing egg.

ADMINISTRATION OF VACCINES

Timing of vaccine administration. Administration of live vaccines at an age earlier than recommended increases the likelihood of a poor response due to maternal antibody. For products that require booster doses for full immunisation, dosing at less than the recommended intervals may result in sub-optimal antibody response. Intervals between doses that are longer than recommended do not impair final antibody levels.

Immunisation Intervals. Different vaccines can usually be given simultaneously although live vaccines (unless a combination product) should be given at different sites. Vaccines should not be mixed in the syringe prior to administration except certain combinations of DTP and Hib vaccines:

i. those provided by the manufacturer in a form to be mixed before administration e.g. Trivax-Hib or ACT Hib DTP.
ii. certain brands of Hib and DTP vaccines which are provided separately may be mixed. It is acceptable to premix ACT Hib and Pasteur Merieux brand DTP and to premix Hibtiter and Evans brand DTP.

If live vaccines are not given simultaneously, it is usually recommended that they are separated by at least 3 week intervals. No interval is required between the administration of live and inactivated vaccines. Live vaccines (except yellow fever) should not be given during the three months after immunoglobulin injection as the response is likely to be impaired.

Route of administration
Oral polio vaccine and oral typhoid vaccine are the only vaccines that are given orally. BCG vaccine is usually given intradermally. In neonates, infants and children less than 5 years of age the percutaneous route, using a multiple puncture technique, is an alternative to the intradermal route for BCG. All other vaccines are given by deep subcutaneous or intramuscular injection. In infants, the antero-lateral aspect of the thigh or upper arm are recommended sites. If the buttock is used, injection into the upper outer quadrant avoids the risk of sciatic nerve damage.

Storage of vaccine
Manufacturer's recommendations on storage must be observed i.e. temperature of 2-8°C. Storage at temperatures below 0°C cause freezing which can lead to deterioration of the vaccine and breakage of the container. If vaccines have been stored at an inappropriate temperature, advice should be obtained from paediatric pharmacists (bleep 1348 or 1376) before they are used.

SCHEDULE FOR IMMUNISATION

Refer to individual monographs for dosing and route of administration.

Vaccine	Age		Comments
DTP❶ and Hib Polio	1st dose 2nd dose 3rd dose	2 months 3 months 4 months	Primary course
MMR	1st dose	12-15 months	Can be given at any age over 12 months
Hib	13 months - 4 years		Only required if not immunised earlier. 1 dose is sufficient.
DT Polio MMR	Booster Booster 2nd dose	3-5 years	3 years after completion of primary course
BCG	Infancy OR 10 - 14 years		For tuberculin negative children only. If <3months of age, tuberculin testing is unnecessary.
Td Polio	} Booster }	13 - 18 years	

DTP   Adsorbed Diphtheria, Tetanus and Pertussis Vaccine
DT   Adsorbed Diphtheria and Tetanus Vaccine
Td   Adsorbed Diphtheria (Low Dose) and Tetanus Vaccine for Adults and Adolescents
MMR = Measles, Mumps and Rubella Vaccine
Hib   = Haemophilus Influenzae B Vaccine
❶   If pertussis vaccine is contra-indicated DT should be given. If pertussis vaccine is subsequently required acellular pertussis vaccine (single antigen) may be used.

PASSIVE IMMUNISATION

Passive immunity is transferred by the injection of human immunoglobulins. These can be divided into two types: human normal immunoglobulin (HNIG) and specific immunoglobulins. HNIG is derived from the pooled plasma of donors and contains antibody to infectious agents currently prevalent in the general population. Specific immunoglobulins are prepared from plasma pooled from donors with high titres of the required antibody as a result of, for example, recent infection or vaccination.

The protection after immunoglobulin is immediate but only lasts a few weeks. Immunoglobulins may interfere with the immune response to live vaccines, which should therefore be given at least 3 weeks before or 3 months after an injection of immunoglobulin. Advice on the availability of human normal immunoglobulin and specific immunoglobulins can be obtained from the paediatric pharmacists (Guy's bleep 1348 or 1376) or drug information centre.

Note: Currently, all immunoglobulins prepared in the UK infer a theoretical risk of transmitting new variant CJD.

HUMAN NORMAL IMMUNOGLOBULIN (HNIG)

HNIG contains antibody to measles, varicella, hepatitis A and other viruses.

Use in Measles

Immunocompromised children who come into contact with measles and infants (<12 months) in whom there is a particular reason to avoid measles (e.g. recent severe illness) may be given HNIG. Infants should subsequently be given MMR vaccine after an interval of at least 3 months.

USE	AGE OF CHILD	DOSE
To prevent an attack	less than 1 year	250mg
	1-2 years	500mg
	3 years and over	750mg
To allow an attenuated	less than 1 year	100mg
attack	1 year and over	250mg

Use in Hepatitis A

HNIG offers short term protection (up to four months) against Hepatitis A infection. It's use should be considered in the following circumstances

i. Contacts of cases of hepatitis A infection and control of outbreaks

ii. As an alternative to the vaccine for those travelling occasionally and for short periods (<3 months) to countries outside Northern & Western Europe, North America, Australia and New Zealand.

USE	AGE OF CHILD	DOSE
To control outbreaks	less than 10 years	250mg
	10 years and over	500mg
Travelling abroad for	less than 10 years	125mg
2 months or less	10 years and over	250mg
Travelling abroad for	less than 10 years	250mg
3-5 months	10 years and over	500mg

SPECIFIC IMMUNOGLOBULINS

These are available for tetanus, hepatitis B and varicella-zoster. **The specific immunoglobulins are often scarce and should be used with discretion.**

HUMAN TETANUS IMMUNOGLOBULIN (HTIG)

HTIG offers immediate protection against tetanus and may be required for the treatment of children with tetanus-prone wounds. The following are considered tetanus-prone wounds:
a) Any wound or burn sustained more than six hours before surgical treatment.
b) Any wound or burn at any interval after injury that shows one or more of the following characteristics:
i. a significant degree of devitalised tissue
ii. puncture-type wound
iii. contact with soil or manure
iv. clinical evidence of sepsis

The following children require HTIG in addition to antibiotics (see page 264) for the immediate treatment of tetanus prone wounds.
a) Unimmunised
b) Immunisation status uncertain
c) Last tetanus vaccine over 10 years ago

Furthermore HTIG may be given to children with an acceptable immunisation history if the risk of infection is considered especially high e.g. stable manure contamination. Children with an unacceptable immunisation history should also receive appropriate tetanus toxoid treatment.

HTIG DOSAGE

Prevention (all ages)	Give 250units intramuscularly **or** 500units if more than 24 hours have elapsed since injury or there is risk of heavy contamination or following burns.
Treatment (all ages)	Give 150units/kg in multiple sites.
AVAILABILITY	HTIG is kept in A&E

HEPATITIS B IMMUNOGLOBULIN (HBIG)

(See page 121).
HBIG gives passive protection against hepatitis B and is normally used in conjunction with hepatitis B vaccine to confer passive/active immunity after exposure.

Neonates
All infants who fulfil the necessary criteria on page 122 should receive HBIG as well as hepatitis B vaccine (see page 121).

Accidental exposure
Children who are accidentally inoculated, or who contaminated their eyes or mouth or fresh cuts or abrasions of the skin, with blood from a known HBsAg positive person may require post exposure prophylaxis. Determine the recipient's hepatitis B vaccine status and consult the Medical Virologist on call. Following accidental exposure HBIG should be given preferably within 48 hours and not later than a week after exposure. See page 121..

VARICELLA ZOSTER IMMUNOGLOBULIN (VZIG)

The use of VZIG is restricted to individuals who fulfil **all** of the necessary criteria on page 223.

IV COMPATIBILITIES

The following drugs are commonly used in the Intensive Care Unit at Guy's and frequent requests regarding the compatibility of concurrent infusions are received. The table below provides guidelines to compatibilities however it is far from complete. Drugs should only be mixed if absolutely necessary, and site of mixing should be checked carefully for signs of colour change or precipitation, particularly for those drugs where compatibility is based only on previous practical experience. Please contact Drug Information (Guy's ext 3594, Lewisham ext 3202, or St Thomas' ext 3069), for further information.

	ACICLOVIR	ADRENALINE	AMINOPHYLLINE	ATRACURIUM	CALCIUM GLUCONATE	DOBUTAMINE	DOPAMINE	FENTANYL	FRUSEMIDE	GLYCERYL TRINITRATE	HEPARIN	HYDRALAZINE	ISOPRENALINE	MIDAZOLAM	MORPHINE	NORADRENALINE	POTASSIUM CHLORIDE	SODIUM BICARBONATE	SODIUM NITROPRUSSIDE	VANCOMYCIN	VECURONIUM
ACICLOVIR	■		I	I		I	I			G	G				I		G	G		G	
ADRENALINE		■	I	G	C	C	G	G	G	G	C			G	G	G	C	I			G
AMINOPHYLLINE	I	I	■	I	G	I	G	C	C	C	C	I	I	G	G	I	G	G		I	G
ATRACURIUM	I	G	I	■		G	G				G			G	G		C			G	G
CALCIUM GLUCONATE		C	G		■	C	P		S		G		P	G		C	C		C	G	
DOBUTAMINE	I	C	I	G	C	■	C	G	I	C	S	S	C	G	C	C	C	I	C		G
DOPAMINE	I	G	G	G	P	C	■	G	I	C	C	P	P	G	G	G	C		C		G
FENTANYL		G	C			G	G	■	S	G	C			G	G	G	C				G
FRUSEMIDE		G	C		S	I	I	S	■	G	C	I	I	I	I	I	G	C	C		I
GLYCERYL TRINITRATE	G	G	C			C	C	G	G	■	G	G		G	C	C	G		G		G
HEPARIN	G	C	C	G	G	S	C	C	C	G	■	C	C	G	C	C	G	C	G	I	G
HYDRALAZINE			I			S	P		I	G	C	■		P	C	I		C			
ISOPRENALINE			I		P	C	P		I		C		■	P	C	I	G		G	C	
MIDAZOLAM		G	G	G	G	G	G	G	G	G	G	P	P	■	G	G	G	C	I	G	C
MORPHINE	I	G	G	G		C	G	G	I	C	C		C	G	■	G	C		G		G
NORADRENALINE		G	I		C	C	G	G	I	C	C	I	I	G	G	■	C	I			G
POTASSIUM CHLORIDE	G	C	G	C	C	C	C	C	G	G	G		G	G	C	C	■	C		G	
SODIUM BICARBONATE	G	I	G			I			C		C	C		C		I	C	■			G
SODIUM NITROPRUSSIDE					C	C	C			G	G		G		G				■		G
VANCOMYCIN	G		I	G	G						I		C	G			G			■	G
VECURONIUM		G	G			G	G	G	I	G	G			C	G	G		G	G	G	■

C = Data showing that solutions are compatible is available.

P = Although the manufacturers do not provide information on compatibilities these solutions have been used in practice without problems. Check for precipitation or colour change during use.

S = Compatible in sodium chloride 0.9% only.

G = Compatible in glucose solutions only.

I = Incompatible.

302

INDEX

INDEX

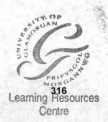